Urinalysis:
A Clinical Guide to
Compassionate Patient Care

Carl A. Osborne, DVM, PhD
Diplomate ACVIM (Internal Medicine)
Minnesota Nephrology/Urology/Urolith Center
Department of Small Animal Clinical Sciences
College of Veterinary Medicine
University of Minnesota
St. Paul, Minnesota

Jerry B. Stevens, DVM, PhD
Professor Emeritus
Department of Pathobiology
College of Veterinary Medicine
University of Minnesota
St. Paul, Minnesota
and
Department of Microbiology, Pathology, and Parasitology
College of Veterinary Medicine
North Carolina State University
Raleigh, North Carolina

With Technical Assistance From:
Lisa K. Ulrich, CVT
    University of Minnesota
Kathleen A. Bird, CVT
    University of Minnesota
Lori A. Koehler, CVT
    University of Minnesota
Laura L. Swanson, CVT
    University of Minnesota
Joanne Holcomb, MT, ASCP
    North Carolina State University

Made possible by an educational grant from Bayer, as
part of its ongoing commitment to help educate practicing
veterinarians worldwide.

Bayer AG
Business Group Animal Health
51368 Leverkusen
Germany

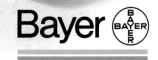

Bayer Corporation
Agricultural Division
Animal Health
Shawnee Mission, Kansas, USA 66201

Library of Congress No. 98-61791
ISBN 1-884254-42-X

The views expressed in this publication represent those of the authors and do not necessarily reflect those of Bayer or Bayer subsidiaries.

This manual is primarily intended as an overview of a scientific topic, as dosages are cited for several pharmacologic agents that may not be the same as those stated on their data sheets in a given country.

In addition, dosages are included for pharmacologic products that may not be licensed for veterinary use in a given country.

Veterinary practitioners/surgeons should consult their local data sheet or equivalent for licensing/prescribing conditions in their particular country.

Queries relating to the enclosed information should be addressed to the Bayer Animal Health Business Group in each individual country.

Printed in U.S.A.

Designed and Published by Veterinary Learning Systems

About the Authors

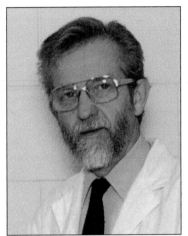

Carl A. Osborne earned his DVM from Purdue University and his PhD from the University of Minnesota. He has been a Diplomate of the American College of Veterinary Internal Medicine since 1972. He currently is professor in the Department of Small Animal Clinical Sciences at the University of Minnesota. He is a member of 24 organizations and is actively involved and has been president of the American College of Veterinary Internal Medicine, Society of Veterinary Nephrology and Urology, World Small Animal Veterinary Association, and Society of International Veterinary Symposia. Dr. Osborne has authored or coauthored three textbooks on urology, nephrology, and urinalysis and more than 650 scientific papers in journals and textbooks. In addition, he has given more than 635 scientific presentations on internal medicine and nephrology/urology to local, state, national, and international veterinary organizations. He is also very committed to the state of veterinary medicine and the ethical responsibility of veterinarians by authoring numerous essays on the art of veterinary medicine.

Dr. Osborne was the 1998 recipient of Hill's Pet Nutrition's Animal Welfare and Humane Ethics Award, presented during the American Animal Hospital Association (AAHA) meeting in March. Upon receiving this award, his words were "Until the day arrives that my lamp of service is extinguished, my goal will be to continue to give my energy and efforts on behalf of others." This recognition of Dr. Osborne is the latest of many awards he has received, including three Norden Distinguished Teaching Awards. He was AAHA's Veterinarian of the Year in 1974, and rarely does a year go by without another organization recognizing his accomplishments and contributions to veterinary medicine.

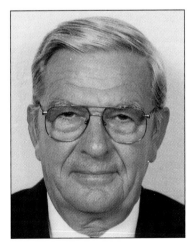

Jerry B. Stevens' outstanding veterinary career started at the University of Minnesota, where he received his BS, DVM, and PhD degrees. He served on the faculty at the University of Minnesota and later at North Carolina State University. Teaching has been an important part of his life, as evidenced by the immense number of graduate students and veterinary students that he worked with, either as teacher, advisor, or committee member. As a mentor, he was at his best. He is currently retired in Belize, Central America.

Dr. Stevens' contributions to the veterinary community are extensive, with research in areas as diverse as liver disease in Bedlington terriers to disease in Atlantic blue crabs. He has authored or co-authored numerous books, book chapters, and scientific publications as well as made presentations both nationally and internationally. As a clinical pathologist, he has had a special interest in improving the quality of diagnostic urinalysis. Although retired, he maintains his research interests in applied clinical pathology.

Preface

ARE YOU A COMPASSIONATE DIAGNOSTICIAN?

What does urinalysis have to do with compassionate patient care? How is the humane quality of compassion linked to our training and experiences as diagnosticians? To foster understanding about the relationship between the ability to diagnose the causes(s) of disease and the ability to incorporate compassion into the diagnostic process, please reflect on the meanings of the terms diagnosis and compassion.

The term **diagnosis** is derived from Greek words meaning to distinguish or discern. Establishment of a diagnosis encompasses determination of the cause(s) of a disease by detection and evaluation of its manifestations. The diagnostic process, including performing and interpreting urinalyses, involves complex cognitive skills acquired by rigorous training and experience.

The term **compassion** is derived from the Latin words "passio" and "cum," which literally mean to suffer with. Thus compassion encompasses our feelings. But more is involved with compassion than our emotions. According to the definition provided by Webster, to be compassionate, two complementary human qualities must be combined. First, we as diagnosticians must have empathetic awareness of the suffering, distress, or troubles of another. Second, we must have an empathetic desire to help correct the problems. Recall that empathy is the projection of our own thoughts and feelings into the thoughts and/or feelings of others in order to better understand them. If we are empathetic, we try to put ourselves in another being's shoes, paws, hooves, or claws. Thus compassion is not a form of pity that is satisfied by mere expression of sorrow. The feeling of sorrow does not transcend to an act of compassion until we make an effort to correct the cause, distress, or suffering of others.

Has the quality of compassion been linked to your training and experiences as a diagnostician? Are you a compassionate diagnostician? Please consider the following viewpoints.

Compassion is linked to our diagnostic abilities in the context of our obligation to attain and maintain professional competence. This association is in reality an application of the Golden Rule. How so? From the perspective that we should strive to provide the quality of diagnostic evaluation that we would desire if we were the patients, rather than the doctors. We need to constantly remind each other that there are some patients we cannot help, but there are none we cannot harm. No patient should be worse for having seen the doctor. Thus an excellent "bedside manner" is not a substitute for professional competency. Would you agree that placing primary emphasis on impressing clients with winsome words to cover misdiagnoses attributable to lack of proper effort or stagnating knowledge is the antithesis of compassion? Isn't it true that our ethical code of practice demands that we not let ill-conceived diagnostic and therapeutic plans jeopardize the welfare of our patients?

But mastering the knowledge and technical skills of the science of veterinary medicine is not enough to make us compassionate diagnosticians. Why not? Because we are not taking care of diseases; rather we are taking care of patients. Most of our clients won't care how much we know unless they also know how much we care. In fact, to some, caring is just as important as curing.

Are all diagnosticians capable of being compassionate at any given time? The answer is no! Why not? Because the quality of human compassion is not instinctive. It can be acquired only by training. Children are not born with it. Only proper training teaches them to become unselfish, self-sacrificing, and altruistic rather than egoistic. Experience is another key factor in enhancing our ability to be compassionate. Most would agree that we generally have the greatest empathy for people or animals whose circumstances we have also experienced. The key point is this! Just as we are expected to attain and maintain our professional competence, we also must attain and maintain humane qualities if we are to be compassionate in a balanced way.

Although the attribute of compassion encompasses many humane facets, three of them are foundation stones in terms of serving clients and helping patients. First, consider the quality of generosity. The root word in generosity is "gen," meaning to create or produce. Applying this perspective to being compassionate diagnosticians, shouldn't we be generous even if our efforts do not always bring us remuneration or prestige? Compassionate generosity is not motivated by a sense of duty or obligation or a desire to acquire prominence. Rather it comes from our hearts. Hippocrates put it this way: "Sometime give your services for nothing ... and if there be an opportunity of serving one who is a stranger in financial straits, give full assistance to such."

Another quality that will help us to maintain our competency as compassionate diagnosticians is kindness. Kindness encompasses the desire to take interest in others and to demonstrate our interest by helpful acts and encouraging words. Compassionate kindness attaches itself to a mission until its purpose in connection with that mission is realized. Kindness by definition should not be motivated solely by self-gain or profit.

Another quality that will help us to be compassionate diagnosticians is humility. As a result of cultivating the strength to be humble, we will properly control the self-centered feeling that our education and professional status make us above or superior to those needing help. Despite our DVM, DMV, VMD, AHT, and PhD degrees, we are all members of a profession whose mission fosters the well-being of others. Our mission is to serve, not to be served. Therefore, if we put compassion into practice when we talk with our clients, we will wisely select words that first do no harm.

Carl A. Osborne

Acknowledgments and Heartfelt Thanks

In this era, completion of textbooks is dependent on the contributions of many individuals. It is with pleasure that we have the opportunity to personally acknowledge them.

Special thanks to Dr. Fernando Vazquez-Rojas and his colleagues at the Animal Health Division of the Bayer Corporation for their vision, trust, encouragement, and support during the past 4 years that this book has been in preparation. We especially appreciate Bayer's sustained commitment to the generation and dissemination of contemporary science to the veterinary profession. In so doing, they help us all fulfill the Veterinarian's Oath, which states in part that we accept improvement in our knowledge and competence as a lifelong obligation.

We also gratefully acknowledge the technical support of Dr. Angela Michaels and Dr. Mary Lou Gantzer of Bayer Diagnostics Division. Angela's and Mary Lou's expertise, especially in urinalysis methodology, has been invaluable. Thanks to both for going the extra mile on behalf of others.

Just as different parts of our bodies must work together to allow us to function effectively and efficiently, so cooperation of different members of an organization foster unity of purpose. This unfailing principle reflects the efforts of the publishing team at Veterinary Learning Systems under the initial leadership of Dr. Beth Thompson. Our heartfelt thanks to Dr. Patricia Franks, who guided this book through the complex process of production. We especially appreciate Pat's patience, empathy, and encouragement when requests for completion of various parts of this book came at times when our mental circuits were in the overload mode. When problems occurred, Pat had the wisdom to fix the fault and not the blame. Warm thanks also to Lilliane Anstee, C. J. Ellis, Cheryl Hobbs (editors), Erin Barnes (Production Manager), Janet Driscoll and Brian Hasenkamp (designers), Karen Oswald (typesetter), and Robin Hipple (indexer) for countless hours of effort that catalyzed the completion of this textbook of urinalysis. A wise sage once penned that writing without thinking is like shooting without aiming. By their skillful use of questions, these wordsmiths kept us on target.

We have incorporated the ideas and contributions of many scientists, researchers, clinical pathologists, and clinicians into this work on urinalysis. Our thanks to all of you, and especially to Drs. Larry Adams, Joseph Bartges, Del Finco, George Lees, Donald Low, Jody Lulich, and David Polzin.

Portions of this book are contained in the publication entitled *Handbook of Canine and Feline Urinalysis*, which we authored in 1981 at the request of Ralston Purina Company, St. Louis. We thank our colleagues at Ralston Purina for their encouragement to write the 1981 textbook and for their permission to include relevant portions of it in this updated text.

Revised and updated portions of information in this book are based on material we authored in the textbook entitled *Canine and Feline Nephrology and Urology* published by Williams & Wilkins Company in 1995. We thank our colleagues at Williams & Wilkins for permission to include relevant topics of our 1995 textbook in this publication.

We have had the opportunity to study the complexity of structural and functional design of the urinary system for more than three decades. What is its origin? Is it owing to our understanding and conscious efforts that the kidneys help to sustain life? In answer to this question, consider the view of Dr. Robert White, a neurosurgeon, who once stated "I am left with no choice but to acknowledge the existence of a superior intellect responsible for the design and development of the incredible brain-mind relationship—something far beyond man's capacity to understand." We echo this acknowledgment as it applies to the production, storage, and elimination of the golden liquid—urine. Design demands a designer. It is with deep respect and appreciation that we pen this closing thought. The "miraclemycin" of our medical armamentarium is Father Design and Mother Time. As their children dedicated to provide health care to others, we vow to strive to augment rather than hinder their efforts.

Carl A. Osborne
Jerry B. Stevens

Foreword

Bayer is proud to sponsor *Urinalysis: A Clinical Guide to Compassionate Patient Care*, which has been written to help veterinary professionals broaden their ability to care for patients. This book contains state-of-the-art information on the best methods for interpreting urinalysis results and for managing urinary tract infections.

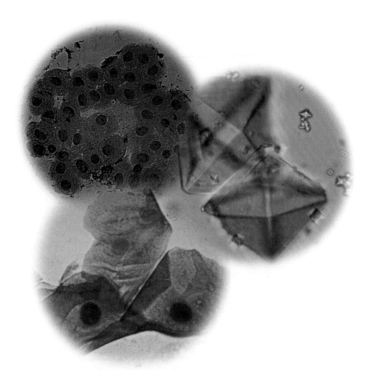

Urinalysis is an important diagnostic tool that provides valuable information about the status of an animal. The study of urine has been the subject of literature since ancient times. Sumerian and Babylonian physicians wrote about changes in the color and character of urine and made suggestions as to diagnosis and treatment as long ago as 4000 BC. During the latter part of the fifth century BC, the great physician Hippocrates wrote, "One can obtain considerable information concerning the general trends by examining the urine." His influence ensured the continued study of urine as a diagnostic tool by medical scholars throughout the centuries.

Today, macroscopic and microscopic examination of urine can provide not only diagnostic and prognostic information but may also be used as an index of therapeutic success. The accurate interpretation of the urine requires an understanding of physiologic processes governing urine formation as well as proper laboratory methods. Drs. Carl A. Osborne and Jerry B. Stevens, internationally recognized leaders in the study of urinalysis, present their knowledge in a practical and usable format.

Bayer has celebrated a century in the medical field and more than 75 years of animal health involvement, with research and development leading to the creation of new products that satisfy the need of veterinary practitioners and surgeons. Bayer's commitment to the veterinary profession, however, goes beyond the introduction of pharmaceuticals, biologicals, and diagnostics. *Urinalysis: A Clinical Guide to Compassionate Patient Care* is one in a series of books sponsored by Bayer that targets areas of clinical relevance in the veterinarian's quest for practical knowledge. This series of publications is an example of our commitment to the veterinary community through our support of independent research in various specialties of veterinary medicine and in the dissemination of information on major areas of scientific interest.

We are deeply grateful to Drs. Osborne and Stevens for the tremendous efforts that led to the production of this book, one that is sure to be considered *the* authoritative guide for many years to come.

Urinalysis: A Clinical Guide to Compassionate Patient Care

Contents

According to Webster's Dictionary, "compassion" is having empathy for the suffering or distress of others and the desire to help. We should express compassion to patients under our care in the form most expected of us, namely professional competence.

C.A.O.

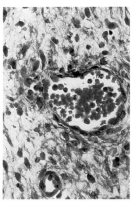

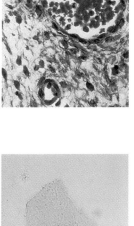

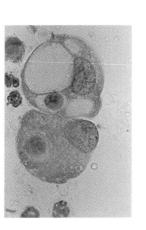

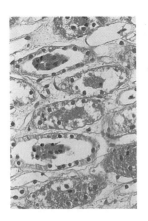

Chapter 5:
Indications for Urinalysis

Chapter 6:
Collection of Urine

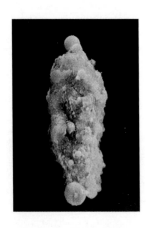

Chapter 7:
"Prophet"-ing More from Urinalysis: Maximizing Reproducible Test Results

Chapter 8:
Macroscopic Urinalysis: Volume, Color, Clarity, and Odor

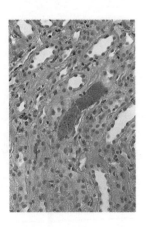

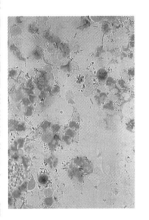

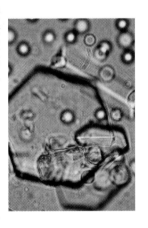

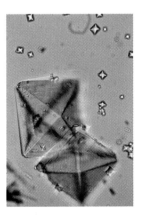

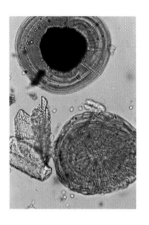

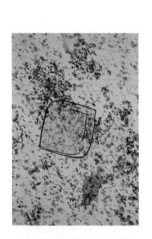

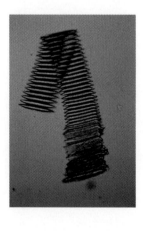

If we as doctors wish to compassionately help our patients, we must do our own thinking in addition to relying on the wisdom of others.

C.A.O.

The Urinary Tract in Health: Definition of Terms and Concepts

Because urinalysis is one of the most important diagnostic tools available to veterinarians, all veterinarians in clinical practice should master laboratory techniques and interpretation of urinalysis.

WHAT IS A COMPLETE ROUTINE URINALYSIS?

In our hospital, a complete routine analysis consists of the evaluation of several physical and chemical properties of urine, estimation of its solute concentration, and microscopic examination of urine sediment (Figure 1-1 and Table 1-1). We recommend that all of these tests be performed because they aid in semiquantitation and localization of abnormal findings and in refinement of problems. For example, interpretation of the results of chemical tests (and sediment examination) is aided by knowledge of urine specific gravity (an indirect index of the volume of urine produced).

The value of microscopic examination of urine sediment in the interpretation of urinalyses is comparable to microscopic examination of blood smears in the interpretation of hemograms. Meaningful interpretation of physical (color, turbidity) and chemical (protein, occult blood, pH) test results of routine urinalyses is dependent on knowledge of the composition of urine sediment. For example, a moderate degree of proteinuria in the absence of significant numbers of red cells and white cells usually indicates proteinuria of glomerular origin. A moderate degree of proteinuria associated with hematuria and pyuria, however, indicates an inflammatory response somewhere along the urinary and/or genital tracts.

QUALITATIVE, SEMIQUANTITATIVE, AND QUANTITATIVE URINALYSES
Overview

Because the concentration of solutes, cells, crystals, and so on varies with the quantity of water being excreted at a particular time, urine samples collected without regard to rate of urine formation (i.e., number of milliliters per unit of time) are only suitable for qualitative and semi-quantitative determinations. Daily variation in urine volume and composition influenced by eating, drinking, metabolism, and various diseases must be considered when interpreting test results. Although pseudoprecision is implied by urine specific gravity values conventionally measured in thousandths of a unit (i.e., 1.001 to 1.060+) and solutes (e.g., glucose, protein) listed as mg/100 ml, such results should not be overinterpreted. Urine samples collected at random are usually suitable for diagnostic screening; however, urine substances obtained during timed intervals may require subsequent testing to clarify the significance of questionable results.

> **Urinalysis is one of the most important diagnostic tools available to veterinarians.**

Quantitative Urinalyses

Collection of urine specimens during a specified period is required to determine quantitatively the excretion rates of some endogenous and exogenous substances as well as to determine the volume of urine produced. For quantitation of endogenous substances (e.g., uric acid, amino acids, hormones, electrolytes), 24 hour urine collections are usually preferred because they eliminate diurnal variations in urine excretion. These urine collections may also be used to verify the existence and/or to determine the magnitude of polyuria.

A metabolism cage is sometimes used to collect all urine formed during a 24 hour interval. In some situations a shorter period may be used, with values prorated to a 24 hour interval. For best results the urinary bladder should be emptied and the urine discarded at the beginning of the collection period. The bladder should be emptied again at the end of the procedure, but the urine should be included in the calculation. The bladder lumen can be flushed with a known volume of saline and/or air and the flushed contents added to the collection vial.

When possible, the patient should be allowed to acclimate to the environment of the metabolism unit for a day or so before beginning the study. This will facilitate more precise measurements.

Reproducible 24 hour collections are notoriously difficult to obtain. The best data are usually obtained by measuring and comparing urine output (and water intake) for each of 2 to 3 days. Quantitation of substances in urine may be obtained by measuring the quantity in a representative aliquot of a well-mixed 24 hour sample and correcting this value for the 24 hour volume (see Chapter 7 for additional information).

Normal 24 hour urine volume is variable and is influenced by:

- Water consumption
- Dietary moisture
- Dietary ingredients that affect urine concentrating capacity
- Environmental conditions
- Activity of the patient

Under normal conditions, 24 hour urine volume for dogs and cats is approximately 20 to 40 ml/kg of their body weight.

For quantitation of exogenous substances, exogenous creatinine clearance, urinary excretion of phenolsulfonphthalein dye, or measurement of endogenous substances whose urinary excretion rate is constant, shorter time intervals are commonly used. The inability of most animals to cooperate in the timing of voiding usually requires use of urinary catheters. Swan-Ganz flow-directed balloon catheters are recommended for timed urine samples to facilitate collecting urine from the bladder. Oral or parenteral administration of appropriate antimicrobial agents at least 8 hours before and 2 to 3 days after catheterization minimizes the likelihood of catheter-induced bacterial urinary tract infections (UTIs).

Fractional Clearance

The concept of fractional clearance is related to the fact that the quantity of a filtered substance that ultimately appears in urine is influenced by the net effect of tubular reabsorption and tubular secretion. Fractional clearance of filtered substances such as electrolytes may be measured in "spot" urine samples. Collection of a timed urine sample is unnecessary.

Using creatinine to measure glomerular filtration rate, the fractional excretion of a filtered substance is calculated by dividing the measured clearance of that substance by the measured clearance of creatinine:

$$FC_x = \frac{U_x V/P_x}{U_{cr}V/P_{cr}} = \frac{U_x P_{cr}}{U_{cr}P_x}$$

where FC = fractional clearance, U_x = urine concentrations of substance x, V = urine volume in milliliters, P_x = plasma concentration of substance x, U_{cr} = urine concentration of creatinine, and P_{cr} = plasma concentration of creatinine.

In normal animals, the fractional excretion of electrolytes is substantially less than 1 because they are conserved to varying degrees following filtration. For example, fractional excretion of calcium is low and that of phosphorus would be high in patients with hyperparathyroidism. Fractional excretion of sodium is aldosterone dependent.

Comparison Between Concentration of Urine Analytes and Concentration of Urine Creatinine

In an attempt to minimize technical difficulties associated with the collection of timed urine samples, the quantity of urinary excretion of various analytes is sometimes evaluated by determining the concentration of the analyte in a "spot" urine sample and then dividing it by the concentration of creatinine in the same spot sample. The reliability of analyte:creatinine ratios is influenced by:

- Whether the rate of production and urinary excretion of creatinine is constant
- Whether the glomerular filtration rate is constant during the general period surrounding the measurement
- Whether the quantity of analyte is excreted in urine at a

URINALYSIS REQUEST/REPORT

Date: _____

_____
Clinician   Student

_____
                         Clinical Problem

Collection Technique
Voided _____   Cysto _____
Midstream Void _____   Cath _____
Manual Compression _____   Table _____
Other Method of Collection _____

Time/Date Collected _____
Time/Date Analyzed _____

Method of Preservation: ☐ Refrigeration
☐ Other _____
Comments _____
Pre Rx Sample _____ ☐ Yes ☐ No
Treatment Sample _____ ☐ Yes ☐ No

Rx Type _____
Diet Fed _____
    ☐ Fasted ☐ Nonfasted ☐ Unknown

[   ] Complete UA

Color _____
Turbidity _____
Specific Gravity [refractometer] _____
                [stick] _____
Leukocytes [stick] _____
Creatinine [stick] _____
Ketones [stick] _____ Acetest _____
Occult Blood [stick] _____ Hematest _____
pH [stick] _____ Meter _____
Glucose [stick] _____ Clinitest _____
Bilirubin [stick] _____ Ictotest _____
Protein [stick] _____ SSA _____
Urobilinogen [stick] _____
Nitrite [stick] _____
Urine Protein:Creatinine Ratio _____
☐ Flocculent after spinning
☐ Milky film after spinning

Special Tests
Acetic Acid   ☐ Dissolve   ☐ Persist
Nitroprusside   ☐ Dissolve   ☐ Persist
NaOH   ☐ Dissolve   ☐ Persist

[   ] Microscopic Exam

5 ml _____ Other (ml) _____
RBCs (/hpf) _____
WBCs (/hpf) _____
Casts (/lpf)   Granular _____
                    Waxy _____
                    Hyaline _____
                    Other _____

Epithelial Cells (/hpf) _____

Comments	Few	Mod	Many

Bacteria (/hpf)

		Few	Mod	Many
Rods		Few	Mod	Many
Cocci		Few	Mod	Many
Other		Few	Mod	Many
Yeast (/hpf)		Few	Mod	Many
Fat (/hpf)		Few	Mod	Many
Sperm (/hpf)		Few	Mod	Many

Crystals (/hpf)

	Few	Mod	Many
Amorph Urate	Few	Mod	Many
Amorph Phos	Few	Mod	Many
Amorph Unk	Few	Mod	Many
Ca Oxalate Di	Few	Mod	Many
Ca Oxalate Mo	Few	Mod	Many
Cystine	Few	Mod	Many
Struvite	Few	Mod	Many
Urate	Few	Mod	Many
Unidentified	Few	Mod	Many

Other/Unidentified Material

	Few	Mod	Many

Unidentified Crystal Drawing or Comments:

Technician _____
Date _____

FIGURE 1-1 *Laboratory form for recording results of a routine urinalysis.*

constant rate during a 24 hour period
■ Whether the effect of glomerular filtration on serum creatinine concentration is constant

Urine protein:creatinine ratios provide a reliable estimate of 24 hour protein excretion.[4] This method is also used to evaluate patients for amino acidurias. For additional details, consult the section on proteinuria in Chapter 10 (Biochemical Analysis of Urine).

With the exception of cortisol, comparison of other analytes in urine to urine creatinine concentration has not consistently proved to be a reliable index of the 24 hour urinary excretion rate. Urine creatinine can be degraded by bacteria if stored at room temperature for an extended period.

OVERVIEW OF URINE FORMATION AND COMPOSITION
Basic Design and Mechanisms

The urinary system is designed to play a major role in maintaining fluid, electrolyte, and acid–base homeostasis by selectively eliminating waste products from the body in soluble form and by producing and degrading some hormones. A conceptual understanding of renal function is an essential prerequisite for determining the optimum times for collecting urine to analyze specific components and interpret results.

The formation of urine by nephrons results from three basic and interrelated processes: glomerular filtration, tubular reabsorption, and tubular secretion. Viewed in a slightly different perspective, the kidney primarily processes some substances by glomerular filtration (e.g., creatinine); some by glomerular filtration and tubular reabsorption (e.g., glucose, allantoin, sodium, and amino acids); some by filtration, absorption, and secretion (e.g., potassium); and some by tubular secretion (e.g., hydrogen ions and ammonia). The combined effect of these functions on the removal of a substance from plasma and the excretion of it in urine is often referred to as *clearance* of the substance. Clearance is equal to the glomerular filtration rate only when the substance is not reabsorbed or secreted by renal tubules. Glomerular filtration, tubular reabsorption, and tubular secretion are significantly influenced by a variety of hormones, including antidiuretic hormone (ADH), aldosterone, parathyroid hormone (PTH) thyrocalcitonin, calcitriol, prostaglandins, calcitonin, and thyroxine.

TABLE 1-1
ANTICIPATED URINALYSIS RESULTS FOR FRESH CANINE AND FELINE URINE

Urine Characteristic	Adult Dogs	Adult Cats
Color	Yellow	Yellow
Appearance	Clear	Clear
Specific gravity		
Minimum	1.001	1.001
Maximum	1.065+	1.080+
Typical range	1.015–1.045	1.035–1.060
Volume (ml/kg body wt/day)	$\cong$20–40+	$\cong$20–30+
pH	4.5–8.5	4.5–8.5
Glucose	Negative	Negative
Ketones	Negative	Negative
Bilirubin	Negative to 2+	Negative
Occult blood	Negative	Negative
Protein	Trace to 1+	Trace
RBCs/hpf	0–5	0–5
WBCs/hpf	0–5	0–5
Casts/lpf	Occasional hyaline	Occasional hyaline
Epithelial cells/hpf	Occasional	Occasional
Fat droplets/hpf	Uncommon	Common
Bacteria/hpf	Negative	Negative
Crystals/hpf	Variable	Variable

hpf = high power field; lpf = low power field.

Glomerular Filtration

The initial phase of urine formation consists of the production of a large quantity of an acellular low protein ultrafiltrate of blood that is filtered through glomeruli. The formation of filtrate from blood (or plasma) is a passive (non–energy-requiring) process for the kidneys. Energy required for glomerular filtration is derived from blood pressure generated by the contraction of the left ventricle and the elasticity of vascular walls. The rate at which kidneys form glomerular filtrate from plasma is called the *glomerular filtration rate* (GFR).

Factors that influence the quality and quantity of glomerular filtrate include the volume of blood in glomerular capillaries, hydrostatic (blood) pressure, colloidal osmotic (or oncotic) pressure of blood in glomerular capillaries, renal interstitial pressure, and renal intratubular hydrostatic pressure (Table 1-2).

The quantity of protein in the glomerular filtrate that is contained in Bowman's space is normally so small that it does not exert an osmotic effect of sufficient magnitude to enhance glomerular filtration. Arterial hydrostatic pressure is the major force that favors glomerular filtration. Forces that oppose glomerular filtration include colloidal osmotic pressure (which arises primarily from nonfiltered protein molecules, especially albumin, in glomerular capillary

> Under normal conditions, 24 hour urine volume for dogs and cats is approximately 20 to 40 ml/kg of their body weight.

plasma), renal intratubular and interstitial pressure, and the selective permeability of glomerular capillary walls.

Glomeruli are designed to function collectively as a sieve that increasingly restricts the passage of macromolecules as they increase in diameter and molecular weight. Most substances in glomerular filtrate have a molecular weight of less than 68,000 D (Table 1-3). Because cells, most proteins (and therefore molecules bound to proteins), and most lipoproteins are too large to pass through glomerular capillary walls, they are retained within the vascular compartment and significant quantities are not present in glomerular filtrate (Table 1-4).

Although the ability of many substances to traverse glomerular capillary walls is related to their size, which is estimated by their molecular weight (the so-called "size selective" factor),

TABLE 1-2

LOCATION OF AZOTEMIA CAUSED BY REDUCED GLOMERULAR FILTRATION

Cause	Classification of Azotemia
Decreased blood volume	Prerenal
Decreased blood pressure	Prerenal
Decreased colloidal osmotic pressure[a]	Prerenal
Decreased vascular patency	Primary renal
Decreased glomerular permeability	Primary renal
Increased renal interstitial pressure	Primary renal
Increased renal intratubular pressure	Primary renal (tubular obstruction)
Increased renal intratubular pressure	Postrenal (obstruction of ureters, bladder, and/or urethra)
Combination of causes	Prerenal and primary renal, postrenal and primary renal, or prerenal and postrenal

[a]Reduction in plasma colloidal osmotic pressure as a result of severe hypoalbuminemia is actually a mechanism of decreased blood volume. It is listed separately for emphasis.

the electrical charge of the substance is also an extremely important variable that influences the degree to which some charged macromolecules are filtered (the so-called "charge selective" factor). The negative charge of glomerular capillary walls impedes the passage of negatively charged (anionic) macromolecules (e.g., albumin), which otherwise would be small enough to be filtered, at least to some degree. Conversely, the negatively charged glomerular capillary wall enhances filtration of some positively charged (cationic) macromolecules. The shape or configuration of macromolecules may also influence their ability to traverse glomerular capillary walls.

Glomerular filtrate is qualitatively similar to plasma in its concentration of electrolytes and macromolecules of relatively low molecular weight. Glomerular filtrate contains the majority (but not all) of the solutes and water that must be eliminated from the body, but in quantities far in excess of those that ultimately appear in urine. It also contains a large quantity of vital metabolites that must be retrieved before urine is eliminated if the body's homeostasis is to be maintained. At first impression, the composition of glomerular filtrate appears to be paradoxical because it might be expected that the glomerular "filter" would retain vital metabolites in plasma and would permit only waste products to escape into the urinary space. Glomeruli effectively restrict the passage of vital blood components such as cells and most proteins but are unable to discriminate between vital metabolites and waste metabolites that are similar in structure and electrical charge. The common denominator of substances that appear in glomerular filtrate does not appear to be their potential value to the body, but rather their molecular characteristics—size, shape, and electrical charge. For the kidneys to regulate body fluid, electrolyte, and acid–base balance, it is essential that both beneficial and worthless metabolites with similar characteristics be subjected to potential loss in urine.

It is conceptually useful to view the consequences of glomerular dysfunction as:

■ Impaired urinary excretion of unwanted metabolites such as urea and creatinine
■ Unwanted urinary excretion of vital metabolites, primarily plasma proteins

Abnormal retention of nonprotein nitrogenous waste products such as urea and creatinine as a result of reduced glomerular filtration is one form of azotemia. As will be discussed, azotemia that occurs as a consequence of decreased GFR may be categorized (or localized) into prerenal, primary renal, and/or postrenal causes.

The formation of urine by nephrons results from three basic but interrelated processes: glomerular filtration, tubular reabsorption, and tubular secretion.

Tubular Reabsorption

Some filtered substances (e.g., creatinine and allantoin) cannot be reused by the body and are not reabsorbed by tubules. Other filtered substances (e.g., amino acids, vitamins, and glucose) are essential for body homeostasis and are almost completely reabsorbed by energy-requiring active tubular transport mechanisms (Table 1-4). The body's requirement for water, electrolytes, and some filtered substances varies, depending on intake, metabolism, and loss of these substances through nonrenal routes. Nephrons regulate conservation and excretion of these substances by active or passive tubular reabsorption. Still other metabolites (e.g.,

TABLE 1-3

COMPARISON OF MOLECULAR WEIGHTS OF SOME METABOLITES AND PLASMA PROTEINS INCLUDED IN AND EXCLUDED FROM GLOMERULAR ULTRAFILTRATE

Substance	Approximate Molecular Weight (D)	Presence in Glomerular Filtrate
Water	18	Present
Sodium	23	Present
Chloride	35.5	Present
Urea	60	Present
Creatinine	113	Present
Glucose	180	Present
$\beta2$-Microglobulin	11,800	Present
Lysozyme (muramidase)	14,400	Present
Myoglobin	17,600	Present
Bence Jones protein (monomer)	22,000	Present
$\alpha1$-Microglobulin	27,000	Present
$\alpha1$-Acid glycoprotein	40,000	Present
Bence Jones protein (dimer)	44,000	Present
Amylase	50,000	Present
Hemoglobin (tetramer)[a]	64,500	Sometimes present
Antithrombin III	65,000	Sometimes present
Albumin	66,000	Sometimes present
Haptoglobin (monomer)	85,000–120,000	Absent
Immunoglobulin G	160,000	Absent
Immunoglobulin A (dimer)	300,000	Absent
Fibrinogen	400,000	Absent
$\alpha2$-Macroglobulin	840,000	Absent
Immunoglobulin M	900,000	Absent

[a]Plasma hemoglobin is normally bound to haptoglobin. Once this binding capacity is saturated, dissociated hemoglobin readily passes through glomerular capillary walls as low molecular weight (32,000 D) dimers.

hydrogen ions, ammonia, potassium, and substances bound to plasma proteins) enter the urine primarily by tubular secretion. Thus, as glomerular filtrate passes through the tubules, it rapidly loses its original identity as tubular reabsorption and tubular secretion selectively modify it according to the body's need. Whereas formation of glomerular filtrate is a passive process for the kidneys, modification of glomerular filtrate by the tubules demands a majority of the energy expended by the kidneys.

Approximately two thirds to three fourths of the total volume of glomerular filtrate is recovered by proximal tubular reabsorption. Whereas proximal tubular reabsorption of water is passive, proximal tubular reabsorption of many substances (e.g., amino acids, calcium, glucose, phosphate, potassium, sodium) is an active process that requires energy. Reabsorption of many metabolites is influenced by hormones.

Some metabolites (including glucose, amino acids, and water-soluble vitamins) are called *threshold substances* because the capacity of tubules to reabsorb them is limited. They are almost totally reabsorbed from glomerular filtrate as long as their concentration is not excessive. If their concentration in blood and thus in glomerular filtrate exceeds the capacity of tubular

transport mechanisms, however, a threshold concentration is reached. Above this concentration, they spill into urine and cause subsequent imbalances (e.g., hyperglycemic glucosuria).

The maximum rate at which an active transport system can reabsorb a particular solute is called its *transport maximum*. The amount of a particular solute transported is proportional to the amount present in tubular filtrate up to the transport maximum of the solute. At higher concentrations the transport mechanism is saturated and there is no appreciable increment in the amount transported.

Tubular Secretion

Filtrate also undergoes considerable modification by tubular reabsorptive and secretory processes in the distal tubules and collecting ducts (Table 1-4). Some clinically significant events that occur in distal nephrons include hydrogen ion secretion, ammonia secretion, potassium secretion, bicarbonate and sodium reabsorption, and urine concentration of dilution. ADH significantly influences water reabsorption in distal nephrons by increasing tubular epithelial cell permeability.

Impaired Tubular Reabsorption or Secretion

Impairment of tubular reabsorption may lead to undesirable loss of varying quantities of metabolites (e.g., calcium, bicarbonate, water-soluble vitamins, or sodium), whereas impairment of tubular secretion may result in retention of some undesirable metabolites (e.g., hydrogen ions or potassium). If they are severe, systemic excesses or deficits in fluid, electrolyte, and acid–base balance may induce polysystemic disease. Correction of systemic water, electrolyte, and acid–base imbalances caused by glomerular and/or tubular dysfunction is a primary goal of symptomatic and supportive management of patients with primary renal failure and uremia.

Hormonal Relationships

Glomerular filtration, tubular reabsorption, and tubular secretion are modified and marvelously integrated by several hormones and other bioactive agents, including renin-angiotensin, catecholamines, ADH, aldosterone, PTH, glucagon, growth hormone, calcitriol, prostaglandins, calcitonin, thyroxin, and a natriuretic factor. In this context, nephrons may be viewed as end organs for multifaceted biologic control systems. It is not surprising therefore that endocrinopathies frequently affect the body's homeostasis adversely by altering renal function.

TABLE 1-4

SUMMARY OF THE PHYSIOLOGIC ACTIVITIES DURING URINE FORMATION

Component	Physiologic Process
■ Glomerulus	Passive formation of ultrafiltrate of plasma devoid of most protein
■ Bowman's capsule	Collection of glomerular filtrate
■ Proximal tubule	Active reabsorption of glucose, proteins and amino acids, vitamins, ascorbic acid, acetoacetate, hydroxybutyrate, uric acid, sodium, potassium, calcium ($\uparrow$ by PTH), phosphate ($\downarrow$ by PTH), sulfate, bicarbonate Passive reabsorption of chloride, water, urea Active secretion of hydrogen ion
■ Henle's loop	Generation of medullary hyperosmolality
—Descending limb	Passive reabsorption of water Passive secretion of sodium, urea
—Thin ascending limb	Passive reabsorption of urea, sodium; impermeable to water
— Thick ascending limb	Active reabsorption of chloride, calcium Passive reabsorption of sodium; impermeable to water, potassium
■ Distal tubule	Active reabsorption of sodium ($\uparrow$ by aldosterone), calcium, HCO$_3$, small amounts of glucose Passive reabsorption of chloride, water ($\uparrow$ by ADH) Active secretion of hydrogen ion, ammonia, uric acid Passive secretion of potassium
■ Collecting ducts	Active reabsorption of sodium ($\uparrow$ by aldosterone) Passive reabsorption of chloride, water ($\uparrow$ by ADH) Active secretion of hydrogen ion Passive secretion of potassium

ADH = antidiuretic hormone; PTH = parathyroid hormone.

Notable examples include pituitary and renal diabetes insipidus, inappropriate secretion of ADH, hyperadrenocorticism, hypoadrenocorticism, diabetes mellitus, hyperthyroidism, and primary and pseudohyperparathyroidism.

In addition to being influenced by various extrarenal hormones, the kidneys *produce* hormones that act on other target organs. The kidneys are involved in the regulation of red cell production by synthesizing and releasing erythropoietin when the oxygen tension of blood perfusing the kidneys is reduced. The kidneys influence calcium phosphorus homeostasis by metabolizing 25-hydroxycholecalciferol, which is formed in the liver, to its most metabolically active form, 1,25-dihydroxycholecalciferol.

The kidneys also *degrade* and/or *excrete* several hormones including PTH, growth hormone, secretin, cholecystokinin, glucagon, gastrin, prolactin, circulating insulin, thyrotropic hormone, and ADH. Failure to degrade hormones as a consequence of renal failure is important in the pathogenesis of the uremic syndrome. Excessive quantities of hormones normally degraded by the kidneys have been added to the impressively long list of so-called *uremic toxins.*

In summary, the kidneys produce and degrade hormones and their function is modified by hormones.

CONCENTRATION AND DILUTION OF URINE

(see also Table 1-5)

Overview of Fundamental Concepts

The kidneys are designed to play a vital role in maintaining fluid balance by regulating the excretion of water. They may conserve water (or concentrate urine) in times of need and eliminate water (or dilute urine) when the body contains excessive fluids.

The fact that the transport of water from one area to another is passive, following gradients established by hydrostatic and osmotic forces, is of fundamental importance in comprehending the processes involved in urine concentration and dilution. Knowing that *concentration* and *dilution* of urine excreted into the renal pelvis are terms comparing final urine composition with that of glomerular filtrate is also of fundamental importance. Urine concentration is associated with tubular conservation of water in excess of solute; urine dilution is associated with conservation of solute in excess of water.

Urine Concentration

Proximal Tubules

Of the approximately 60 L of glomerular filtrate formed by an adult 20 lb dog each day, less than 1% (approximately ½ L) is normally eliminated as urine. Almost 75% of the water is passively reabsorbed by proximal tubules after active reabsorption of such solutes as sodium, calcium, phosphorus, glucose, and others (Table 1-4). Because the relative quantities of water and solute reabsorbed by proximal tubules are more or less equal, the osmolality (Osm) and specific gravity (SG) of modified filtrate at their terminal portions is roughly the same as that of glomerular filtrate (SG = ≅1.008 to 1.012; Osm = ≅300 mOsm/kg). Proximal tubular reabsorption of water is often referred to as *obligatory water reabsorption* because it is not influenced by mechanisms specifically directed toward modulation of fluid balance.

Even though proximal tubules do not play a primary role in water balance, they may affect the volume and concentration of final urine if pharmacologic (osmotic diuretics) or patholog-

TABLE 1-5

GLOSSARY OF TERMS RELATED TO URINE CONCENTRATION AND DILUTION

- **Baruria**—Urine of high specific gravity and high osmolality.

- **Concentration of urine**—Tubular modification of glomerular filtrate so that more water than solute is removed. The specific gravity of glomerular filtrate is approximately 1.008 to 1.012, while the osmolality is approximately 300 mOsm/kg. Concentrated urine has a higher specific gravity and higher osmolality than glomerular filtrate (Figures 1-3 and 1-4).

- **Dilution of urine**—Tubular modification of glomerular filtrate so that more solute than water is removed. Dilute urine has a lower specific gravity and lower osmolality than does glomerular filtrate.

- **Hypersthenuria**—Urine of high specific gravity and high osmolality.

- **Isosthenuria**—Urine with a specific gravity and osmolality similar to those of plasma and glomerular filtrate. Severe impairment in the ability to concentrate or dilute glomerular filtrate according to body need is sometimes called *fixed specific gravity*.

- **Osmolality**—The property of a solution that is dependent on the concentration of osmotically active particles in solution. For osmolality the unit of solvent measurement is mass (kilograms), and therefore osmolality is expressed as mOsm/kg of solution. For osmolarity the unit of solvent measurement is volume (liter), and therefore osmolarity is expressed as mOsm/L of solution.

- **Urine specific gravity**—Measurement of the density of urine compared with that of pure water. Urine specific gravity is the ratio of the weight of urine to the weight of an equal volume of water, both measured at the same temperature. Because specific gravity is a ratio, it is not followed by a unit of measurement.

ic (e.g., hyperglycemic glucosuria, Fanconi's syndrome) mechanisms impede the usual quantity of solute (and therefore water) from being reabsorbed. Interference with proximal tubular reabsorption may overwhelm the reabsorptive capacity of distal portions of nephrons. The mechanism of the resultant pharmacologic or pathologic polyuria is commonly referred to as *osmotic diuresis* (as opposed to water diuresis).

Distal Nephron

The quantity of water removed from modified filtrate by the distal nephron is influenced by body water balance. Recall that the loops of Henle and vasa recta have a structure that is responsible for generating and maintaining a gradient of increasing solute concentration (especially sodium, chloride, and urea)

from the outer portion (adjacent to the cortex) to the inner portion (adjacent to the renal pelvis; Figures 1-2 and 1-3).

Applied Anatomy

The anatomic configuration and function of medullary tubules (loops of Henle, distal tubules, and collecting ducts) and vessels (vasa recta) responsible for hyperosmolality of renal medullary interstitial tissue is collectively called the *countercurrent system*. Conceptual understanding of this system is a fundamental prerequisite to the meaningful evaluation of patients with disorders of urine concentration and dilution. The name countercurrent system depicts the fact that the hairpin shape of the loops of Henle and vasa recta allows filtrate inflow to (1) run parallel to, (2) in close proximity to, and (3) in an opposite direction to that of filtrate outflow. The anatomic arrangement of a Henle's loop multiplies the osmotic gradient actively generated by this structure as it moves toward the renal pelvis (Figure 1-2). Henle's loops are called *countercurrent multipliers* because they multiply the renal interstitial solute gradient from the corticomedullary junction to the region adjacent to the renal pelvis. Vasa recta are often called *countercurrent exchangers*. In addition to providing nutrients to structures in the renal medulla, they remove water and excess solute reabsorbed by the distal tubules and collecting ducts. Because of the relatively slow rate of blood flow in vasa recta, solutes passively diffuse out of portions leaving the medulla and into portions of vessels traveling toward the renal pelvis. Conversely, water passively diffuses out of descending vessels and into ascending vessels. Hyperosmolality is maintained because solutes tend to circulate in the medulla, whereas water tends to bypass it.

Applied Physiology

In the thin descending limb of the loops of Henle, water passively leaves the tubular lumens, attracted by the ever increasing gradient of solutes in medullary interstitial tissue generated by the countercurrent system. As a result, intraluminal solute increases in concentration. At the turn of the loop, tubular filtrate is almost as hyperosmotic as the adjacent medullary interstitium because water has been removed in excess of solute (in dogs SG = $\cong$1.060 and Osm = $\cong$2400 mOsm/kg; in cats SG = $\cong$1.080 and Osm = $\cong$3000 mOsm/kg). Solute (sodium, chloride) is actively transported from the thick ascending portion of a Henle's loop, but an equivalent amount of water cannot passively follow (Table 1-4 and Figure 1-3). Separation of sodium, chloride, and water at this site is important in the establishment of medullary interstitial hyperosmolality. Because solute is removed from tubular lumens in excess of water, the fluid that enters the distal tubular lumens of dogs is hypoosmotic.[1] In contrast to glomerular filtrate (and plasma), the fluid that enters the distal tubular lumens of cats is isoosmotic.[2] In the process of moving through the loops of Henle, an additional 5% of the original volume of glomerular filtrate is removed. So-called loop or saluretic diuretics (furosemide and ethacrynic acid) induce diuresis (at least in part) by inhibiting active chloride transport by the thick ascending limbs of Henle's loops.

ADH (vasopressin) is an important component of the urine concentration mechanism because it influences the permeabili-

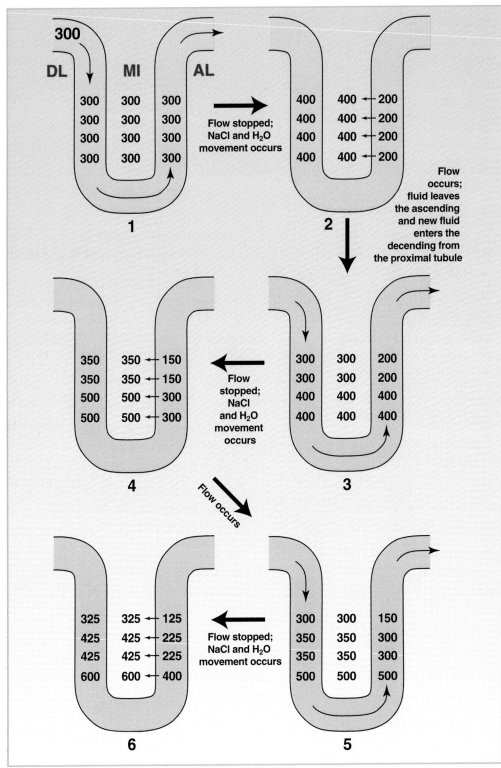

FIGURE 1-2 *Hypothetical illustration of how the loop of Henle functions to produce a progressively increasing osmotic gradient in the medullary interstitium (MI). (1) Osmolality in the descending limb (DL) and the ascending limb (AL) of Henle's loop is isotonic at 300 milliosmoles (mOsm). (2) Transport pumps in the AL move sodium and chloride into the MI, increasing the mOsm to 400. Equilibration of mOsm occurs between the DL and the MI. (3) Isotonic fluid from the proximal tubule continues to flow into the DL, and the hypotonic fluid flows out of the AL into the distal tubule. (4) The process described in step 2 of active transport of sodium and chloride out of the AL into the MI continues; equilibration of mOsm occurs between the DL and the MI. (5) Step 3 is repeated. (6) Step 2 is repeated. As a result, the difference in mOsm between the base and the tip of Henle's loop is 275, which is greater than the 200 mOsm maximum gradient generated at any level of Henle's loop. By increasing the length of Henle's loop, this effect is multiplied so that the difference in mOsm between base and tip of Henle's loop can be more than 2000 mOsm in dogs and more than 2500 mOsm in cats.*

ty of distal tubular and collecting duct epithelium to water. Provided sufficient medullary solute concentration can create an osmotic gradient between the interstitium and tubular lumens and provided sufficient ADH can increase the permeability of epithelial cells of the distal nephrons to water, more water than solute will migrate from tubular lumens to the medullary interstitium (Figures 1-3 through 1-5). Consequently, in contrast to glomerular filtrate, the remaining tubular fluid will contain more solute than water. Of the remaining 20% of the volume of the original glomerular filtrate, approximately 15% is reabsorbed by the distal tubules and more than 4% is reabsorbed by collecting ducts. During states of maximum water conservation (or antidiuresis), the specific gravity of final urine of dogs may equal or slightly exceed 1.060 (≅2400 mOsm/kg; Figure 1-4). Maximum antidiuresis in cats may be associated with the formation of final urine with a specific gravity equal to or slightly greater than 1.080 (≅3000 mOsm/kg). It is hypothesized that cats have a greater capacity to maximally concentrate urine than do dogs, by virtue of the longer loops of Henle and longer vasa recta, because their countercurrent system has the ability to generate a higher medullary solute concentration than dogs. Other factors may also be involved, however.[5]

The purpose of the countercurrent system is to generate and maintain a sufficiently high concentration of solutes (primarily sodium, chloride, and urea) in the renal medullary interstitium to attract water from a region of lower solute concentration (distal tubular and collecting duct lumens). The importance of urea in the countercurrent system is illustrated by the fact that dogs fed a high protein diet are better able to maximally concentrate urine than are dogs fed a low protein diet.[3] Impaired synthesis of urea as a consequence of some forms of generalized hepatic disease (cirrhosis and portal vascular shunts) may be responsible, at least in part, for the polyuria commonly asso-

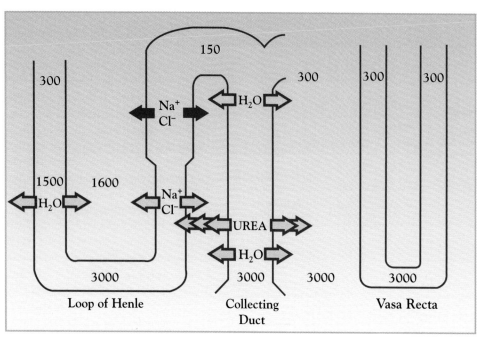

FIGURE 1-3 *Schematic representation of the urine-concentrating mechanism in the feline medulla. Numbers represent milliosmoles per liter. Solute in the descending loop of Henle is concentrated by passive movement of water into the hyperosmolar interstitium. The ascending limb is impermeable to water, but NaCl moves into the interstitium passively (open arrows) in the inner medulla and by active transport (solid arrows) in the outer medulla, creating dilute urine in the distal tubule (150 mOsm/kg). Water may be reabsorbed in both the outer and inner medulla if ADH renders collecting duct cells permeable to water. Urea passively reabsorbed in the inner medulla in the presence of ADH contributes to interstitial hyperosmolarity. The vasa recta provide nutrition to the medulla and remove quantities of solute and water beyond those necessary to maintain normal interstitial volume and osmolality. (Modified from Finco DR: Kidney function, in Kaneko JJ (ed): Clinical Biochemistry of Domestic Animals. San Diego, Academic Press, 1989, p 506.)*

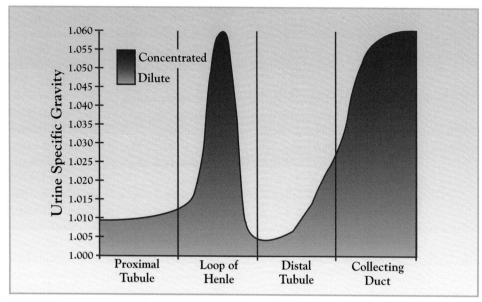

FIGURE 1-4 *Schematic representation of changes in specific gravity of canine urine as it passes through the nephron during a state of maximum antidiuresis.*

ciated with these disorders. Likewise, excessive loss of sodium, chloride, or urea from the medullary interstitium (so-called medullary solute washout) would be associated with impaired ability to concentrate urine. It seems logical to hypothesize that excessive loss of sodium in urine as a consequence of hypoadrenocorticism may reduce renal medullary solute concentration

sufficiently to account (at least in part) for the impaired ability to concentrate urine commonly observed in association with this endocrinopathy. Likewise, impaired function of a sufficient population of nephrons as a consequence of primary glomerular, tubular, interstitial, or vascular disorders will interfere with the generation of renal medullary hyperosmolality by the loops of Henle. Obligatory polyuria and compensatory polydipsia are well-known consequences.

Urine Dilution

In the absence of ADH, relatively little water is removed from the lumens of distal tubules and collecting ducts. However, active transport of solutes (such as sodium) from the lumens of distal nephrons still occurs. As a consequence, more solute than water is removed from tubular lumens, and such urine is said to be dilute (or hyposthenuric) compared with glomerular filtrate (and plasma; Figure 1-5). The rate at which water is excreted without solute during the production of hypotonic urine is called *free water clearance*. The specific gravity (and osmolality) of dilute urine (SG = 1.001 to ≅1.006; Osm = 50 to ≅275 mOsm/kg) would be less than that of glomerular filtrate.

Pharmacologic agents (e.g., ethanol, morphine) or pathologic disorders (central diabetes insipidus, renal diabetes insipidus) that interfere with the production, release, or action of ADH on distal nephrons are commonly associated with profound polyuria. This form of diuresis is commonly called *obligatory water diuresis* (as opposed to osmotic diuresis). A compensatory water diuresis may occur in association with so-called *psychogenic* (or primary) *polydipsia*.

Impaired Urine Concentration and Dilution

In dogs, generalized renal disease of sufficient severity to impair approximately two thirds or more of nephron function impairs urine concentration and dilution. If damage to nephrons is extensive, the specific gravity may become "fixed" at approximately 1.008 to 1.012 (so-called *isosthenuria*). Although the specific gravity of urine in such patients is similar to that of glomerular filtrate, it should not be inferred that the tubules have completely lost the ability to modify it. The vast majority of water and metabolites filtered by glomeruli of such

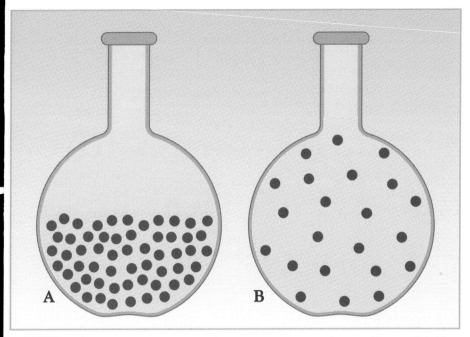

FIGURE 1-5 *Schematic representation of urine concentration and urine dilution.* (**A**) *Urine concentration is characterized by removal of more water than solute from glomerular filtrate. The result is a reduced volume of urine containing a relatively high concentration of solute (higher than that of glomerular filtrate).* (**B**) *Urine dilution is characterized by removal of more solute than water from glomerular filtrate. The result is an increased volume of urine containing a relatively low concentration of solute (lower than that of glomerular filtrate).*

patients must be recovered if life is to be sustained. Lack of detectable glucose in the urine of most patients with primary renal failure and isosthenuria illustrates the point. For another illustration, the fact that polyuria occurs in azotemic patients with glomerular filtration that is 75% or less of normal is sometimes viewed as a paradox. Shouldn't the volume of urine formed also be 25% or less of normal? The confusion can readily be resolved by comparing the daily volume of glomerular filtrate in a 20 lb dog (60 L) with that formed by a patient with primary polyuric renal failure (75% of 60 L, or 15 L) and by comparing the daily volume of urine produced by a normal individual (approximately 0.5 L) with that produced by the patient with polyuric renal failure (approximately 2 L). Even though the volume of glomerular filtrate formed as a consequence of renal failure is 25% of normal (15 L), impaired ability of the tubules to modify the filtrate results in polyuria characterized by a fourfold increase in urine volume.

Final Composition of Urine

The urinary system is designed to eliminate body wastes in liquid form. Urine that is eliminated from the body contains a variable number and quantity of soluble organic and inorganic substances cleared from blood by the kidneys to maintain homeostasis. Urine also contains substances that inhibit crystal formation (e.g., Tamm-Horsfall mucoprotein), crystal aggregation (e.g., nephrocalcin), and bacterial UTIs (e.g., immunoglobulin A).

The composition of normal urine varies widely, being influenced by many factors including species, age, body metabolism and endocrine function, environment, physical activity, and type of diet and amount of water consumed. Test results that may be expected when evaluating normal randomly collected and voided urine samples by commercially manufactured dipsticks are listed in Table 1-6.

Although not contained in glomerular filtrate, voided urine may contain a few red blood cells, a few white cells, a few tubular, transitional, and squamous epithelial cells, occasional hyaline or granular casts, a variety of crystals, and occasional bacteria, spermatozoa, and fat droplets.

TABLE 1-6

URINE COMPOSITION: NORMAL FINDINGS

- **Albumin**—Negative; trace to 1+ in highly concentrated samples

- **Bilirubin**—Dogs, negative to 1+; cats, negative

- **Blood, occult**—Negative; positive results may be caused by trauma induced by collection method (catheterization, cystocentesis, or digital compression of the urinary bladder)

- **Glucose**—Negative

- **Ketones**—Negative

- **Nitrite**—Test pad unreliable in dogs and cats

- **pH**—5.5 to 8.5

- **Protein**—Negative; trace to 1+ in highly concentrated samples

- **Specific gravity**—Test pad unreliable in dogs and cats

- **Urobilinogen**—Negative

- **White cells (leukocyte esterase)**—Test pad unreliable in cats and insensitive in dogs

REFERENCES AND SUGGESTED READINGS

1. Clapp JR, Robinson RR: Osmolality of distal tubular fluid in the dog. *J Clin Invest* 45:1847–1853, 1966.
2. Finco DR: Kidney function, in Kaneka JJ (ed): *Clinical Biochemistry of Domestic Animals*, ed 4. New York, Academic Press, 1989.
3. Jolliffe N, Smith HW: The excretion of urine in the dog. *Am Physiol* 98:572–577, 1931.
4. Lulich JP, Osborne CA: Interpretation of urine protein-creatinine ratios in dogs with glomerular and nonglomerular disorders. *Compend Contin Educ Pract Vet* 12:59–72, 1990.
5. Schmidt-Nielsen B: Urinary concentrating processes in vertebrates. *Yale J Biol Med* 52:545–561, 1979.

Chapter 2

The compassionate principle that guides our actions must be the welfare of our patients first ... and last.

C.A.O.

Renal Disease, Renal Failure, and Uremia: Definition of Terms and Concepts

I.	**Renal Disease**
II.	**Renal Failure (Insufficiency)**
III.	**Azotemia**
IV.	**Uremia**
V.	**Differentiation Between Renal Disease and Renal Failure**

Confusion and misunderstanding often occur when two people attempt to communicate using two different languages. More commonly, confusion arises between individuals using the same language but attaching different meanings or different definitions to what appears to be a universally accepted term (such as renal disease). Confusion caused by use of the terms *renal disease, renal failure, azotemia,* and *uremia* as synonyms may result in misdiagnosis and formulation of inappropriate or even contraindicated therapy.

RENAL DISEASE

The term *renal disease* should not be considered synonymous with the terms *renal failure* and *uremia* unless it is described as generalized renal disease. The key point is that, depending on the quantity of renal parenchyma affected and the severity and duration of lesions, renal disease(s) may or may not cause renal failure or uremia. The clinical relevance of the difference between renal disease and renal failure is emphasized by the fact that symptomatic and supportive therapies designed to correct fluid, electrolyte, acid–base, nutrient, and endocrine imbalances in patients with renal failure typically are not appropriate for patients with renal disease without renal dysfunction. Patients with adequate renal function do not need dietary modification, phosphorus-binding agents, alkalinizing agents, supplemental erythropoietin, supplemental vitamin D, or supplemental vitamins.

Renal disease may affect glomeruli, tubules, interstitial tissue, and/or vessels. Some renal diseases may be associated with dysfunction (e.g., some forms of nephrogenic diabetes insipidus and renal tubular acidosis) or biochemical abnormalities (e.g., cystinuria) without detectable renal morphologic alterations. Others may be associated with morphologic renal disease (anomalies, infections, endogenous or exogenous toxin-induced lesions, immune-mediated lesions, damage caused by hypercalcemia and other mineral imbalances, traumatic lesions) that affects one or both kidneys. The specific cause(s) of renal disease(s) may or may not be known; however, quantitative information about renal function (or dysfunction) is not defined. Renal disease(s) may regress, persist, or advance. Unfortunately, many renal diseases escape detection until they become so generalized that they induce clinical signs resulting from serious impairment of renal function.

RENAL FAILURE (INSUFFICIENCY)

Failure is defined as an inability to perform. The term *renal failure* (or renal insufficiency) typically has been used to imply that two thirds to three quarters or more of the functional capacity of the nephrons of both kidneys has been impaired. It often is used to connote a less severe state of renal dysfunction (or renal insufficiency) that is not (yet) associated with polysystemic clinical manifestations (i.e., uremia). Studies in dogs revealed that impaired ability to concentrate and dilute urine caused by primary renal disease was not detected by evaluation of urine specific gravity until about two thirds of the nephrons of both kidneys were surgically extirpated. Although the serum concentrations of urea nitrogen and creatinine vary inversely with glomerular filtration rate (GFR), primary renal azotemia and retention of other metabolites normally excreted by the kidneys are usually not recognized until the functional capacity of 70% to 75% of the nephrons is affected (Table 2-1).

Renal function *adequate* for homeostasis does not require that *all* nephrons be functional. The concept that adequate renal function is not synonymous with total renal function is of importance in understanding the difference between renal disease and renal failure; making meaningful prognoses; and formulating specific, supportive, and symptomatic therapy.

Renal failure is analogous to liver failure or heart failure in that a level of organ dysfunction is described rather than a specific disease entity. The kidneys are designed to perform multiple functions, including selective elimination of waste products of metabolism from the body, synthesis of a variety of hormones, and degradation of a variety of hormones. Failure to perform these functions may not be an all or none phenomenon (Table 2-1). For example, in patients with slowly progressive renal diseases, failure to appropriately concentrate or dilute urine according to body need typically precedes failure to eliminate waste products of metabolism of such magnitude that it causes azotemia. In turn, laboratory detection of impaired ability to eliminate waste products of metabolism (e.g., urea and creatinine) and to maintain electrolyte and nonelectrolyte solute balance within normal limits typically precedes the onset of polysystemic clinical signs of renal dysfunction.

Clinical signs and polysystemic disorders caused by deficits and excesses in water, electrolyte, acid-base, endocrine, and nutrient balance are not invariably present in patients with primary renal failure (i.e., not all patients with primary renal failure are uremic). This is related, at least in part, to the reserve capacity of the kidneys and the ability of unaffected nephrons to undergo compensatory hypertrophy and hyperplasia. Polysystemic signs of renal failure (i.e., uremia), including vomiting, diarrhea, depression, anorexia, dehydration, and weight loss, usually do not occur until more than three quarters of the total nephron population has been functionally impaired.

TABLE 2-1

COMPARISON OF THE LEVEL OF NEPHRON FUNCTION ASSOCIATED WITH TYPICAL MANIFESTATIONS OF RENAL DYSFUNCTION

Type of Impaired Function	Amount of Nephron Dysfunction
Altered glomerular capillary permeability to plasma proteins	Variable[a]
Impaired tubular concentration or dilution of glomerular filtrate	At least two thirds in dogs, and even more in cats
Azotemia and hyperphosphatemia caused by impaired GFR	At least three quarters
Impaired synthesis of erythropoietin and 1,25–vitamin D	Greater than three quarters
Polysystemic signs of uremia	Greater than three quarters

GFR = glomerular filtration rate.
[a]Glomerular proteinuria may occur in patients with normal GFR, normal tubular reabsorption, and normal tubular secretion. It may also occur when these functions are mildly or severely altered.

AZOTEMIA

Azotemia is defined as an abnormal concentration of urea, creatinine, and other nonprotein nitrogenous substances in blood, plasma, or serum. Azotemia is a laboratory finding with several fundamentally different causes. Because nonprotein nitrogenous compounds (including urea and creatinine) are endogenous substances, abnormally elevated concentrations in serum may be caused by (1) an increased rate of production (of urea by the liver or of creatinine by muscles), (2) by a decreased rate of loss (primarily by the kidneys), or (3) both of these mechanisms.

Because azotemia may be caused by factors that are not directly related to the urinary system and by abnormalities of the lower urinary tract not directly related to the kidney, azotemia should not be used as a synonym for renal failure or uremia. Although the concentrations of serum urea nitrogen and creatinine are commonly used as crude indices of GFR, meaningful interpretation of these parameters depends on recognition and evaluation of prerenal, primary renal, and postrenal factors that may reduce GFR (Tables 1-2 and 2-2).

UREMIA

Uremia is defined as (1) abnormal quantities of urine constituents in blood caused by primary generalized renal disease *and* (2) the polysystemic toxic syndrome that occurs as a result of abnormal renal function (Figures 2-1 through 2-5). When the structural and functional integrity of both kidneys has been compromised to a sufficient degree that polysystemic signs of renal failure are clinically manifested, the relatively predictable complex of uremia appears, regardless of the underlying cause. In some instances, uremic crises may suddenly be precipitated by prerenal disorders (e.g., congestive heart failure, acute pancreatitis, hypoa-

TABLE 2-2

EXAMPLES OF DIFFERENT CAUSES OF AZOTEMIA IN DOGS

Factors	Prerenal Causes		Postrenal Causes	Primary Renal Causes					
	Pancreatitis (7-yr-old male Boston terrier)	Hypoadreno-corticism (3-yr-old female greyhound)	Urethral Obstruction (9-yr-old male miniature poodle)	Hypercalcemic Polyuric Nephropathy (5-yr-old female mixed breed)	Ischemic Oliguric Renal Failure (11-yr-old female beagle)	Early Glomerular Disease with Glomerulo-tubular Imbalance, Amyloidosis (7-yr-old female Great Dane)	Advanced Polyuric Glomerular Amyloidosis (5-yr-old male beagle)	Chronic Polyuric Escherichia coli pyelonephritis (10-yr-old female Siamese cat)
Serum								
Urea nitrogen (mg/dl)	65	75	54	75	207	50	148	74
Creatinine (mg/dl)	2.1	2.5	2.0	4.5	16.2	2.0	5.1	6.1
Sodium (mEq/L)	147	136	151	159	133	144	146	152
Potassium (mEq/L)	4.9	7.1	4.1	4.4	6.0	3.1	3.8	4.8
Na:K ratio	>25:1	<25:1	>25:1	>25:1	<25:1	>25:1	>25:1	>25:1
Calcium (mg/dl)	10.0	11.5	9.0	14.7	9.1	9.8	7.0[a]	9.5
Amylase	7 × normal	Normal	ND	2 × normal	ND	2 × normal	Normal	Normal
Urine								
Volume	Decreased	Decreased	Absent	Increased	Decreased	Normal	Increased	Increased
Specific gravity	1.047	1.017	1.021	1.014	1.010	1.024	1.011	1.018
pH	6.0	6.0	8.0	6.0	5.5	6.5	5.5	6.0
Protein	Negative	Negative	4+	Negative	1+	3+	4+	Trace
Casts/lpf	Moderate granular	Few granular	Negative	Negative	Negative	Occasional hyaline	Rare hyaline	Negative
RBCs/hpf	0–1	Occasional	TNTC	Negative	2–3	Negative	Negative	Negative
WBCs/hpf	0–1	Negative	TNTC	Negative	0–1	Negative	Negative	1–2
Crystals/hpf	Negative	Negative	Struvite	Negative	Negative	Negative	Negative	Negative

hpf = high power field; lpf = low power field; ND = not determined; TNTC = too numerous to count.

[a] Associated with a marked reduction in the total concentration of serum protein and albumin.

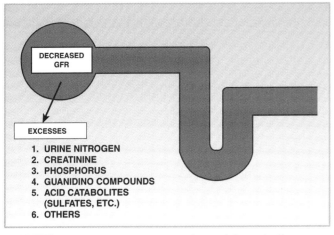

FIGURE 2-1 *Various diseases that cause decreased glomerular filtration rate result in excessive systemic accumulation of substances normally eliminated by the kidneys. Excesses of these substances contribute to uremic signs.*

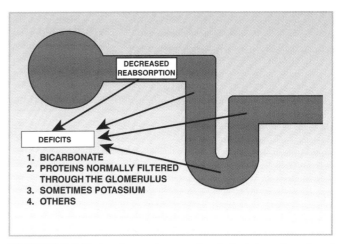

FIGURE 2-2 *Various diseases that cause impaired tubular reabsorption of vital substances filtered by glomeruli result in systemic deficits that contribute to uremic signs.*

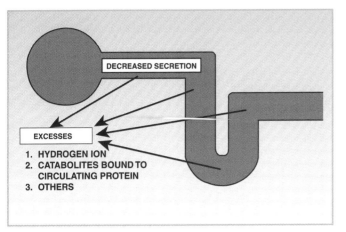

FIGURE 2-3 *Various diseases that cause impaired tubular secretion result in systemic excesses of substances normally eliminated in urine. Excesses of these substances contribute to uremic signs.*

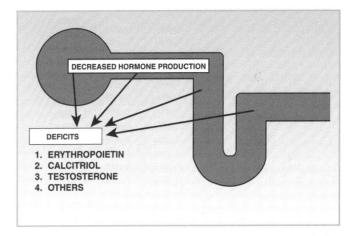

FIGURE 2-4 *Various diseases that impair production of hormones lead to systemic deficits that contribute to signs of uremia.*

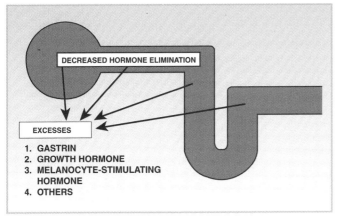

FIGURE 2-5 *Various diseases that impair elimination of hormones by the kidneys result in systemic excesses that contribute to signs of uremia.*

drenocorticism) or, less commonly, postrenal disorders (urethral obstruction, displacement of the urinary bladder into a perineal hernia) in patients with previously compensated primary renal failure (Table 1-2).

Uremia is characterized by multiple physiologic and metabolic alterations that result from renal insufficiency. Renal insufficiency may be caused by numerous disease processes that have in common impairment of at least three quarters of the function of both kidneys. Depending on the biologic behavior of the disease in question, primary renal failure may be reversible or irreversible, acute or chronic, and oliguric and/or polyuric.

As mentioned, renal disease may precede renal failure; likewise, renal failure may precede uremia. In some patients, renal disease may not progress to a state of renal failure. In others, prerenal events may precipitate a uremic crisis in patients with chronic renal failure. In untreated patients uremia is always accompanied by renal disease, renal failure, and azotemia.

DIFFERENTIATION BETWEEN RENAL DISEASE AND RENAL FAILURE

The differentiation between renal disease and renal failure (with or without uremia) may be facilitated by understanding that not all diagnostic procedures used to detect disorders of the urinary system provide information about the capacity of the renal functional and that differentiating inflammatory dis-

TABLE 2-3

DIAGNOSTIC PROCEDURES COMMONLY USED TO DETECT AND LOCALIZE DISORDERS OF THE URINARY SYSTEM

Method	Renal Function	Localized to Kidney	Localized to Urinary System
Urea nitrogen (serum or plasma)	GFR	No[a]	No
Creatinine (serum or plasma)	GFR	No[a]	No
Exogenous iohexol clearance	GFR	No	No
Specific gravity (urine)	Tubular reabsorption	No[a]	No
Osmolality (urine)	Tubular reabsorption	No[a]	No
Phenolsulfonphthalein (urine excretion)	Renal blood flow, tubular secretion	No[a]	No
Sodium sulfanilate (plasma retention)	GFR	No[a]	No
Intravenous urography	Crude index of renal blood flow and GFR	Yes	Yes
Ultrasonography	No	Yes	Yes
Water deprivation and vasopressin response tests	Tubular function	No[a]	No
Renal tubular epithelial cells	No	No[b]	No
Urinary casts	No	Yes	—
Renal biopsy	No	Yes	—
Significant bacteriuria	No	No	Yes[c]
Proteinuria	No	No[d]	No
Pyuria	No	No[b]	Yes[c]
Hematuria	No	No[b]	Yes[c]

GFR = glomerular filtration rate.
[a]Alterations in renal function are not always caused by diseases localized to the kidneys.
[b]Unless present in urinary casts.
[c]Assuming that urine is not contaminated by the genital tract.
[d]Large quantities of protein in absence of RBCs and WBCs suggest glomerular disease.

eases of the lower urinary tract from those affecting the upper urinary tract is not always possible (Table 2-3). For example, the detection of a significant number of casts in urine sediment provides reliable evidence of renal tubular involvement because casts form in the loops of Henle, distal tubules, and collecting ducts. It cannot be inferred that detection of large numbers of casts is indicative of renal failure, however, because their presence or absence cannot be correlated with the degree or renal dysfunction (if any).

Differentiation between renal disease and renal failure has clinical significance when gastrointestinal, endocrine, pancreatic, and hepatic diseases causing clinical signs similar to those associated with uremia (i.e., vomiting, diarrhea, polydipsia, dehydration, depression, anorexia, and weight loss) secondarily induce prerenal azotemia and/or ischemic tubular disease characterized by formation of variable numbers of epithelial, granular, and waxy casts (Table 2-3). Although extrarenal fluid loss and subsequent reduction in renal perfusion may be of sufficient magnitude to damage some nephrons and cause prere-

nal azotemia, detection of concentrated urine (specific gravity >1.030 in dogs and >1.035 to 1.040 in cats) indicates a population of functioning nephrons adequate to prevent signs caused by primary renal failure (Tables 2-2 and 2-3 and Figure 1-4). Effort should be made to rapidly restore renal perfusion, however, because progressive destruction of nephrons may induce primary ischemic renal failure.

SUPPLEMENTAL READING

DiBartola SP: Clinical approach and laboratory evaluation of renal disease, in Ettinger SJ, Feldman EC (eds): *Textbook of Veterinary Internal Medicine*. Philadelphia, WB Saunders, 1995, pp 1706–1719.

Grauer GF, Lane IF: Acute renal failure, in Ettinger SJ, Feldman EC (eds): *Textbook of Veterinary Internal Medicine*. Philadelphia, WB Saunders, 1995, pp 1720–1733.

Osborne CA, Finco DR: *Canine and Feline Nephrology and Urology*. Baltimore, Williams & Wilkins, 1995.

Polzin DJ, Osborne CA, Bartges JW, et al: Chronic renal failure, in Ettinger SJ, Feldman EC (eds): *Textbook of Veterinary Internal Medicine*. Philadelphia, WB Saunders, 1995, pp 1734–1760.

Chapter 3

Compassion is having empathy for the suffering or distress of others and the desire to help (Webster's Dictionary). We should express compassion to patients under our care in the form most expected of us, namely professional competence.

C.A.O.

Bacteriuria and Urinary Tract Infections: Definition of Terms and Concepts

I.   **Clinical Significance of Bacterial Urinary Tract Infections***

II. **Definition of Terms in Context of Urinary Tract Infections**
   A. Bacteriuria in Context of UTI
   B. Pyuria in Context of UTI
   C. Urine pH in Context of UTI
   D. Specific Gravity in Context of UTI
   E. Inflammation Versus Bacterial Infection in Context of UTI

III. **Bacterial Urinary Tract Infections**
   A. Overview
   B. Pathogenesis
      1. Uncomplicated (Simple) Infections

2. Complicated Infections
3. Recurrent Bacterial Infections
   a. Relapsing Infections
   b. Recurrent Reinfections
   c. Superinfections

IV. **Diagnostic Urine Culture**
   A. Overview
   B. Urine Collection Methods
   C. Timing of Urine Collection and Sample Preservation
   D. Significance of Qualitative Urine Cultures
   E. Concept of Significant Bacteriuria and Quantitative Urine Cultures
      1. Conceptual Overview
      2. Quantitative Urine Cultures

*For therapeutic antibiotic recommendations, see Appendix C.

CLINICAL SIGNIFICANCE OF BACTERIAL URINARY TRACT INFECTIONS

Bacterial urinary tract infection (UTI), a common cause of urinary tract disease in dogs, is estimated to affect 14% of all dogs during their lifetime and 10% of dogs admitted to veterinary hospitals.[24–26] In one autopsy study the infection rate was reported to be 6% in males and 27% in females.[3] Infections most commonly affected dogs less than 2 years or older than 6 years of age.

Data retrospectively derived from the Purdue Veterinary Medical Data Base revealed the following trends. Between January 1, 1980, and September 30, 1995, lower urinary tract diseases were diagnosed in 3% (24,087 of 809,849) of dogs admitted to veterinary colleges in North America that are registered with the Purdue Center. Of the 24,087 cases of lower urinary tract disease recorded, 57.4% (13,817) occurred in female dogs and 42.6% (10,270) occurred in male dogs. In these 24,087 dogs, urinary incontinence (23.7%), urolithiasis (21.3%), UTIs (19.4%), and neoplasia (7.3%) were diagnosed most often. The prevalence of UTI was 19.4% for all dogs, with females accounting for 23% and males accounting for 14.6%.[30]

In contrast, results of several investigations of feline lower urinary tract disease indicate that the initial episode in young to middle-aged cats (1 to 10 years of age) is associated with bacterial UTI in only 1% to 3% of the patients.[5,10,22,31] This observation is supported by retrospective evaluation of data from 24 Colleges of Veterinary Medicine in North America compiled by workers at the Veterinary Data Base, Purdue University. From 1980 to 1997, lower urinary tract disease (LUTD) was diagnosed in 10.3% (22,378 of 216,833) of cats admitted to 24 teaching hospitals (cases were counted only once irrespective of the number of readmissions). Of the 22,378 cats with LUTD, bacterial UTI was diagnosed in 5% and bacterial cystitis was diagnosed in 3%. Of 22,378 cats diagnosed with LUTD at 24 colleges of veterinary medicine, 2% were less than 1 year old. These data indicate that lower urinary tract disease is uncommon in immature cats. However, when we encounter LUTD in immature cats, we have a high index of suspicion of bacterial UTI associated with functional or anatomic defects. Although bacterial UTI was uncommonly encountered in young adult cats, the prevalence of UTI increased with age.

In one retrospective study, the prevalence of bacterial UTIs in geriatric cats (10 years of age and older) with lower urinary tract disease was greater than 50%.[7] Approximately two thirds of the cats with bacterial UTI also had a diagnosis of renal failure.

Once established, bacterial UTI may be associated with one or more sequelae (Table 3-1). However, early detection followed by proper treatment and follow-up evaluation will minimize the occurrence and severity of these sequelae.

No pathognomonic history, physical examination, radiographic, or ultrasonographic findings have been associated with bacterial UTI. A definitive diagnosis requires urinalysis and urine culture to confirm the presence of pathogenic bacteria.

DEFINITION OF TERMS IN CONTEXT OF URINARY TRACT INFECTIONS
Bacteriuria in Context of UTI

Bacteriuria is the presence of bacteria in urine. It is not synonymous with UTI for the following reasons:

- Urine normally is sterile until it reaches the mid-urethra. The urethra of dogs and cats, however, contains a resident population of bacteria, with the greatest at the distal end of the urethra (Table 3-2). The normal flora of bacteria must be considered when interpreting the results of urine cultures, especially if samples are collected during voiding or by catheterization. Most of these organisms are gram positive. The significance of bacteria in voided or catheterized urine samples should be interpreted with caution because samples collected by these methods may be contaminated with bacteria normally residing in the distal urethra and genital tracts.
- Urine may be contaminated with bacteria after it is removed from the patient and before it is cultured. Some bacteria may multiply at a rate that doubles their numbers every 45 minutes.

Bacteria may be difficult to identify by light microscopic examination of urine. In addition, nonbacterial look-alikes may be confused with bacteria. Although detection of structures that look like bacteria in urine sediment suggests UTI, the diagnosis should be verified by urine culture.

TABLE 3-1
POTENTIAL SEQUELAE TO UNTREATED BACTERIAL URINARY TRACT INFECTIONS

1. **Lower Urinary Tract Dysfunction (Acute or Chronic)**
   a. Dysuria; pollakiuria
   b. "Urge" incontinence
   c. Damage to the detrusor muscle
   d. Damage to the urethra
2. **Prostatitis (Acute or Chronic)**
3. **Infertility**
4. **Struvite Urolithiasis and Its Sequelae**
5. **Renal Dysfunction (Acute or Chronic)**
   a. Pyelonephritis
   b. Renal failure
   c. Septicemia (especially in patients with concomitant obstruction to urine outflow)
6. **Anemia of Chronic Inflammation**
7. **Lumbosacral Diskospondylitis**

Detection of a significant number of bacteria in association with pyuria indicates that the inflammatory lesion is active and has been caused or complicated by bacterial infection. Because bacteria are more difficult to observe than white cells in sediment, pyuria may appear to be unassociated with bacteriuria. Not detecting bacteria in urine sediment does not exclude their presence. Approximately 10,000 rod-shaped bacteria per milliliter of urine are required for visualization by light microscopy in unstained preparations of urine sediment. Cocci may not be consistently detected if fewer than 100,000 ml are present.[13,14] Gram's stain or new methylene blue stain may aid in detection of bacteria.

Detection of bacteria within the cytoplasm of phagocytes found in fresh urine sediment suggests in vivo phagocytosis rather than contamination of urine sample during collection or analysis.

Occasionally, patients develop *asymptomatic bacteriuria*, which is verification of significant bacteriuria unaccompanied by signs referable to urinary tract disease. The term is synonymous with *covert bacteriuria*. Asymptomatic or covert bacteriuria is sometimes encountered in dogs given glucocorticoids or with hyperadrenocorticism. In other cases, the suspected predisposing cause is impossible to identify.

Pyuria in Context of UTI

Pyuria is the presence of white cells in urine. A significant number of white cells in urine usually represents a normal protective response by the body to an irritant. Pyuria and infection are not synonymous because pyuria may occur with inflammation attributable to both infectious and noninfectious causes.

When performing a urinalysis to rule in or rule out bacterial UTI, evaluation of urine sediment for white cells should be done using standard techniques. Dipstick leukocyte assays alone are not satisfactory (see the section on leukocyte esterase tests in Chapter 10).[15,34] In dogs, leukocyte test pads frequently yield false-negative results,

Not detecting bacteria in urine sediment does not exclude their presence.

TABLE 3-2

BACTERIA DETECTED IN THE UROGENITAL TRACT OF NORMAL MALE AND FEMALE DOGS[6,13,14,28]

Genus	Distal Urethra (Males)	Prepuce	Vagina
Acinetobacter		+	+
Bacteroides			+
Bacillus		+	+
Citrobacter			+
Corynebacterium	+	+	+
Enterococcus			+
Enterobacter			+
Escherichia	+	+	+
Flavobacterium	+	+	+
Haemophilus	+	+	+
Klebsiella	+	+	+
Micrococcus			+
Moraxella		+	+
Mycoplasma	+	+	+
Neisseria			+
Pasteurella		+	+
Proteus		+	+
Pseudomonas			+
Staphylococus	+	+	+
Streptococcus	+	+	+
Ureaplasma	+	+	+

even when pyuria is present. Although the test is specific for white cells in dogs, it is insensitive. In most cats, leukocyte test pads yield false-positive results in the absence of pyuria. Therefore, the test is of no value in cats.

A significant number of white cells (which may be associated with red blood cells [RBCs] and protein) in a properly collected urine sample suggest an active inflammatory lesion of the urinary tract. The inflammatory lesion may or may not be associated with infectious agents.

Although the normal range of white cells (neutrophils) in urine sediment prepared from a 5 ml aliquot of urine has been reported to be from 0 to 3 white cells per high power field (hpf; 400×) in samples collected by cystocentesis, a value of 0 to 8 WBCs/hpf has been reported in catheterized or midstream voided samples.[23] In this context it becomes readily apparent that there is no absolute cutoff point between an upper limit of the "normal" number of white cells and a lower limit of the "abnormal" number of white cells. Several variables that influence numbers should be considered when interpreting the significance of white cells in urine sediment (Tables 11-6 and 11-9).

Detection of a significant number of bacteria in association with pyuria indicates that the inflammatory lesion is active and has been caused or complicated by bacterial infection (Figure 3-1).

Observation of white cell casts indicates renal tubular involvement in the inflammatory and/or infectious process. White cell casts may undergo degeneration to become granular casts. In our experience, white cell casts are not commonly associated with proven bacterial UTI. Absence of white cells or granular casts does not exclude renal involvement in the inflammatory process.

For additional details, consult the section describing white cells in Chapter 11.

Urine pH in Context of UTI

Although the detection of persistently alkaline urine may be considered to be an indication for further diagnostic study, it should not be considered synonymous with UTI. Several in vivo factors other than bacterial degradation of urea to ammonia affect urine pH.

Urine pH will be persistently alkaline if a UTI is caused or complicated by urease-producing bacteria (especially Staphylococcus, Proteus, and Ureaplasma species). An alkaline urine pH in the absence of pyuria, hematuria, and proteinuria, however, is usually a normal finding.

Because many bacterial uropathogens are not urea splitters, urine pH may not be altered by production of ammonia from urea. Acid or neutral urine pH values do not rule out the possibility of UTI.

Specific Gravity in Context of UTI

Impaired capacity to concentrate urine, with or without azotemia, may be detected in dogs and cats with bilateral generalized infection of the kidneys.[32] Impaired urine concentration capacity may complicate recognition of UTI by "diluting" the magnitude of pyuria and bacteriuria detected by urinalysis.

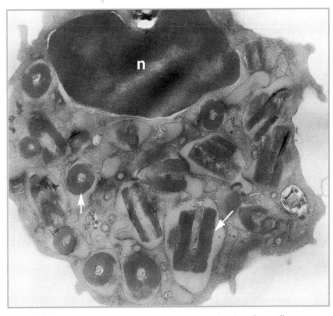

FIGURE 3-1 Transmission electron micrograph of a white cell containing bacteria (arrows). These structures were contained in a matrix-crystalling urethral plug removed from a 2-year-old neutered male domestic shorthair cat. n = nucleus of white cell. (16,000× = original magnification.)

Inflammation Versus Bacterial Infection in Context of UTI

It is essential to distinguish between inflammation and bacterial infection related to urinary tract disease (Table 3-3). In addition to bacterial infection, many diverse noninfectious disease processes, including neoplasia and urolithiasis, result in inflammatory lesions of the urinary tract characterized by exudation of RBCs, white cells, and protein into urine. The resultant hematuria, pyuria, and proteinuria suggest inflammatory urinary tract disease but do not indicate its etiology or location within the urinary tract.

Although detection of bacteria in fresh urine sediment should prompt consideration of UTI, it should be verified by urine culture (Table 3-4). In addition to urine culture, renal function tests, radiographic and ultrasonographic studies, endoscopy, urodynamic studies, and biopsy procedures often provide the additional information necessary to localize the disease process and establish its cause (Table 3-5).[32]

Detection of infection should be established by urine culture because diagnosis based solely on recognition of inflammatory cells in urinalysis will result in overdiagnosis of infection. Conversely, absence of hematuria, pyuria, and proteinuria does not rule out the existence of infection because it can occur without stimulating a detectable inflammatory response.

BACTERIAL URINARY TRACT INFECTIONS
Overview

Bacterial UTI encompasses a variety of clinical entities with a common denominator of microbial invasion of any of the urinary tract components (Table 3-6). UTI is usually caused by ascending migration of bacteria that are inhabitants of the microflora of the lower genitourinary and intestinal tracts.[9a,27a]

Infection may predominate at a single site (e.g., the kidney [pyelonephritis], ureter [ureteritis], bladder [cystitis], urethra [urethritis], or prostate [prostatitis]), affect two or more of these sites, or it may be restricted to the urine (bacteriuria). Although terms such as pyelonephritis, cystitis, and urethritis are commonly used, they reflect localized expressions of UTIs that can potentially affect the entire urinary tract. The important point is that the entire urinary system is at risk for invasion after any of its parts has been colonized with bacteria.

Pathogenesis

Although the pathogenesis of UTIs is still somewhat obscure, it is known that infection depends on the balance between the virulence of uropathic infectious agents (analo-

TABLE 3-3
CHECKLIST OF POSSIBLE CAUSES OF INFLAMMATION DETECTED BY URINALYSIS BUT UNASSOCIATED WITH MICROSCOPIC BACTERIURIA

1. Noninfectious disease of the urinary tract
2. Numbers of bacteria in urine too few for consistent detection by conventional light microscopy (bacterial rods < 10,000/ml, bacterial cocci < 100,000/ml at high power magnification)
3. Male dogs with prostatitis
4. Infection caused by mycoplasma, ureaplasma, or viruses
5. Administration of antimicrobial agents before performing urinalysis

TABLE 3-4
CHECKLIST OF FACTORS THAT MAY EXPLAIN STERILE BACTERIAL URINE CULTURES WHEN BACTERIA WERE OBSERVED IN URINE SEDIMENT

1. Nonviable microbes in urine at the time of collection (host defenses, antimicrobial agents)
2. Urinalysis performed on a sample that was contaminated after collection and improperly preserved
3. Death of fastidious uropathogens between the time of sample collection and urine culture
4. Improper preservation of urine sample
5. Improper culture technique
6. Mistaken identity of structures resembling bacteria in urine sediment

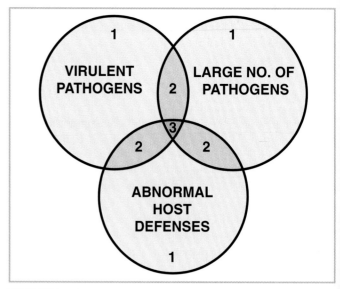

FIGURE 3-2 *Schematic illustration of various combinations of risk factors for urinary tract infections. **1** = lower risk of infection if only one of these factors is present; **2** = higher risk of infection if any combination of two of these factors is present; **3** = highest risk of infection when all three of these factors are present.*

gous to seeds) and host resistance (analogous to soil; Tables 3-7 and 3-8; Figure 3-2).[32] Evidence obtained in recent years indicates that the growth of microbial seeds is enhanced if suitable soil characterized by increased host susceptibility is present.

TABLE 3-5

ABNORMALITIES THAT MAY AID IN LOCALIZATION OF BACTERIAL URINARY TRACT INFECTIONS

Sites of Infection	History	Physical Examination	Laboratory Results	Radiology and Ultrasonography
Lower urinary tract	Dysuria; pollakiuria Urge incontinence Signs of abnormal detrussor reflex (overflow incontinence; residual urine) Gross hematuria at end of micturition No systemic signs of infection Recent catheterization; urethrostomy	Small, painful, thickened bladder (unless urethra obstructed) Palpable masses in urethra or bladder Flaccid bladder wall; residual urine in bladder lumen Abnormal micturition reflex ± Palpation of uroliths	Normal CBC Urinalysis = pyuria, hematuria, proteinuria, bacteriuria Urine culture = significant bacteriuria	Kidneys usually not enlarged Structural abnormalities of lower urinary tract ± Urocystoliths and/or urethroliths ± Only thickening of bladder wall and irregularity of mucosa Rarely intramural gas formation (emphysematous cystitis)
Upper urinary tract	Polyuria and polydipsia ± Signs of systemic infection ± Signs of renal failure	± No detectable abnormalities ± Fever and other signs of systemic infection ± Abdominal (renal) pain Kidney size is normal or increased	± Leukocytosis Urinalysis (variable) = pyuria, hematuria, proteinuria, bacteriuria, WBC or granular casts Impaired concentration ± Azotemia and other abnormalities typical of renal failure	Increase in kidney size ± Abnormal kidney shape ± Nephrolithiasis ± Dilated renal pelves; dilated pelvic diverticula ± Evidence of outflow obstruction
Acute prostatitis or prostatic abscess	Urethral discharge independent of micturition Signs of systemic infection ± Reluctance to defecate or micturate ± Hindlimb lameness or locomotor difficulty	± Fever and other signs of systemic infection ± Painful prostate and/or painful abdomen ± Enlarged or asymmetrical prostate	± Leukocytosis Urinalysis = pyuria, hematuria, proteinuria, bacteriuria Cytology = infectious inflammation	± Indistinct cranial border; enlargement ± Cysts ± Reflux of contrast agent into prostate
Chronic prostatitis	Recurrent UTIs Urethral discharge independent of micturition ± Dysuria	Often no detectable abnormalities ± Enlarged or asymmetrical prostate	Normal CBC Similar to acute prostatitis	± Similar to acute prostatitis ± Abnormal prostatic urethra ± Mineralization

Thus, one should have a high index of suspicion of host defense dysfunction in patients with bacterial UTI, especially if the infection is persistent or recurrent. Use of antimicrobial agents to eliminate uropathogens remains the cornerstone of therapy; however, the status of host defense mechanisms is also an important factor in the pathogenesis of UTIs (Tables 3-8 and 3-9). In other words, in addition to focusing on microbial pathogens (seeds), which traditionally have been accepted as the primary cause of UTI, abnormalities in host defenses (soil) representing major predisposing factors to UTIs must be considered.

A UTI is not a definitive diagnostic entity. Because bacterial UTI encompasses a spectrum of underlying predisposing factors,

diagnostic and therapeutic requirements vary from case to case. Conceptual understanding of the interaction of various host defense mechanisms with pathogenic microbes permits the development of a diagnostically and therapeutically significant classification of UTIs. The common denominator of this classification (the presence or absence of detectable abnormalities in host defense mechanisms) allows differentiation of complicated UTIs from uncomplicated (or simple) UTIs (Table 3-9).[32]

Uncomplicated (Simple) Infections

Uncomplicated UTI is defined as an infection in which no underlying structural, neurologic, or functional abnormality can

TABLE 3-6

DIFFERENT CLASSIFICATIONS OF URINARY TRACT INFECTIONS

I. BY LOCATION
 A. Upper urinary tract infection
  1. Pyelonephritis
   a. Unilateral
   b. Bilateral
  2. Pyelitis
  3. Ureteritis
  4. Combinations of 1, 2, and 3
 B. Lower urinary tract infection
  1. Cystitis
  2. Urethritis
  3. Prostatitis
  4. Combinations of 1, 2, and 3

II. BY COMPLEXITY
 A. Uncomplicated (Simple) UTI
 B. Complicated UTI

III. BY DURATION
 A. Acute UTI
 B. Subacute UTI
 C. Chronic UTI

IV. BY PATHOGEN
 A. Bacterial UTI
  1. Gram positive
  2. Gram negative
 B. Viral UTI

 C. Fungal UTI
 D. Spirochete UTI
  1. Leptospiral
  2. Borreliosis
 D. Parasitic UTI
 E. Rickettsial UTI
 F. Ureaplasmal/mycoplasmal UTI

V. BY RESPONSE TO TREATMENT
 A. Reinfection
 B. Persistent infection
 C. Relapsing infection
 D. Superinfection

Modified from Barsanti JA: Genitourinary infections, in Greene CE (ed): *Infectious Diseases of the Dog and Cat*, ed 2. Philadelphia, WB Saunders, 1998, p 629.

TABLE 3-7

SOME FACTORS THAT MAY ENHANCE THE VIRULENCE OF UROPATHOGENIC BACTERIA

A. *Escherichia coli*
 1. Certain O (somatic) antigens
  a. Outer polysaccharide portion of bacterial envelope
  b. Smooth colony morphology on culture plate
  c. Indirect marker of virulence (human studies)

 2. Certain K (capsular) antigens
  a. The capsule surrounds the bacterium
  b. May inhibit phagocytosis and complement-mediated bactericidal activity
  c. Increased resistance to inflammation favors persistence of bacteria in tissue

 3. Adhesive fimbriae (pili) (Figure 3-3)
  a. Proteinaceous filamentous organelles that protrude from the surface of the bacterium
  b. Specific types of fimbriae (p–fimbriae) enhance the ability of a bacterium to remain adherent to uroepithelium, despite cleansing action of the urinary system

 4. Hemolysin
  a. Increases amount of free iron available for bacterial growth
  b. May cause tissue damage

 5. Aerobactin
  a. Iron binding protein
  b. Facilitates bacterial growth

 6. R–plasmids
  a. Promotes resistance to antimicrobial agents

 7. Resistance to serum bactericidal activity

 8. Short generation time in urine

B. *Proteus, Staphylococcus*, some *Klebsiella*
 1. Adherence factors

 2. Urease
  a. Bacterial enzyme that hydrolyzes urea to ammonia
  b. Ammonia directly injures epithelium
  c. Urease fosters production of magnesium ammonium phosphate uroliths

 3. R–plasmids

 4. Production of protective biofilms (slime layer)

 5. Production of nucleases and proteases

C. *Pseudomonas*
 1. Heavy mucoid polysaccharide capsule
  a. Prevents antibody coating

 2. R–Plasmids

be identified. Although useful, this classification may be misleading because it implies that bacterial infection is always the primary abnormality. This may be the situation if normal host defenses are overwhelmed by a large inoculum of pathogens; however, most bacteria survive and multiply only when host defenses are compromised. UTI encompasses a transient or per-

sistent defect in the patient's innate defense mechanisms, even though the underlying cause may escape detection.

The clinical relevance of identifying uncomplicated UTI is that the infection is more likely to be caused by a transient, self-limiting, and potentially reversible abnormality in host defenses than one that is caused by identifiable abnormalities

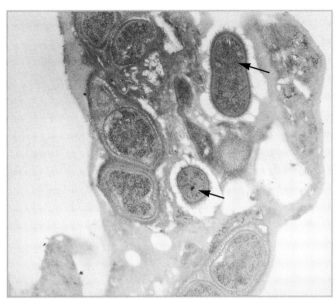

FIGURE 3-3 *Transmission electron micrograph of bacteria (arrows) thought to be* Escherichia coli *contained in the matrix of a struvite urolith formed by a 3-year-old neutered female domestic shorthair cat. Note the fimbriae protruding from the surface of the bacteria. (16,000× = original magnification.)*

in local host defenses (complicated UTI). Therefore, there is usually a better prognosis for recovery.

Complicated Infections

Complicated UTI occurs as a result of bacterial invasion of the urinary system secondary to an identifiable disease that interferes with defense mechanisms. Causes of complicated UTI include interference with micturition, anatomic defects, alterations in urothelium, altered volume, voiding frequency, and impaired immunocompetence (Table 3-9). Clinical signs of UTI are often the first evidence of underlying congenital or acquired abnormalities. In general, the underlying cause must be removed or corrected if secondary bacterial infection is to be completely eradicated. Failure or inability to do so is a common cause of recurrent UTIs (relapse, reinfection, or superinfection.

Recurrent Bacterial Infections

Recurrence of clinical and/or laboratory signs of UTIs after withdrawal of therapy may be classified as relapses, reinfections, or superinfections. Classification of recurrences is determined by comparing results of follow-up urine cultures to results of initial diagnostic urine cultures (Appendix C, Table C-9). It is impossible to dif-ferentiate relapsing recurrences from reinfections without comparing results from bacterial culture of urine obtained before initiation of therapy to those from bacterial cultures of urine obtained during and/or after withdrawal of therapy.

Relapsing Infections

Relapses (persistent infections) are defined as recurrences caused by the same species and serologic strain of microorganism within several days to a few weeks of the date of cessation of therapy. Relapses represent antimicrobial treatment failures associated with one or more causes and affect both male and female dogs and cats throughout their lifespan (Table 3-10).[32] The pathogenesis of relapsing UTI likely involves failure to completely eliminate pathogenic bacteria before antimicrobial therapy is withdrawn. Relapses have the potential to cause significant morbidity if mismanaged.

Recurrent Reinfections

Reinfections are defined as recurrent infections caused by a different pathogen(s). If tissues of the urinary tract have had time to heal from the infection, reinfections often occur at a longer interval following cessation of therapy than do relapses. Reinfection may be associated with several causes (Table 3-11) but typically represent superficial invasion of the tissues surrounding the lumen of the urinary tract.[32] Reinfections appear to be more common in female dogs and young to middle-aged cats with lower urinary tract disease.

TABLE 3-8

NATURAL AND ACQUIRED HOST DEFENSES OF THE URINARY TRACT

I. NORMAL MICTURITION
  A. Adequate urine volume
  B. Frequent voiding
  C. Complete voiding

II. ANATOMIC STRUCTURES
  A. Urethral high pressure zones
  B. Surface characteristics of urethral urothelium
  C. Urethral peristalsis
  D. Prostatic secretions (antibacterial fraction and immunoglobulins)
  E. Length of urethra
  F. Ureterovesical flap valves
  G. Ureteral peristalsis
  H. Glomerular mesangial cells (?)
  I. Extensive renal blood supply and flow
  J. Others (?)

III. MUCOSAL DEFENSE BARRIERS
  A. Antibody production
  B. Surface layer (hydrophilic glycosaminoglycans)
  C. Intrinsic mucosal antimicrobial properties
  D. Exfoliation of cells
  E. Bacterial interferences by commensal microbes (normal flora of distal urethra and distal genital tract)
  F. Others(?)

IV. ANTIMICROBIAL PROPERTIES OF URINE
  A. Extremes (high or low) of urine pH
  B. Hyperosmolality
  C. High concentration of urea
  D. Organic acids
  E. Small molecular weight carbohydrates
  F. Tamm–Horsfall mucoprotein
  G. Leukocyte esterase (cats?)
  H. Others (?)

V. SYSTEMIC IMMUNOCOMPETENCE
  A. Cell-mediated immunity
  B. Humoral-mediated immunity

TABLE 3-9

CLASSIFICATION OF SOME IDENTIFIABLE PREDISPOSING CAUSES OF COMPLICATED UTIs

I. INTERFERENCE WITH NORMAL MICTURITION
   A. Mechanical obstruction to outflow
      1. Uroliths and strictures (especially of urethra)
      2. Herniated urinary bladder
      3. Prostatic cysts, abscesses, or neoplasms
      4. Obstructing urothelial neoplasms

   B. Incomplete emptying of excretory pathway
      1. Damaged innervation
         a. Vertebral fractures, luxations, subluxations
         b. Intervertebral disc disease
         c. Vertebral osteomyelitis
         d. Neoplasia
         e. Vertebral or spinal cord anomalies
         f. Reflex dyssynergia
      2. Anatomic defects
         a. Diverticula of urethra, bladder, ureters, renal pelves (especially persistent urachal diverticula)
         b. Vesicoureteral reflux

II. ANATOMIC DEFECTS
   A. Congenital or inherited
      1. Urethral anomalies
      2. Ectopic ureters

      3. Persistent urachal diverticula
      4. Primary vesicoureteral reflux

   B. Acquired
      1. Diseases of the urinary tract, especially lower portions
      2. Secondary vesicoureteral reflux
      3. Urethrostomy, trigonal–colonic anastomosis, and other surgical diversion procedures

III. ALTERATION OF UROTHELIUM
   A. Trauma
      1. External force
      2. Palpation
      3. Catheterization and other instrumentation
      4. Urolithiasis

   B. Metaplasia
      1. Administration of estrogens
      2. Estrogen-producing Sertoli cell neoplasms

   C. Neoplasia

   D. Urinary excretion of cytotoxic drugs, such as cyclophosphamide

   E. Alteration of normal flora of the distal urethra, prepuce, and vagina

   F. Other

IV. ALTERATIONS IN THE VOLUME, FREQUENCY, OR COMPOSITION OF URINE
   A. Decreased urine volume
      1. Negative water balance
         a. Decreased water consumption
         b. Vomiting and/or diarrhea
      2. Primary oliguric renal failure

   B. Voluntary or involuntary retention

   C. Glucosuria

   D. Formation of dilute urine[a]

V. IMPAIRED IMMUNOCOMPETENCE
   A. Diseases
      1. Congenital immunodeficiency (?)
      2. Acquired
         a. Hyperadrenocorticism (?)
         b. Uremia

   B. Corticosteroids; immunosuppressant drugs

[a]Formation of dilute urine predisposes the patient to lower UTI but may prevent or minimize bacterial infections of the renal medulla.

Superinfections

Superinfections are defined as infections with an additional organism during the course of antimicrobial treatment. They are most likely to occur in association with indwelling urethral catheters. They also occur as sequelae to urinary diversion techniques in which the urinary tract communicates with the intestinal tract or when proximal portions of the urethra, urinary bladder, or kidneys communicate directly with the exterior (as with antepubic urethrostomy, tube cystostomy, or percutaneous nephropyelostomy).

Consult Appendix C (Treatment of Bacterial Urinary Tract Infections) for recommendations about management of recurrent bacterial UTIs.

DIAGNOSTIC URINE CULTURE
Overview

Urine culture is the gold standard for diagnosis of UTIs. In addition, bacterial pathogens are accurately identified. Diagnosis of bacterial UTIs solely on the basis of clinical signs usually results in overdiagnosis. Failure to perform urine cultures or to interpret the results of urine cultures correctly may lead to both diagnostic errors and therapeutic failures.

Diagnostic urine cultures and antimicrobial susceptibility tests are highly recommended when antimicrobial therapy fails to ameliorate clinical signs or any time UTIs recur. Antimicrobial therapy should be withdrawn for 3 to 5 days prior to collecting urine for culture.

In dogs and cats, therapy for bacterial UTI is often initiated without the benefit of culture results. When this form of empirical therapy is considered, it is important to remember the following:

■ Because several different bacterial species may cause UTIs in dogs or cats, reliable prediction of the causative bacterial pathogen or the antimicrobial agent to which it might be susceptible is not possible (Tables 3-12 amd 3-13).

TABLE 3-10

CHECKLIST OF POTENTIAL CAUSES OF PERSISTENT (RELAPSE) INFECTION WITH SAME TYPE OF BACTERIA

1. Use of improper antimicrobial susceptibility tests and/or misinterpretation of results

2. Mixed infections with more than one type of pathogen in which all pathogens were not eradicated by antimicrobial therapy

3. Failure to prescribe antimicrobial agents for a sufficient period to eradicate pathogens (a relapse or persistent infection occurs)

4. Failure to prescribe a proper dosage and/or maintenance interval for an antimicrobial agent that would otherwise be effective

5. Lack of compliance characterized by the failure or inability of owners to administer the prescribed dose of antimicrobial agent(s) at the proper maintenance intervals and for sufficient duration

6. Use of ineffective drugs
   a. Ineffective against uropathogens
   b. Failure to attain therapeutic concentration in urine
   c. Failure to achieve therapeutic concentrations at infection sites (especially kidneys, prostate gland, and infection–induced uroliths)
   d. Inappropriate use of combinations of drugs that interfere with their ability to eradicate bacteria

7. Failure of the patient to absorb a portion or all of an orally administered drug because of ingesta, gastrointestinal dysfunction, or interaction with other drugs

8. Premature assessment of therapeutic response

9. Initiation of therapy at an advanced state in the evolution of the disease

10. Acquired drug-resistant bacteria, including L–forms

11. Host factors detrimental to drug efficacy

TABLE 3-11

CHECKLIST OF POTENTIAL CAUSES OF REINFECTION WITH DIFFERENT BACTERIA

1. Invalid culture results caused by
   a. Contamination of specimen during collection, transport, storage, or handling
   b. Improper technique of bacterial culture of urine

2. Continued dysfunction of host defense mechanisms (Tables 3-8 and 3-9)

3. Failure to recognize and eliminate a predisposing cause

4. Iatrogenic infection, especially associated with catheterization

5. Sequelae to surgical techniques that have impaired host defense function, especially urethrostomy and urine diversion procedures

6. Spontaneous reinfection

to collect urine samples for bacterial culture by cystocentesis to eliminate problems of differentiating contaminants from pathogens. Although detection of bacteria in urine samples collected by cystocentesis is highly indicative of bacterial UTI, further information is required to localize the site(s) of infection (Table 3-5).

The urinary bladders of patients with irritative cystitis may be too small to safely collect urine by cystocentesis. In this circumstance, inducing diuresis with parenteral fluids or furosemide is acceptable to facilitate diagnostic culture of urine collected by cystocentesis. However, diuresis will reduce quantitative culture counts. Urine formation enhanced with parenteral fluids or furosemide is not suitable for diagnostic urinalysis.

If dysuria and pollakiuria prevent collection of urine by cystocentesis, it may be necessary to collect midstream urine samples for culture during voiding or use catheterization. In these situations, the external genitalia of males and females must be rinsed with an appropriate cleansing solution before urine is obtained. It may be necessary to clip the hair surrounding the vulva of some long-haired female dogs.

We do not routinely use catheters for urine collection to avoid iatrogenic UTI. If catheters are used, they must be in good condition and sterilized.

Only sterilized collection containers should be used, and the containers should have tight-fitting lids. Sterile containers may be obtained by sterilizing Dixie cups in ethylene oxide gas, or they may be purchased from commercial manufacturers.

If the results of quantitative urine culture of noncatheterized midstream or catheterized urine samples are equivocal following serial cultures, collection of urine by cystocentesis should again be considered.

Detection of bacteria in urine aseptically collected by cys-

■ Bacterial urinary tract pathogens may have acquired resistance to many commonly used antimicrobial agents.

Even if antimicrobial susceptibility tests are not performed, differentiating bacteria into gram-positive, gram-negative, or gram-mixed populations can facilitate selection of an effective antimicrobial agent. In some patients both bacterial culture and antimicrobial susceptibility tests are essential (Table 3-14). Consult Appendix C (Treatment of Bacterial Urinary Tract Infections) for recommendations.

Urine Collection Methods

For qualitative and quantitative bacterial culture, we prefer

TABLE 3-12

OCCURRENCE OF DIFFERENT BACTERIA IN DOGS WITH UTIs[a]

Pathogen	Bilberstein[8] (n=102)	Finco et al[11] (n=27)	Ihrke et al[16] (n=27)	Kivisto et al[18] (n=187)	Ling et al[27] (n=1400)	Wooley and Blue[35] (n=655)	Ling[26] (n=?) Male	Ling[26] (n=?) Female
Bordetella bronchiseptica	0%	0%	3.7%	0%	0%	0%	NR	NR
Enterobacter spp.	0%	5.9%	0%	3%	2.6%	3.3%	2%	3%
Escherichia coli	11.8%	36%	59%	67%	37.8%	20.1%	46%	42%
Klebsiella pneumoniae	2.9%	5%	7%	0%	8.1%	3.4%	8%	12%
Proteus mirabilis	10.8%	32%	11%	3%	12.4%	15.4%	12%	6%
Pseudomonas aeruginosa	2.9%	2.7%	0%	0%	3.4%	6.9%	3%	3%
Staphylococcus spp.	56.9%	19%	11%	21%	14.5%	9.6%	12%	12%
Streptococcus spp.	9.8%	9%	22%	6%	10.7%	10.6%	14%	11%

NR = not reported.
[a]The percentages in some columns add to more than 100% because of multiple isolates per specimen.

TABLE 3-13

PREVALENCE OF DIFFERENT TYPES OF BACTERIA ISOLATED FROM CATS WITH LOWER URINARY TRACT DISEASE

Bacteria	% of Known Isolates* (n = 762)	% of Known Isolates[†] (n = 255)
Escherichia coli	62	47
Staphylococcus spp.	16	18
Streptococcus/ Enterococcus spp.	8	13
Proteus spp.	5	4
Klebsiella spp.	5	4
Pseudomonas spp.	4	1
Pasteurella spp.	<1	2
Enterobacter	<1	1
Mycoplasma	NR	2

NR = not reported.
*Data from Purdue University Veterinary Medical Data Base, October 1998.
[†]Data from Davidson AP, Ling GV, Stevens F, et al: Urinary tract infections in cats: A retrospective survey. *Calif Vet* 5:32–34, 1992.

tocentesis, even in low numbers, indicates UTI. However, false-positive results may occur if the needle penetrates a loop of intestine during cystocentesis or if the sample is contaminated during transfer to culture media.

Timing of Urine Collection and Sample Preservation

If diagnostic bacterial cultures are to be performed, urine should be collected for culture before antibacterial therapy is initiated. If antimicrobial therapy has already been instituted, it should be discontinued for approximately 3 to 5 days before urine culture to minimize inhibition of in vivo and in vitro bacterial growth.

Because urine may be a good culture medium at room temperature (bacterial counts may double every 20 to 45 minutes), it should be cultured within 15 to 30 minutes from the time of collection if significant results are to be consistently obtained.[2] Culturing fresh urine samples also is important because destruction of some fastidious bacteria may occur within an hour of collection. If culturing freshly collected urine samples is not possible, the samples should be immediately refrigerated after collection. Refrigerated samples may be stored for up to 6 hours without significant additional growth of bacteria.[33] However, fastidious organisms may be killed in the urine environment if refrigeration storage time is prolonged. Alternatively, commercially manufactured collection tubes containing preservatives (B-D Urine C & Transport Kit) combined with refrigeration may be used to preserve specimens for up to 72 hours.[1] Freezing urine samples may destroy bacteria.

Significance of Qualitative Urine Cultures

Qualitative urine culture includes the isolation and identification of bacteria in urine, but does not include quantitation of bacterial numbers.

Although urine contained in the urinary bladder is normally sterile, urine that passes through the urethra and genital tract may become contaminated with resident bacteria normally present in these locations (Table 3-15). Gram-positive bacteria appear to be common inhabitants of the canine urethra. The significance of bacteria in midstream

TABLE 3-14

INDICATIONS FOR ANTIMICROBIAL SUSCEPTIBILITY TESTS

1. Confirmed complicated UTI (see Table 3-9)
2. Frequent recurrences of UTI (see Tables 3-10 and 3-11)
3. Clinical signs persist for more than 5 to 7 days after empiric therapy was initiated or become substantially more severe any time after initiation of therapy
4. Antimicrobial treatment within past 3 weeks
5. Recent transurethral catheterization
6. Patient at high risk of morbidity associated with UTI
   a. Urinary outflow obstruction
   b. Uremia
   c. Diabetes mellitus
   d. Neurogenic bladder
   e. Hyperadrenocorticism
   f. Glucocorticoid treatment

TABLE 3-15

SOME FACTORS INFLUENCING INTERPRETATION OF QUALITATIVE BACTERIAL CULTURES OF URINE

1. Method of urine collection?
2. Time lapse between urine collection and culture?
3. Method of preservation if urine is not cultured within 30 minutes?
4. Pure or mixed culture of bacteria?
   In dogs:
   —One isolate   in about 80% of UTI
   —Two isolates   in only 17% of UTI
   —Three isolates   in only 3% of UTI
   In cats:
   —One isolate   in about 85% of UTI
   —More than one isolate in about 15% of UTI
5. Magnitude of inflammatory response (if any) detected by urinalysis?
6. Detection of bacteria in uncontaminated fresh unspun urine?

(first portion of stream not included) urine samples or in samples obtained by manual compression of the bladder is often difficult to interpret because these bacteria may be pathogens or contaminants. Even catheterized samples may be contaminated as the catheter passes through the lower genital tract and urethral lumen. For this reason, urine culture techniques should include estimates of the number of bacteria present in each milliliter of urine (quantitative culture) in addition to identification of bacterial organisms (qualitative culture).

Although qualitative culture is theoretically satisfactory when urine samples are obtained by cystocentesis, an element of doubt may exist concerning minor bacterial contamination from the skin or during transfer of urine for the culture. For this reason quantitative urine culture also is recommended for samples collected by cystocentesis.

Several factors should be considered when interpreting the significance of qualitative bacterial cultures of urine (Table 3-15). Isolation of a single species is of special interest since approximately 80% of UTIs in dogs are caused by a single species of pathogen, 17% are caused by two species, and 3% are caused by three species.[1,26] Therefore identification of multiple species of bacteria should arouse suspicion that one or more of them represent contaminants.

Concept of Significant Bacteriuria and Quantitative Urine Cultures
Conceptual Overview

Quantitative urine culture includes determination of the number of bacteria (colony-forming units) per unit of volume

in addition to isolation and identification of bacteria. It is the preferred method of diagnostic culture for urine samples obtained by any collection method.

The concept of significant bacteriuria was introduced to aid differentiation between harmless bacterial contaminants of urine and pathogenic organisms causing infectious disease of the urinary system. This concept is based on probability and the observation that a high bacterial count in a properly collected and cultured urine sample indicates the probability of UTI. Small numbers of bacteria obtained from untreated patients usually indicate contamination. When interpreting quantitative bacterial cultures, several variables should be considered.

In humans, urine bacterial counts in excess of 100,000 organisms of a single species per milliliter of urine are considered to be significant.[17] From 10,000 to 100,000 bacteria of a single species per milliliter are isolated in catheterized or midstream urine samples is interpreted as suspected bacterial infection. Urine from patients with suspected bacteriuria should be cultured a second time. If the same organism is isolated at a similar or higher concentration, the presence of bacterial infection is confirmed because reproducible results would not be expected as a result of contamination. The presence of fewer than 10,000 bacteria per milliliter in midstream or catheterized urine samples usually represents contaminants.

Although controlled experiments with statistical analyses have not been performed, clinical studies of quantitative urine culture (utilizing the calibrated loop technique) performed at the University Veterinary Hospital of the University of Minnesota and elsewhere[4,10] have revealed that noncatheterized

TABLE 3-16

INTERPRETATION OF QUANTITATIVE URINE CULTURES IN DOGS AND CATS[a]

Collection Method	Significant		Suspicious		Contaminant	
	Dogs	Cats	Dogs	Cats	Dogs	Cats
Cystocentesis	≥1,000[b]	≥1,000	100–1,000	100–1,000	≤100	≤100
Catheterization	≥10,000	≥1,000	1,000–10,000	100–1,000	≤1,000	≤100
Voluntary voiding	≥100,000[c]	≥10,000	10,000–90,000	1,000–10,000	≤10,000	≤1,000
Manual compression	≥100,000[c]	≥10,000	10,000–90,000	1,000–10,000	≤10,000	≤1,000

[a]The data represent generalities. On occasion, bacterial UTI may be detected in dogs and cats with fewer numbers of organisms (i.e., false-negative results).
[b]Numbers represent colony-forming units of bacteria per milliliter of urine.
[c]Caution: Contamination of midstream samples may result in colony counts of 10,000/ml or greater in some dogs and cats (i.e., false-positive results). Therefore, they should not be used for routine diagnostic culture of urine from dogs or cats.

midstream urine samples and catheterized urine samples obtained from dogs with clinical, laboratory, and radiographic evidence of UTI usually contained more than 100,000 bacteria per milliliter. Urine obtained from most dogs without UTIs was either sterile or contained fewer than 10,000 bacteria per milliliter of urine (Table 3-16); however, counts of 100,000 bacteria per milliliter occurred with sufficient frequency to make this form of urine collection unsatisfactory for routine diagnostic bacterial culture.

Bacterial UTI may be present in patients with fewer than 10,000 bacteria per milliliter of urine and should be suspected in this circumstance if patients have characteristic clinical and urinalysis findings. Bacterial contamination of voided and catheterized samples is more likely to occur in female than male dogs and cats.[9]

The lower limit of organisms that indicates significant bacteriuria in feline urine cultures has not been determined. It may be less than those in humans and dogs, however, because feline urine is apparently less conducive to bacterial growth than is urine of dogs or humans (Table 3-16). In addition, other factors may influence the results of quantitative culture of urine for bacteria (Table 3-17).

Detection of even a low number of bacteria in urine aseptically collected by cystocentesis indicates UTI. However, false-positive results may occur if the needle penetrates a loop of intestine during cystocentesis or if the sample is contaminated during transfer to a culture medium.

Quantitative Urine Cultures

The most accurate methods of quantitative bacterial culture of urine are obtained by dilution pour plate methods. Unfortunately, this method is relatively time consuming and therefore has not been adopted as a routine procedure by most veterinarians.

A less time-consuming technique involves the use of cali-

TABLE 3-17

CHECKLIST OF FACTORS THAT MAY INFLUENCE THE NUMBER OF BACTERIAL COLONY-FORMING UNITS OBTAINED BY QUANTITATIVE URINE CULTURE

1. **Species** (dog, cat, other; see Table 3-16)
2. **Collection method** (see Table 3-16)
3. **Time elapsed between collection and culture of urine**
4. **Method of preservation** (if any)
5. **Variables related to ability of bacteria to grow in vitro**
6. **Frequency of micturition**
7. **Magnitude of diuresis (concentration or dilution)**
8. **Site(s) of bacterial infection**
9. **Administration of antimicrobial agents prior to bacterial culture**

brated bacteriologic inoculating loops (available from Scientific Products, McGraw Park, IL) or microliter mechanical pipettes[22] that deliver exactly 0.01 or 0.001 ml of urine to culture plates. To facilitate qualitative and quantitative cultures, urine is streaked over the surface of both blood agar and MacConkey's agar by conventional methods. The plates are incubated upside down for 18 to 24 hours at 37°C and then exam-

TABLE 3-18

ABNORMALITIES THAT MAY AID IN LOCALIZATION OF BACTERIAL UTIs[a]

Pathogen	Gram's Stain	Appearance On	
		Blood Agar	MacConkey Agar
Escherichia coli	Negative rods	Smooth gray colonies; may be hemolytic	Pink-red colonies (usually lactose positive)
Enterobacter spp.	Negative rods	Smooth gray-white colonies	Pink-red colonies (lactose positive)
Enterococcus spp.	Positive cocci	Small smooth white colonies; ± partial hemolysis	No growth
Klebsiella spp.	Negative rods	Mucoid gray-white colonies	Pink-red mucoid colonies (usually lactose positive)
Proteus mirabilis	Negative rods	Usually swarm rather than form isolated colonies	Colorless to tan (transparent) colonies (lactose negative)
Pseudomonas spp.	Negative rods	Gray to green colonies; fruity or ammonia odor; often hemolytic	Colorless to greenish tan (transparent) colonies (lactose negative)
Staphylococcus spp.	Positive cocci	Small white or yellow colonies; often hemolytic	No growth
Streptococcus spp.	Positive cocci	Small, often tiny pinpoint colonies; partial hemolysis or complete hemolysis	No growth

[a]Adapted from Biberstein EL: Calif Vet 31:10–17, 1997, and Ling GE: JAVMA 185:1162–1164, 1984.

teria. However, all individuals can recognize the fact that growth does not occur on culture plates. Therefore we recommend that veterinarians culture urine on microbiology plates using calibrated loops. If no growth occurs after incubation at 37°C for 18 to 30 hours or if only a small number of bacteria grows (contaminants), further efforts to identify bacterial species are unwarranted. If a significant number of bacteria (colony-forming units) is isolated, the microbiologic plates can be sent to commercial laboratories for species identification and antimicrobial susceptibility tests. Alternatively, bacteria from selected colonies of the microbiologic plate could be collected on a swab and sent to commercial laboratories in a transport medium. Use of commercially manufactured screening culture kits designed to obtain quantitative bacterial counts may also be used.[19,20]

REFERENCES AND SUGGESTED READINGS

1. Allen TA, Jones RL, Purvance J: Microbiologic evaluation of canine urine: Direct microscopic examination and preservation of specimen quality for culture. JAVMA 190:1289–1291, 1987.
2. Asscher AW: Urine as a medium for bacterial growth. Lancet 2:1037–1041, 1966.
3. Barsanti JA, Johnson CA: Genitourinary infections, in Greene CE (ed): Infectious Diseases of the Dog and Cat, ed 2. Philadelphia, WB Saunders, 1998, pp 626–646.
4. Barsanti JA, Blue J, Edmunds J: Urinary tract infections due to indwelling bladder catheters in dogs and cats. JAVMA 187:384–388, 1985.
5. Barsanti JA, Finco DR, Shotts EB, et al: Feline urologic syndrome: Further investigation into etiology. JAAHA 18:391–395, 1982.
6. Barsanti JA, Johnson CA: Genitourinary infections, in Greene CE (ed): Infectious Diseases of the Dog and Cat, ed 1. Philadelphia, WB Saunders, 1990, pp 157–183.
7. Bartges JW: Lower urinary tract disease in older cats: What's common? What's not? Proceedings of a Symposium on Health & Nutrition of Geriatric Dogs & Cats sponsored by Hill's Pet Nutrition, Orlando, FL, 1996.
8. Biberstein EL: Urinary tract infections in dogs: Microbiological diagnosis. Calif Vet 31:10–17, 1977.
9. Comer KM, Ling GV: Results of urinalysis and bacterial culture of canine urine obtained by antepubic cystocentesis, catheterization, and midstream voided methods. JAVMA 179:891–895, 1981.
10. Chew DJ, DiBartola SP: Diagnosis and pathophysiology of renal disease, in Ettinger SJ (ed): Textbook of Veterinary Internal Medicine, ed 3, vol 2. Philadelphia, WB Saunders, 1989, pp 1893–1961.
11. Finco DR, Shotts EB, Crowell WA: Evaluation of methods for localization of urinary tract infection in the female dog. Am J Vet Res 40:707–712, 1979.

ined for bacterial growth. Blood agar will support growth of most aerobic organisms encountered in patients with UTI. MacConkey agar provides information that aids in tentative identification of bacteria and prevents "swarming" of Proteus microbes (Table 3-18).

Although pour plate and loop dilution techniques provide accurate results, they have several disadvantages. Transporting urine specimens to a commercial microbiology laboratory results in an increase in time between urine collections and culture and therefore increases the risk for erroneous results, especially if the samples are not properly refrigerated. Delay in obtaining results from a commercial laboratory may delay initiation of appropriate therapy. In addition, the cost of laboratory-performed quantitative urine cultures may be significant, especially if serial cultures from the same patient are required.

Many veterinarians do not perform urine cultures because of the time and expertise required to specifically identify bac-

12. Gaastra W, van Oosterom RA, Pieters EW, et al: Isolation and characterization of dog uropathogenic *Proteus mirabilis* strains. *Vet Microbiol* 48:57–71, 1996.

13. Hinman F: Meatal colonization in bitches. *Trans Am Assoc Genitourin Surg* 68:73, 1977.

14. Hirsch DC, Wiger N: The bacterial flora of the normal canine vagina compared with that of vaginal exudates. *J Small Anim Pract* 18:25–30, 1977.

15. Holan KM, Kruger JM, Gibbons SN, et al: Clinical evaluaton of a leukocyte esterase test–strip for detection of feline pyuria. *Vet Clin Pathol* 6:126–131, 1997.

16. Ihrke PJ, Norton AL, Ling GV, Stannard AA: Urinary tract infection associated with long–term corticosteroid administration in dogs with chronic skin diseases. *JAVMA* 186:43–46, 1985.

17. Kass EM: The role of asymptomatic bacteriuria in the pathogenesis of pyelonephritis, in Quinn EL, Kass EM (eds): *Biology of Pyelonephritis.* Boston, Little Brown and Co, 1960.

18. Kivisto AK, Vasenius H, Lindberg LA, et al: Desorption assay. A function in vitro test for measuring the adhesion of *E. coli* on the urinary tract epithelium (of dogs). *Invest Urol* 15:412–415, 1978.

19. Klausner JS, Osborne CA, Stevens JB: Screening tests for the detection of significant bacteriuria, in Kirk RW (ed): *Current Veterinary Therapy VII.* Philadelphia, WB Saunders, 1980.

20. Klausner JS, Osborne CA, Stevens JB: Clinical evaluation of commercial reagent strips for detection of significant bacteriuria in dogs and cats. *Am J Vet Res* 37:714–722, 1976.

21. Lees GE: Epidemiology of naturally occurring feline bacterial urinary tract infections. *Vet Clin North Am* 14:471–479, 1984.

22. Lees GE, Rogers KS, Wolf AM: Diseases of the lower urinary tract, in Sherding RG (ed): *The Cat: Diseases and Clinical Management.* New York, Churchill Livingstone, 1989, pp 1397–1454.

23. Ling GV, Kaneko JJ: Microscopic examination of canine urine sediment. *Calif Vet* 30:14–18, 1976.

24. Ling GV: Therapeutic strategies involving antimicrobial treatment of the canine urinary tract. *JAVMA* 185:1162–1164, 1984.

25. Ling GV: Urinary tract infections, in Prescott JF, Baggot JD (eds): *Antimicrobial Therapy in Veterinary Medicine,* ed 2. Ames, IA, Iowa State University Press, 1993, pp 349–370.

26. Ling GV: *Lower Urinary Tract Diseases of Dogs and Cats.* St. Louis, The CV Mosby Co, 1995.

27. Ling GV, Bibersten EL, Hirsh DC: Bacterial pathogens associated with urinary tract infections. *Vet Clin North Am* 9:617–630, 1979.

28. Ling GV, Ruby AL: Aerobic bacterial flora of the prepuce, urethra and vagina of normal adult dogs. *Am J Vet Res* 39:695–698, 1978.

29. Low DA, Braaten BA, Ling GV, et al: Isolation and comparison of *Escherichia coli* strains from canine and human patients with urinary tract infections. *Infect Immun* 56:2601–2609, 1988.

30. Lulich JP, Osborne CA: The impact of age on lower urinary tract disease of dogs. Proceedings of a Symposium on Health & Nutrition of Geriatric Dogs & Cats sponsored by Hill's Pet Nutrition, Orlando, FL, 1996.

31. Osborne CA, Kruger JM, Johnston GR, Polzin DJ: Feline lower urinary tract disorders, in Ettinger SJ (ed): *Textbook of Veterinary Internal Medicine,* ed 3, vol 2. Philadelphia, WB Saunders, 1989, pp 2057–2082.

32. Osborne CA, Lees GE: Bacterial infections of the canine and feline urinary tract, in Osborne CA, Finco DR (eds): *Canine and Feline Nephrology and Urology.* Malvern, PA, Williams & Wilkins, 1995, pp 759–797.

33. Padilla J, Osborne CA, Ward GE: Effects of storage time and temperature on quantitative culture of canine urine. *JAVMA* 178:1077–1081, 1981.

34. Vail DM, Allen TA, Weiser CA: Applicability of leucocyte esterase test strip in detection of canine pyuria. *JAVMA* 189:1451–1433, 1986.

35. Wooley RE, Blue JL: Bacterial isolations from canine and feline urine. *Mod Vet Pract* 57:535–538, 1976.

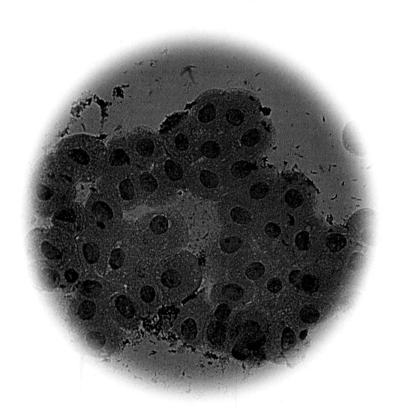

Chapter 4

The miraclemycin of our medical armamentarium is father design and mother time. As their children, we must strive to compassionately augment rather than hinder their efforts.
C.A.O.

Diagnostic Perspectives and Axioms

ANATOMY OF A DIAGNOSIS

If a client were to ask you to describe the processes involved in diagnosing various illnesses, how would you respond? Are there different types of diagnosis? If so, what do they mean?

We would begin to answer these questions in this fashion. The most reliable way to solve a problem is to first define it (see Seven Clinical Axioms of Diagnosis and Treatment and Table 4-1). In terms of solving the problem of illness, the diagnosis is used as the definition.

The noun *diagnosis* is derived from a Greek word meaning to distinguish or discern, and the verb *discern* conveys the concept of an ability to recognize and understand the difference between two or more things. A diagnosis encompasses defining the cause(s) of disease(s) by detecting and evaluating the body's manifestations of the disease. Discerning the underlying cause(s) of clinical signs of illness is not always easy because body systems and organs manifest the effects of a variety of different causes of disease in a limited number of ways. For example, the signs of pruritus, vomiting, diarrhea, polyuria, and the like may represent different causes that require different solutions. Ability to reliably establish the different causes of various illnesses requires specialized knowledge and the experience to apply that knowledge wisely in a fashion that benefits the patient.

Logically, the process of diagnosis should begin by collecting relevant clinical information. A diagnosis (or conclusion) is then formulated on the basis of that information. However, it is one thing to make a diagnosis and another to substantiate it! Many clients have experienced symptoms similar to the clinical sign they observe in their pets. Based on their experience, they may have a preconceived idea of the underlying cause(s) and therefore how the pet's illness should be treated. If we begin the diagnostic process with a preconceived notion about the cause of a patient's illness, however, we have a tendency to ask questions and perform diagnostic procedures that support our preconceptions. This is called bias. If we are not careful in how we collect information, our biases may cause us to make an erroneous diagnosis (i.e., an erroneous conclusion).

SEVEN CLINICAL AXIOMS OF DIAGNOSIS AND TREATMENT (Table 4-1)

An axiom is a statement universally accepted as true.

TABLE 4-1
SEVEN CLINICAL AXIOMS OF DIAGNOSIS AND TREATMENT

1. There is a fundametal different between:
   a. Knowledge (facts)
   b. Wisdom (ability to apply knowledge)

2. There is a fundamental difference between:
   a. Problem definition
   b. Problem solution

3. There is a fundamental difference between:
   a. Observations
   b. Interpretations of observations

4. There is a fundamental difference between:
   a. Possibilities
   b. Probabilities

5. There is a fundamental difference between:
   a. Disease
   b. Failure

6. There is a fundamental difference between:
   a. Events induced by the disease(s)
   b. Compensatory responses to disease-induced events

7. There is a fundamental difference between:
   a. Specific treatment
   b. Supportive treatment
   c. Symptomatic treatment
   d. Palliative treatment
   e. Inappropriate treatment

1. There Is a Fundamental Difference Between Knowledge and Wisdom

Knowledge is fact. Knowledge consists of familiarity with information gained by study and observation (i.e., empirical experience or investigation). Unfortunately, most of us have been taught to overemphasize the accumulation of new knowledge to a point where we neglect the development of wisdom.

Wisdom consists of a combination of knowledge and judgment, thereby encompassing the ability to use knowledge successfully. It implies sufficient breadth of knowledge and depth of understanding to provide sound judgment. Although essential, facts (knowledge) by themselves are rarely of useful value. Facts are not science, just as the dictionary is not literature. In the context of diagnosing and treating diseases, facts become useful only to the extent that they can be applied to define and solve problems. If we have knowledge but we are unable to apply it, we lack wisdom.

2. There Is a Fundamental Difference Between Problem Definition and Problem Solution

The ability to define a patient's medical problems without overstating them is a crucial first step in the diagnostic process because problems must be defined before they can be solved.

No veterinarian has or ever will be trained to single-handedly solve all types of medical problems. No one can recall enough knowledge and be proficient in sufficient techniques to guarantee the ability to provide the best care to every patient. Veterinarians can be trained to identify problems accurately, however. They can and should be master "problem definers."

Accurate definition of a patient's clinical problems allows us in our role as diagnosticians to more efficiently utilize resources (journals, books, consultations, referrals) that help to resolve diagnostic and therapeutic problems. A problem well defined is half solved.

3. There Is a Fundamental Difference Between Observations and Interpretations

Discernment of the difference between observations (facts) and interpretations of observations (inferences) is critical to our conceptual understanding of the anatomy of a diagnosis. As veterinarians, we frequently interview clients who confuse observations and interpretations when they describe the medical condition of their pets. A classic example is to misinterpret the observation of tenesmus as constipation in a male cat with urethral obstruction. This error in reasoning is not limited to clients, however. It affects all of us at one time or another. For example, when asking for specific laboratory data (such as the hematocrit value), we may be told that it is normal (an interpretation). However, a hematocrit value of 37% (an observation), which may be normal in a well-hydrated sedentary patient, may be abnormal in a severely dehydrated patient. Although observations or interpretations may be erroneous, in our experience misinterpretation of a correct observation is the most common pattern of error.

The point is that a misinterpreted problem is the worst of all problems. Why? Because if misinterpretations are unknowingly accepted as facts, misdiagnosis followed by misprognosis and formulation of ineffective or contraindicated therapy may result. This is indeed ironic because a patient's condition may worsen as a consequence of our role as veterinarians.

4. There Is a Fundamental Difference Between Possibilities and Probabilities

The need to discern the difference between diagnostic possibilities and diagnostic probabilities is another key medical axiom. In general, the collection and interpretation of relevant clinical data allow us to reduce numerous diagnostic possibilities to a few probabilities or one probability.

Diagnosis may be derived by the process of exclusion (rule out) or by the process of inclusion (rule in). Even after a large quantity of relevant data has been collected, however, many diagnostic probabilities continue to represent educated opinion rather than fact. The point is that absence of clinical evidence of suspected diseases is not always synonymous with evidence of the absence of these diseases. As a corollary, detection of evidence consistent with a specific type of disease is not always pathognomonic for that disease. It follows that as veterinarians, we should convey to our clients that our diagnoses, prognoses, and treatment recommendations are not infallible. The practice of veterinary medicine requires judgment in the absence of certainty.

5. There Is a Fundamental Difference Between Disease and Failure

Discernment of the conceptual difference between organ disease and organ failure is also fundamental to proper diagnostic refinement. Organ function that is *adequate* to sustain homeostasis is often not synonymous with *total* organ function. For example, patients with only one kidney have adequate renal function to live a *normal* life without manifestations of renal dysfunction. Even when slowly progressive irreversible lesions occur, signs of organ failure do not develop if adequate quantities of functional parenchyma (e.g., nephrons, hepatic lobules) remain to sustain homeostasis. This concept is the basis for distinguishing organ disease (such as cardiac valvular insufficiency) from organ failure (such as altered circulation associated with abnormal cardiac rate and rhythm, which ultimately occur as a result of irreversible progressive cardiac valvular insufficiency). The approach to managing a patient with cardiac valvular insufficiency and adequate cardiac function is very different from management designed for a patient with cardiac valvular insufficiency and congestive heart failure.

6. There Is a Fundamental Difference Between Clinical Signs Induced by Diseases and the Body's Compensatory Response to Disease-Induced Signs

Clinical manifestations of disease can be subdivided into two classes:

- Signs directly induced by the disease, such as impaired urine concentrating capacity and obligatory polyuria associated with damage to the countercurrent system in patients with bilateral bacterial pyelonephritis
- The body's compensatory response to these signs, such as compensatory polydipsia needed to maintain fluid balance because of obligatory polyuria, compensatory inflammation in response to damaged tissue, fever in response to systemic infectious agents, polychromasia and reticulocytosis in response to anemia, and hyperparathormonemia in response to hypocalcemia

It follows that making a diagnosis of infection solely on the basis of pyuria would be an overdiagnosis because pyuria may be a compensatory response to both infectious and noninfectious diseases.

7. There Is a Fundamental Difference Between Specific, Supportive, Symptomatic, and Palliative Treatment Protocols

Specific treatment is given to eliminate, destroy, or modify the primary cause(s) of renal disease. Examples of specific treatment include prescribing antimicrobial agents to combat bacterial infections of the kidneys or antidotes to counteract toxins and relieving urinary tract obstruction to correct postrenal azotemia.

Supportive treatment consists of therapy

> A misinterpreted problem is the worst of all problems.

> Organ function that is *adequate* to sustain homeostasis is often not synonymous with *total* organ function.

that modifies or eliminates abnormalities that occur secondary to primary diseases. Treatment designed to correct fluid, electrolyte, acid–base, endocrine, and nutrient imbalances caused by primary renal failure is an example of supportive therapy. Successful specific therapy of the underlying causes of organ failure usually depends on successful supportive therapy designed to correct the consequences of impaired organ function.

Symptomatic treatment consists of therapy designed to eliminate or suppress clinical signs. Examples of symptomatic treatment include administering antiemetics to control vomiting or antihypertensive drugs to control high blood pressure.

Palliative treatment consists of therapy chosen to ameliorate the clinical signs associated with progressive diseases for which the underlying cause cannot be cured.

Inappropriate treatment consists of therapy for which the associated risks outweigh the probable benefits. Treatment of illnesses is founded on the intent of the doctor to help the patient. Good intent, however, does not always result in a beneficial outcome. Some patients cannot be helped, but there are none we cannot harm.

KEY POINT: Drugs used to eliminate, control, or prevent various diseases also have the potential to induce disease. A majority of pharmacokinetic and toxicity studies have been limited to studies in healthy animals, despite the fact that many drugs are given to patients with disease and/or dysfunction of one or more body systems. For example, the kidneys play vital roles in the absorption, biotransformation, and elimination of any drugs, including antimicrobials. If doses of pharmacologic agents designed for patients with normal renal function are repeatedly given to patients with renal dysfunction, the likelihood of adverse drug reactions is enhanced. In one study, the frequency of adverse drug reactions was 95% in patients with serum urea nitrogen levels below 20 mg/dl but 25% in patients with serum urea nitrogen levels greater than 40 mg/dl.[5] To the unsuspecting therapist and client, such adverse drug reactions may be erroneously attributed to progression of the underlying disease or regarded as an unusual manifestation of the underlying disorder.

All forms of treatment should be given only after considering the potential benefits to the patient and the potential morbidity and mortality. If drugs that depend on the kidneys or liver for metabolism and/or elimination are needed to treat patients in renal or hepatic failure, their dose or maintenance interval should be adjusted to maintain comparable plasma drug concentrations known to be safe and effective in patients with normal function.

BALANCING TREATMENT GOALS OF VETERINARIANS AND CLIENTS

Once the goal of therapy is defined, the feasibility of such therapy must be assessed. In many situations the final choice will represent a balance between the optimum therapy for the problem(s), availability of optimum therapy, and type of therapy our clients can or are willing to purchase. There must be no misunderstanding about what is wanted and what is given. In a symbolic way, we must determine whether a client wants "a dog, horse, cow, cat" or "this dog, horse, cow, cat" while trying to be the patient's advocate.

GENERAL PRIORITIES FOR CLINICAL INVESTIGATIONS
Diagnosis by Rule Out
Overview

Traditionally, diagnostic plans encompass the formulation of differential or tentative diagnosis rule outs (R/Os) or rule ins (R/Is) and choices of tests to prove or disprove various hypotheses. However, the consideration of tentative differentials is premature unless the problems have been accurately defined, verified, and (if possible) localized. These beginning steps of diagnosis are a part of an overall priority of clinical investigation (Table 4-2).

Verification

It is often necessary to verify the presence and nature of problems identified by clients. Conceptually, verification of problems is the first priority of diagnostic evaluation (Table 4-2). Failure to verify clinical problems is among the most common and fundamental causes of misdiagnosis. Clients often make inaccurate observations that, if accepted without verification, may lead to a great deal of nonproductive activity in pursuit of nonexistent disorders. This may also result in a costly and time-consuming series of diagnostic and therapeutic plans before errors are identified.

For example, if polyuria is identified as an owner's complaint in the problem list, the first diagnostic plan should be to confirm polyuria by observation and/or evaluation of urine specific gravity or osmolality. In other situations, a client's observations may be accurate (e.g., "My male cat has been straining to eliminate"), but the interpretation may be erroneous (e.g., "My cat is constipated," when in reality the cat has a urethral obstruction). The key point is that diagnostic consideration should first be given to verifying the owner's statement about constipation.

Based on accurate definition and verification of problems from data collected from various sources (the patient's history, physical examination, and various preliminary laboratory tests and diagnostic procedures), we recommend that clinical problems be classified into one of four progressive levels of diagnostic refinement (Table 4-2). Listed from the lowest to the highest level of refinement, problems may be defined (or diagnosed) as:

■ **Unquantified (subjective) sign or clinical finding** (e.g., depression, polydipsia, polyuria, vomiting)—The distinguishing factor in this category is the subjectivity of the finding. It is "soft" data because it is unlikely to be reproducible. If these types of problems are mild and transient, treatment my not be warranted; however, if they are severe, recur intermittently, persist, or are progressive, further

TABLE 4-2
THE FOUR PRIORITIES OF CLINICAL INVESTIGATION

I. First Priority: Verification of Problems
   A. Especially important for historic problems such as polyuria, tenesmus, vomiting, diarrhea, and so forth
   B. Also of importance for transient intermittent problems

II. Second Priority: Localization of Problems
   A. Striving to localize problems to a body system or organ
   B. Localization may also be used to categorize the underlying pathophysiologic characteristics of the disease
   C. Examples include
       1. Prerenal, intrarenal renal, and postrenal azotemia
       2. Primary or secondary gastrointestinal disease
       3. Regenerative or nonregenerative anemia
       4. Preglomerular, glomerular, or postglomerular proteinuria
       5. Neurogenic versus nonneurogenic incontinence
       6. Physiologic versus pathologic versus pharmacologic polyuria

III. Third Priority: Consideration of Probable Pathophysiologic Cause(s) of Disease (DAMNIT)
   A. D = Degenerative, Developmental, Demented (psychologic or behavioral)
   B. A = Anomaly, Allergic, Autoimmune
   C. M = Metabolic, Mechanical
   D. N = Nutritional, Neoplastic (benign or malignant)
   E. I = Inflammatory (infectious or noninfectious), Immune, Ischemic, Inherited, Iatrogenic, Idiopathic
   F. T = Toxicity (endogenous or exogenous), Trauma (internal or external)

IV. Fourth Priority: Establishing Specific Cause(s) of Disease

information is often warranted to identify their source and cause and to formulate a prognosis and treatment plan.

■ **Reproducible (objective) diagnostic findings** (e.g., mild proteinuria, urine:protein creatinine ratio of 5.7, palpable splenic mass, a hematocrit of 19 associated with marked polychromasia, serum potassium concentration of 7.4 mEq/L)—Because findings in this category are reproducible, they are sometimes called "hard" data. If these problems are mild and transient, treatment may not be warranted; however, if they are severe, intermittently recurrent, persistent, or progressive, further information is usually warranted to identify their source and cause and to formulate a prognosis and treatment plan. In addition, it may be useful to repeat appropriate diagnostic procedures to determine if the abnormality (e.g., elevated in serum urea nitrogen concentration) is getting better, getting worse, or remaining the same and to determine the rate of change in the abnormality.

■ **Pathophysiologic syndromes** (e.g., chronic polyuric azotemic renal failure, congestive heart failure, hepatic encephalopathy, nephrotic syndrome, malabsorption syndrome; Table 4-2)—Problem refinement of this degree requires integration of signs induced by the disease (e.g., polyuria) and the body's compensatory responses to the effects of disease (e.g., polydipsia). Pathophysiologic syndromes may be recognized without knowledge of their underlying cause(s). Patients with various pathophysiologic syndromes of unknown cause often benefit from supportive and symptomatic therapy (e.g., correction of deficits and excesses in fluid, electrolyte, nutrient, acid–base, and endocrine imbalances in patients with polyuric renal failure).

■ **Specific diagnostic entities** (e.g., immune complex protein-losing glomerulonephropathy and nephrotic syndrome caused by *Borrelia burgdorferi*, splenic hemangiosarcoma with metastases to the peritoneum, omentum, lungs, and heart, congenital intrahepatic portovascular shunt with encephalopathy, and ammonium urate urocystoliths):

KEY POINT: It is not necessary or even desirable to expend the resources or expose the patient to unnecessary risks associated with invasive diagnostic techniques to determine the specific cause of all illnesses. Examples at one end of the disease severity spectrum include self-limiting noncommunicable infectious diseases and self-limiting noninfectious diseases, such as transient vomiting and diarrhea associated with dietary indiscretion. Examples at the other end of the disease severity spectrum include end-stage organ (hepatic, renal) failure in which the disease has advanced beyond the possibility of recovery even if the underlying cause could be identified and eliminated.

Thought and practice are required to construct an accurately refined problem list (Tables 4-3 to 4-5). When integrating problems to their highest degree of refinement, it is important to consider that clinical manifestations of disease are usually a combination of (1) signs induced by the disease (such as bacteriuria associated with infection of the urinary tract) and (2) the body's compensatory response to these problems (such as pyuria and perhaps proteinuria and hematuria caused by host inflammation to

> Clients often make inaccurate observations that, if accepted without verification, may lead to considerable nonproductive activity in pursuit of nonexistent disorders.

> It is not necessary or even desirable to expend the resources or expose the patient to unnecessary risks associated with invasive diagnostic techniques to determine the specific cause of all illnesses.

eradicate bacteriuria and repair damaged tissues).

Localization

Localization of problems to an organ or body system should follow their verification (Table 4-2). This is the second in the sequence of priorities of diagnostic evaluation. For example, if a patient is examined because of gross hematuria but no other abnormalities are initially identified, the problem should be listed as gross hematuria. Additional information is required to determine its location(s) (kidneys, ureters, urinary bladder, urethra, genital tract) and cause(s) (anomalies, neoplasia, infection, uroliths, exogenous or endogenous toxins, coagulopathies). In contrast, if hematuria occurs independent of micturition and is associated with a palpable lesion of the urethra, the problem should logically be defined as a urethral lesion associated with gross hematuria.

Pathophysiologic Mechanisms

Following localization of problems to a body system or organ, it is helpful to consider basic pathophysiologic mechanisms when trying to determine probable (rather than possible) causes of each problem. This is the third priority of clinical investigation. The acronym DAMNIT is often useful for this purpose (Table 4-2). Because this acronym encompasses familiar pathophysiologic disease processes, with routine use we will find it easy to apply to our diagnostic method. When utilized in conjunction with the patient history, physical examination, and other diagnostic data, the DAMNIT acronym facilitates rapid and reproducible formulation of probable rule outs (or tentative differentials) for each patient's undiagnosed problems. As an iterative memory aid, some of the pathophysiologic mechanisms listed with different letters in the DAMNIT acronym overlap (i.e., autoimmune and immune, developmental, anomaly, and inherited).

In the context of identifying pathophysiologic mechanisms likely to be causing the clinical problems, the most probable cause(s) of these problem(s) should be ruled in or ruled out by implementing appropriate diagnostic plans.

Specific Diagnosis

After considering basic pathophysiologic mechanisms of disease, the next logical step is to consider the most probable specific cause(s) of the problem (Table 4-2). Knowledge of the specific cause(s) of a patient's disease(s) is of more than academic interest because knowledge of the specific cause often permits:

■ A more accurate prognosis (or forecast) of the biologic behavior of the illness

■ Assessment of the ability of the body to

TABLE 4-3
DEFINING PROBLEMS AT AN APPROPRIATE LEVEL OF REFINEMENT

Example 1

Unrefined
1. Palpable bladder mass
2. Hematuria
3. Dysuria
4. Proteinuria
5. Pyuria
6. Significant bacteriuria

Refined
Disease of the urinary bladder associated with:
1. Palpable mass
2. Primary or secondary infection of the urinary tract (significant bacteriuria)
3. Dysuria
4. Inflammation of the urinary tract (pyuria, proteinuria, hematuria)

Example 2

Unrefined
1. Polyuria
2. Polydipsia
3. Dehydration
4. Inappropriate urine specific gravity (1.015)
5. Proteinuria
6. Pyuria
7. Significant bacteriuria
8. Azotemia

Refined
Dysfunction of the kidney associated with:
1. Impaired ability to concentrate urine (specific gravity = 1.015), polyuria, and compensatory polydipsia
2. Reduced glomerular filtration rate (azotemia)
3. Primary or secondary infection of the urinary tract (significant bacteriuria) associated with inflammation (pyuria and proteinuria)
4. Dehydration

TABLE 4-4
PROPER VERSUS OVERSTATED DEFINITION

Unrefined Problems
1. Dysuria
2. Abnormal urine odor
3. Bacteriuria
4. Pyuria
5. Hematuria
6. Proteinuria

Properly Defined Problem List
Disease of the urinary tract associated with:
1. Primary or secondary bacterial infection (significant bacteriuria)
2. Inflammation of the urinary tract (proteinuria, pyuria, hematuria)

Overstated Problem List
1. Bacterial cystitis

TABLE 4-5
PROPER DEFINITION VERSUS OVERSTATED CAUSES OF VOMITING

Proper Definition
Secondary gastrointestinal disease associated with:
1. Vomiting
2. Dehydration
3. Impaired ability to concentrate urine (specific gravity = 1.018)
4. Azotemia
5. Hyperkalemia
6. Increased packed-cell volume

Overstated Definition
Oliguric primary renal failure[a] characterized by:
1. Vomiting
2. Dehydration
3. Impaired ability to concentrate urine
4. Azotemia
5. Hyperkalemia
6. Hemoconcentration

[a]Similar signs may be caused by hypoadrenocorticism.

functionally compensate for irreversible damage to various biologic functions

■ Assessment of the availability of specific therapy (in contrast to supportive and symptomatic therapy) to eliminate or halt progression of the underlying cause(s) of the disease

■ Assessment of the need for supportive and/or symptomatic therapy of associated dysfunctions

The suspected specific causes should be arranged in order of priority so that the most probable causes are investigated first, while the least probable causes are considered last (if it becomes necessary to consider them at all). At this phase of clinical investigation, the diagnostic plans should clearly identify what cause(s) is to be ruled out or ruled in and should clearly specify tests or procedures (e.g., laboratory data, radiographic data, biopsy data, exploratory surgery) to be used to accomplish this goal.

The specific tests and procedures chosen to evaluate each problem and the rate and frequency with which they are determined are greatly influenced by the status of the patient. If the problem is life threatening, probable diagnostic differentials (rule outs) may need to be investigated simultaneously, that is, in parallel. For example, if a critically ill patient is admitted because of rapidly progressive vomiting, dehydration, polyuria, and extreme depression, it will be necessary to obtain laboratory and radiographic data to simultaneously (in parallel) prove or disprove primary renal failure, diabetic ketoacidosis, hepatic failure, and pyometra. If these probable causes are prioritized and investigated one at a time (i.e., in series), the patient may die before a specific diagnosis is established. In contrast, if these problems are not as severe, are not as life threatening, and do not appear to be progressing at a rapid rate, the most probable hypothesized cause (e.g., primary renal failure) should be pursued first. If clinical data rule out the disease that the clinician considered to be the most probable cause (e.g., primary renal failure), the second most probable cause (e.g., diabetic ketoacidosis) should be pursued and so on.

Summary

One of the most frequent errors that we make in our role as diagnosticians is prematurely guessing specific causes of our patients' problems (i.e., jumping to conclusions) (1) without **verifying** the existence of problems (especially those identified by owners), (2) without **localizing** problems to the appropriate body system or organ, and (3) without considering **basic pathophysiologic disease mechanisms** that might be involved. If we habitually bypass these important components of problem solving, we will become overly dependent on establishing a diagnosis on the basis of textbook descriptions or our previous personal experience. As a result, our ability to recognize specific causes of diseases that we have not previously encountered will be hindered. This concept is of fundamental importance because, in fact, most textbook descriptions are abstracts of prototypical features of diseases that uncommonly coexist in each patient. Just as no two individuals are exactly alike in health, neither are any two exactly alike in disease.

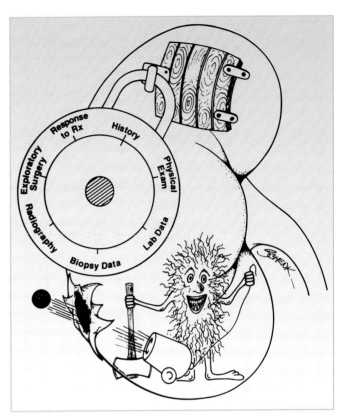

FIGURE 4-1 *Schematic illustration of the combination lock concept of diagnostic method. The specific components and sequence in which they are used vary from patient to patient and from disease to disease. (From Osborne CA: The problem oriented medical system. Vet Clin North Am 13:745–790, 1983.)*

An Effective Combination to Establishing Clinical Diagnoses
The Elusive Key to Diagnosis

The concept of a *key* pathognomonic finding that can unlock the door to a specific diagnosis is unrealistic. Rarely does a single historical event, physical examination finding, laboratory test result, or radiograph finding provide information of sufficient specificity to warrant a specific diagnosis. Likewise, memorization of textbook descriptions of characteristic clinical findings of specific diseases is not consistently effective. Why? Because the same disease typically induces a variety of clinical and laboratory manifestations of different degrees of severity in different patients.

Opening the Combination Lock to a Diagnosis

A more useful analogy is to consider that determining the underlying cause of an illness is more like opening a combination lock than a key lock (Figures 4-1 and 4-2). The history is usually one numeral of the combination; the physical examination is another; and laboratory tests, radiography and ultrasonography, endoscopy, and biopsy procedures are often additional numerals. Depending on the disease, there may be other numerals as well. Response to various types of drugs, hormones, or diets and exploratory surgery are additional examples that may be a part of the sequence of numerals needed to open the combination lock concealing the underlying cause of an illness. But more than knowledge of the numbers

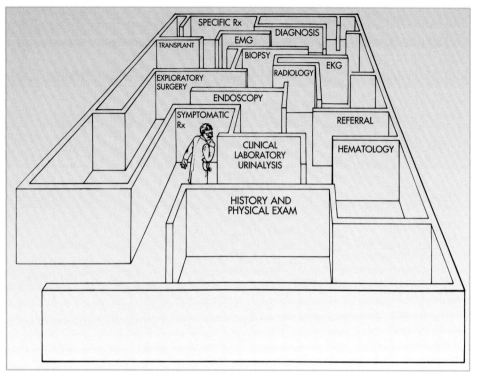

FIGURE 4-2 *Schematic illustration of the diagnostic and therapeutic maze that veterinarians encounter if they try to resolve a patient's problems by recalling textbook descriptions of diseases and unstructured personal experience. (Adapted from Osborne CA: The problem oriented medical system. Vet Clin North Am 13:745–790, 1983.)*

for the combination is required to open the lock. As is the case with any combination lock, the bolt cannot be released without knowing the proper consecutive sequence of numerals (e.g., 7 to the right; 10 to the left; 59 to the right; 41 to the left).

The problem-oriented system of diagnosis, prognosis, and therapy is an action-oriented protocol that provides a conceptually simple, logical, and effective format for determining the identity and exact sequence for the combination of data that directs us toward recognition of the causes of various diseases. Refer to p. 39 for additional details on the problem-oriented system.

PROGNOSIS: SENTENCING GUIDELINES FOR PATIENTS
Definitions

The word *prognosis* is derived from Greek words (pro, "before"; gnosis, "to know") and means a forecast of the probable outcome of abnormalities associated with one or more diseases. *Dorland's Medical Dictionary* defines prognosis as "a forecast as to the probable outcome of an attack of disease" or "the prospect as to recovery from a disease as indicated by the nature and symptoms of the case." Synonyms for the term prognosis include prediction, foretelling, and forecast. As

with most aspects of patient care, a prognosis requires judgment in the absence of certainty. For some patients the prognosis is lifesaving; for others, it is a death sentence. It is therefore appropriate to ask, "How reliable are our prognoses?"

To permit meaningful exchange of knowledge, every scientific discipline must define its terms. We recommend terminology that lends itself to quantification of the probability of a predicted outcome (Table 4-6).

Short-Term versus Long-Term Prognosis

The prognosis for each problem affecting patients should be consistently subcategorized according to predicted events in the immediate future (short-term prognosis) and to the probability of resolving morphologic and functional abnormalities in the distant future (long-term prognosis). For example, the short-term survival prognosis for subclinical glomerular amyloidosis characterized by proteinuria is good to excellent; however, the long-term survival prognosis of patients with glomerular amyloidosis has, to date, been poor to grave. In contrast, the short-term survival prognosis for postrenal azotemia caused by urethral obstruction with a urolith and characterized by profound metabolic acidosis, severe hyperkalemia, and marked hypothermia may be guarded to poor; removal of the urolith combined with appropriate supportive and symptomatic therapy, however, may be associated with good to excellent chances for long-term survival.

Other concepts that should be considered when formulating prognoses are summarized in Table 4-7. What about the concept of aging and its relationship to prognosis? Aging is associated with a decline in total function (or functional reserve) of several organs (e.g., the kidneys) and systems (e.g., the immune system). Thus, the short- and long-term prognoses for complete recovery of geriatric patients from various metabolic, degenerative, neoplastic, traumatic, infectious, and toxic dis-

TABLE 4-6
DEFINITION OF PROGNOSTIC TERMS

Term	Prediction of Recovery	
	Qualitative	Quantitative
Excellent	Highly probable	75%–100%
Good	Probable	50%–75%
Guarded	Unpredictable	50%
Poor	Improbable	25%–50%
Grave	Highly improbable	0%–25%

TABLE 4-7

CONCEPTS THAT MAY INFLUENCE PROGNOSIS

1. Observations versus interpretations
2. Possibilities versus probabilities
3. Level of problem refinement
4. Organ disease versus organ failure
5. Adequate versus total organ function
6. Age (in the context that advanced age is not synonymous with an unfavorable prognosis)
7. Nonprogressive disease versus progressive, irreversible disease and dysfunction
8. Clinical signs directly attributable to the underlying disease versus clinical signs attributed to the body's compensatory responses to the disease
9. Concomitant but unrelated diseases that influence the body's compensatory responses and/or selection of treatment
10. Short-term versus long-term prognosis
11. Specific versus supportive or symptomatic treatment
12. Disease-induced versus treatment-induced illness

eases may be less favorable than those for younger patients with similar disorders. This generality, however, should not be used as the primary basis for recommending "benign neglect" or euthanasia. Aged patients often regain and maintain adequate function of various organs and systems to sustain a good quality of life.

Communication of Prognostic Expectations With Clients

Once a prognosis has been established and a therapeutic plan has been formulated, follow-up evaluations of the course of the disease and its response to therapy (if any) are recommended. Clients should be informed in sufficient detail of the veterinarian's prediction of the progress of the case so that they can recognize deviations from the expected and have some perspective on the significance of the deviations. Veterinarians should also convey to their clients that their opinions, judgments, diagnosis, and prognosis are not infallible and that if significant changes from the expected are observed, the clients should call or return the pet for reevaluation.

THE PROBLEM-ORIENTED MEDICAL SYSTEM

The problem-oriented veterinary medical system is a simple, structured, and reproducible set of rules and directions that guides our care of patients. This system favors the ana-

lytic mode of diagnosis rather than the memorization mode. In our role as veterinary diagnosticians, this guidance system helps us efficiently and effectively direct medical action toward the primary goals of defining and resolving our patients' problems. The problem-oriented system also can guide us in formulating therapy and monitoring patient response to therapy.

The problem-oriented system, consisting basically of four related phases of medical action, encompasses the fundamentals of problem solving that are practical for general practitioners, body system or discipline specialists, or clinicians affiliated with university veterinary teaching hospitals. The system is founded on the basic steps of all investigations, whether they be research laboratory oriented or patient oriented. In research laboratories, experiments are designed to prove or refine a hypothesis (a proposition that must be proved).

The four phases of scientific method are:

1. Collecting an initial body of information
2. Formulating hypotheses to explain observations
3. Conducting experiments to prove or disprove hypotheses
4. Interpretating results and determining whether additional studies are needed (Table 4-8)

The same four phases of scientific endeavor represent the problem-oriented veterinary medical system; only the names are changed (Table 4-8). Listed in order of use they are:

1. Collecting information (so-called data base)
2. Defining the problems (so-called problem list)
3. Devising plans to further refine the causes of problems and to treat the problems (so-called initial plans)
4. Interpreting and recording additional information generated by initial plans; decisions are also made on whether additional plans are necessary (so-called follow-up plans or progress notes)

As is the situation with the research scientist, consistent success of practicing veterinarians in defining and solving

TABLE 4-8

COMPARISON OF SIMILARITIES OF THE FOUR PHASES OF SCIENTIFIC METHOD WITH THE FOUR PHASES OF MEDICAL ACTION OF THE PROBLEM-ORIENTED SYSTEM

Scientific Method	Problem-Oriented Method	Layperson's Terms
1. Collect information	1. Initial data base	1. Collect information
2. Form hypotheses	2. Define problems	2. Decide what is wrong
3. Conduct experiments	3. Form and implement plans	3. Figure out what to do and do it
4. Interpret results	4. Follow up interpretation and additional plans	4. Analyze results

TABLE 4-9

COMPARISON OF FEATURES OF THE PROBLEM-ORIENTED MEDICAL RECORD WITH THE CHAOTIC MEDICAL RECORD

Problem-Oriented Medical Record	*Chaotic Medical Record*
Defined data collection	Data collection varies from patient to patient
Complete problem list	No problem list
Diagnostic and therapeutic plans correspond to each problem	Diagnostic and therapeutic plans may or may not correspond to each separate problem
Additional diagnostic and/or therapeutic plans correspond to each separate problem	Additional diagnostic and therapeutic plans deal randomly with the patient's problems
Data in records are readily accessible and retrievable	Data in records often inaccessible or too time-consuming to obtain

patients' problems depends on consistently collecting, recording, organizing, and interpreting clinical data. The problem-oriented medical system provides a blueprint that all members of the veterinary practice can follow in their efforts to provide proper, timely, and cost-efficient care.

The problem-oriented veterinary medical record is the focal point of the problem-oriented veterinary medical system in that relevant information is visibly linked to specific problems. It is the antithesis of the chaotic veterinary medical record (Table 4-9).

In summary, the problem-oriented system is a practical clinical method that can help guide us in our efforts to unlock the door to the correct diagnosis.

CONCLUDING CAVEATS

We must use caution not to misdiagnose an illness by guessing the underlying cause based on inadequate or questionable evidence (Figure 4-2). Each diagnosis should be stated at the level of diagnostic refinement that can be reasonably justified according to current knowledge about the patient. Why? Because an overstated diagnosis may lead to a plan of management that ultimately results in a worse outcome than the untreated illness. But no patient should be worse for having seen the doctor.

The Greek term *iatros* means physician and is derived from the word *iasthai*, which means to heal or cure. In the context of pathophysiologic mechanisms of disease, what is the significance of the term iatrogenic (Table 4-2)? The term iatrogenic means *physician induced*. The fact that the term iatrogenic is listed as a pathophysiologic mechanism of disease emphasizes that there are some patients we cannot help, but there are none we cannot harm.

REFERENCES AND SUGGESTED READINGS

1. Hurst JW: How to implement the Weed system. *Arch Intern Med* 128:456–462, 1971.
2. Osborne CA: The problem oriented medical system. Improved knowledge, wisdom and understanding of patient care. *Vet Clin North Am* 13:745-790, 1983.
3. Osborne CA: Don't just do something—stand there: An exposition of Hippocrates admonition: "First do no harm." *Compend Contin Educ Pract Vet* 13:1248–1262, 1991.
4. Saidla JE: Problem oriented veterinary medical record, in Ettinger SJ (ed): *Textbook of Veterinary Internal Medicine: Diseases of the Dog and Cat.* Philadelphia, WB Saunders, 1983, pp 29–37.
5. Smith JW, Seidl LG, Cluff LE: Studies on the epidemiology of adverse drug reactions. V. Clinical factors influencing susceptibility. *Ann Intern Med* 65:629-640, 1966.
6. Stogdale L: The problem oriented record for medical practice. *Vet Med* 79(7):901-910, 1984.
7. Weed LL: *Medical Records, Medical Education, and Patient Care.* Chicago, Year Book Medical Publishers, 1971.

Chapter 5

If there is compassion…keep an eye not only on your own personal interests, but also take personal interest in the needs of others.

After Phillipians 2:1-4

Indications for Urinalysis

WHEN IS URINALYSIS INDICATED?

The primary indications for routine urinalysis are:

- As an aid in the search for the diagnosis of various diseases
- To screen patients for asymptomatic disease
- To monitor the biologic behavior of diseases in order to determine whether they are
  —Reversible
  —Irreversible but nonprogressive
  —Irreversible and progressive
- To monitor the efficacy and safety of therapy

URINALYSIS AS AN AID TO SEARCH FOR THE DIAGNOSIS OF DISEASE

Urinalysis is often a component of in-depth searching protocols (so-called problem-specific data bases) designed to evaluate the cause and status of specific syndromes affecting the urinary system and other body systems.

Disorders of the Urinary System

For patients in which urinary disease is suspected, a complete urinalysis should be considered to collect data that can help verify or eliminate diagnostic possibilities formulated on the basis of observations obtained from the history and physical examination.

Examples of some findings associated with untreated urinary diseases include:

- **Primary renal failure**—Varying degrees of impaired ability to concentrate and dilute urine in response to appropriate stimuli, low pH, sometimes proteinuria, sometimes glucosuria, sometimes bacteriuria and an inflammatory response
- **Renal disease**—Sometimes casts, proteinuria, hematuria, pyuria, bacteriuria, and glucosuria.
- **Bacterial urinary tract infection**—Significant bacteriuria typically associated with varying degrees of pyuria, hematuria, and proteinuria
- **Renal tubular acidosis**—Impaired ability to acidify urine or conserve bicarbonate in response to appropriate stimuli
- **Fanconi syndrome**—Normoglycemia, glucosuria, aminoaciduria, proteinuria, and renal tubular acidosis
- **Cystinuria**—Precipitation of cystine crystals that may grow to form uroliths, especially in concentrated acid urine
- **Neoplasia**—Sometimes exfoliated neoplastic cells in urine sediment; varying degrees of pyuria, hematuria, and proteinuria; and sometimes bacteriuria
- **Calcium oxalate urolithiasis**—Often calcium oxalate crystalluria, acid urine pH, varying degrees of hematuria, proteinuria, and pyuria

Nonurinary Disorders

Urinalysis can also be helpful in defining and verifying problems in patients with nonurinary disorders. Like complete blood counts, a urinalysis produces results that provide information about the integrity of many body systems. For this reason, we routinely include urinalysis and hemograms as a part of the initial evaluation (so-called minimum data base) of patients with illness of unknown cause that require hospitalization or frequent outpatient evaluation if hospitalization is not feasible. The detection of abnormal findings by urinalysis may dictate the need for further evaluation. Because the results frequently indicate the system(s) or organ(s) affected, they often influence the selection of additional diagnostic tests or procedures.

Urinalysis findings that may be associated with extraurinary diseases include:

- **Diabetes mellitus**—Hyperglycemia, glucosuria, sometimes ketonuria, and sometimes evidence of bacterial urinary tract infection
- **Central diabetes insipidus**—Hyposthenuria
- **Hepatic failure**—Sometimes bilirubinuria; sometimes ammonium urate, tyrosine, and other crystals; and sometimes impaired urine concentration
- **Severe hemolytic disease**—Hemoglobinuria, hyperurobilinoginuria
- **Prerenal azotemia**—Formation of concentrated urine (also called baruria or hypersthenuria)
- **Systemic acidosis (acidemia)**—Frequently, formation of acid urine

URINALYSIS TO SCREEN PATIENTS FOR ASYMPTOMATIC DISEASE

Screening examinations can detect treatable diseases without subjecting a patient to excessive risk. They should not be associated with false-positive results that lead to costly follow-up diagnostic evaluations.

Urinalysis has been accepted as a cost-effective screening procedure during routine health examinations because changes in the composition of urine can often be detected early during the asymptomatic phase of many illnesses. The macroscopic portion of a urinalysis costs little and is technically easy to perform. If the macroscopic examination of urine obtained from a healthy animal is normal, the sediment is also likely to be normal. Therefore, some veterinarians may choose not to include microscopic evaluation of urine sediment as part of routine screening evaluations. The decision to include the more time-consuming, and therefore more expensive, microscopic examination of urine sediment as a screening method could be based on exposure to disease risk factors for the population being evaluated.

> Urinalysis can be helpful in defining and verifying problems in patients with nonurinary disorders.

Because the kidneys play an important role in maintaining homeostasis, abnormalities that have the potential to alter blood composition are often first manifest as abnormalities in urine. For example, when screening geriatric dogs for evidence of renal dysfunction, impaired urine concentration can often be detected before the onset of azotemia (Table 2-1). Urinalysis may also be valuable for detecting early stages of glomerular disease since persistent proteinuria in the absence of hematuria and pyuria may be a more sensitive index of glomerular damage than qualitative (serum urea nitrogen and creatinine concentrations) or quantitative measurement (clearance techniques) of glomerular filtration rate. Likewise, urinalysis is valuable for screening patients at high risk for urolithiasis since in vivo crystalluria (microliths) precedes formation of many types of uroliths (macroliths).

If an abnormality is detected by screening urinalysis, more diagnostic evaluation usually is required to evaluate the problem. For example, if freshly voided urine is turbid or has an abnormal color or odor or the macroscopic reagent test strips are positive for occult blood, protein, or glucose, evaluation of urine sediment is recommended.

URINALYSIS TO MONITOR THE BIOLOGIC BEHAVIOR OF DISEASE

Once a disease becomes established, there are three possible outcomes. The disease may be reversible or irreversible. If it is irreversible, it may be nonprogressive or progressive. Stated in another way, diseases can get better, get worse, or remain the same. With the aid of urinalysis, monitoring the course of each disease and the rate at which changes occur helps to refine prognosis and therapy.

URINALYSIS TO MONITOR THE EFFECTIVENESS AND SAFETY OF THERAPY

Serial urinalyses can be used to monitor patient response to therapy and to detect relapses or recurrences of various diseases (Table 5-1). Urinalysis may also be used to monitor the safety of drugs. For example, evidence of gentamicin-induced nephrotoxicity may be provided by serial evaluation of urine sediment for casts, monitoring urine specific gravity for evidence of impaired tubular function, and watching for development of normoglycemic glucosuria. In addition, serially collected urine samples may be monitored for increases in urine enzyme concentrations (γ-glutamyl transpeptidase [GGT]; N-acetyl-β-D-glucosaminidase [NAG]).

Single determinations of most laboratory tests indicate the status or functional competence of the organ or body system at the time the tests were performed. Single evaluation of many laboratory tests, including urinalyses, is

> Reevaluation of appropriate components of a urinalysis often indicates the trend of the abnormality.

TABLE 5-1

URINALYSIS AND URINE CULTURE RESULTS OF A 10-YEAR-OLD MALE SIAMESE BEFORE AND DURING ANTIBIOTIC TREATMENT FOR URINARY TRACT INFECTION

Factor[a,b]	Day																
	1[c]	14	32	43	57	63	71	107	139	170	211	245	287	337	369	477	725
Specific gravity	1.018	1.016	1.013	1.013	1.015	1.014	1.015	1.016	1.018	1.017	1.016	1.020	1.016	1.016	1.017	1.020	1.020
pH	6.0	6.0	6.0	6.0	6.0	6.0	6.0	6.0	6.5	6.0	6.0	6.0	6.0	6.0	6.0	6.0	6.0
Protein[d]	Trace	0	Trace	Trace	Trace	Trace	Trace	Trace	Trace	Trace	2+	Trace	1+	1+	Trace	Trace	1+
RBC/hpf	0	0	Occ.	Occ.	Occ.	Occ.	0	0	0	0	0	0	2–3	0	0	0	Occ.
WBC/hpf	1–2	0	40–50	60–65	20–25	15–20	3–4	0	0	0	0	0	0	0	0	0	0
Quantitative culture (colony)	E. coli (>10⁵)	0	E. coli (>10⁵)	E. coli (2000)	E. coli (800)	E. coli (>10⁵)	0	0	0	0	0	0	0	0	0	0	0

From Osborne CA: Control of chronic relapsing feline bacterial pyelonephritis with the aid of enrofloxacin. *Proceedings of the First International Baytril Symposium*, Bonn, 1992, p 28.

hpf = high power field (×450).

[a]Samples were collected by cystocentesis.

[b]Glucose, acetone, and bilirubin were not detected in any sample.

[c]Therapy with amoxicillin was initiated on day 1 and discontinued on day 107. Therapy with enrofloxacin was initiated on day 57. Therapy with enrofloxacin was initiated on day 63 and discontinued on day 107. Preventative therapy with enrofloxacin was initiated on day 107.

[d]Values represent semiquantitative evaluations based on a scale of 0 to 4; urine volume was not considered.

analogous to obtaining a patient's temperature once. In either situation, whether an abnormality remains unchanged, increases or decreases in severity, or the rate at which change is occurring cannot be determined. Reevaluation of appropriate components of urinalysis often indicates the trend of the abnormality. Detection of remission or exacerbation of abnormal test results by serially performed tests often provides a reliable index of prognosis and/or efficacy of treatment.

VALUE OF NORMAL VERSUS ABNORMAL URINALYSIS RESULTS

Urinalysis results provide information that helps practitioners evaluate the integrity of the urinary and other body systems. The value of test results that indicate an abnormality is obvious. Normal test results are also valuable

> Knowledge that physiologic processes are functioning adequately provides objective information with which to exclude them as a cause of clinical signs.

because they indicate that selected physiologic processes governing the formation of urine (including selective permeability of glomeruli, tubular reabsorption of some metabolites and tubular secretion of others) are functioning adequately (Table 5-1). Knowledge that physiologic processes are functioning adequately provides objective information with which to exclude them as a cause of clinical signs.

Whether a particular value is normal or abnormal is often influenced by the diet being consumed, condition of the patient at the time the sample was collected, the method of collection, type (if any) of preservation used, the laboratory method used, and whether diagnostic or therapeutic agents were given before the sample was collected. Therefore, these variables should be considered when interpreting test results.

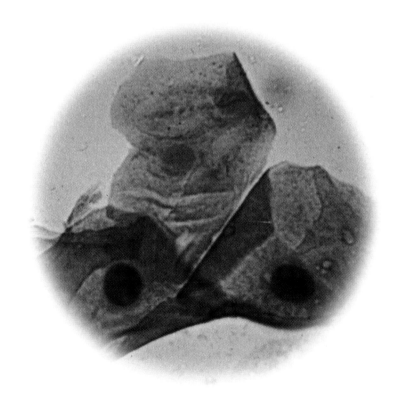

Chapter 6

Compassionate doctors encourage others, especially during difficult times. The root term in encourage is the Latin term "cor" meaning heart. To encourage means to give from the heart.

C.A.O.

Collection of Urine

PERSPECTIVES

In addition to techniques of analysis and interpretation of results, collection of urine is an integral part of urinalysis. The method of collection and the collection container itself may influence test results and their interpretation (see Chapter 7 for additional information).

Patients should be protected from iatrogenic complications associated with collection techniques, including trauma to the urinary tract and urinary tract infection (UTI). In addition, strive to collect a sample whose in vitro characteristics are similar to its in vivo characteristics.

COLLECTION CONTAINERS

Disposable and reusable containers designed specifically for collection of urine from humans may be obtained from a variety of medical supply houses. We routinely use disposable plastic cups.[a] These cups are clean, readily available, and inexpensive and have tight-fitting lids. They may be sterilized with ethylene oxide gas. Use of containers improvised by owners are not recommended since they often contain contaminants (detergents, food, cosmetics, etc.) that may interfere with enzymatic and chemical tests.

Use of transparent containers made of glass or plastic facilitate observation of macroscopic characteristics of urine. If urinalysis cannot be performed within 30 minutes following collection, however, opaque containers should be considered to minimize photochemical degradation of urine constituents by bright light.

Urine obtained for bacterial culture must be collected in sterilized syringes or sterilized containers with tight-fitting lids. Sterilized containers may be obtained by:

■ Sterilizing disposable plastic cups in ethylene oxide gas
■ Sterilizing glass or metal drinking cups in an autoclave
■ Purchasing them from commercial manufacturers

Samples collected by catheterization or cystocentesis may be transported and stored in the collection syringe. Samples collected by placing commercially manufactured absorbent sponges in the urine stream during the voiding phase of micturition and then squeezing urine from the sponge into a collection bag or container may be satisfactory for chemical testing, but they are not reliable for evaluation of urine sediment since cells, casts, and crystals may become trapped in the sponge.

COLLECTION OF TABLETOP URINE SAMPLES (Figure 6-1)

Patients with lower urinary tract disease often have reduced bladder capacity and urge incontinence. As a result, collection of urine into a cup during the voiding phase of micturition or by cystocentesis is difficult. Frequently, small quantities of urine are voided before they can be collected.

Collection of urine for analysis from smooth, clean tabletops may be facilitated with the aid of a needle and syringe. Urine samples collected in this fashion are satisfactory for screening urinalysis, provided they are analyzed soon after col-

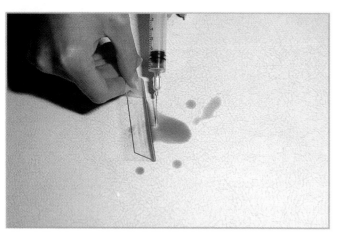

FIGURE 6-1 *Position of a microscope slide to facilitate aspiration of pooled urine voided on a table. As the tilted slide is advanced, the pooled urine was aspirated into a syringe through a hypodermic needle.*

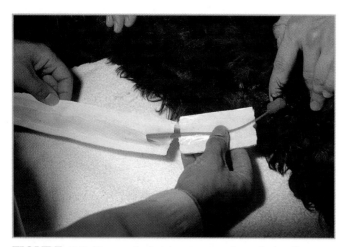

FIGURE 6-2 *Transurethral catheterization of a male dog illustrating proper retraction of the prepuce, and advancement of a flexible catheter without contaminating it with hands. An inexpensive sleeve to manipulate the catheter was made by cutting away the tip of the package, and then cutting an appropriately sized section from the body of the package to manipulate the catheter.*

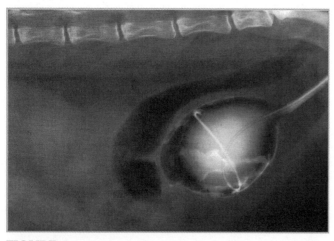

FIGURE 6-3 *Double contrast cystogram of an adult female dog illustrating overinsertion of the urinary catheter. This error is a common cause of trauma which in turn (1) alters the result of urinalysis and (2) predisposes the patient to iatrogenic urinary tract infection.*

TABLE 6-1

NORMAL VOIDING: ADVANTAGES AND DISADVANTAGES

ADVANTAGES
- It is not associated with any risk of complications to the patient.
- It can be used by clients.

DISADVANTAGES
- Samples are frequently contaminated with cells, bacteria, and other debris located in the genital tract or on the skin and hair. Voided samples are usually unsatisfactory for culture of urine for bacteria.
- Samples may be contaminated by substances in the external environment.
- The patient will not always void at the will of the client or veterinarian.

lection. The value of the results will be influenced by the cleanness of the table from which the sample was collected. Contamination of the sample with disinfectants used to clean the tabletop may interfere with chemical tests.

COLLECTION TECHNIQUES

Urine may be removed from the bladder by:

- Natural voiding
- Manual compression of the urinary bladder
- Transurethral catheterization
- Cystocentesis

Regardless of the method used, proper technique should be used to prevent iatrogenic trauma to the urethra and urinary bladder and iatrogenic UTI.

The significance of debris, cells, or organisms in urine sediment should always be interpreted with knowledge of the method of collection. This should be included on the form used to record urinalysis results (see Chapter 1, Figure 1-1).

NORMAL VOIDING

The primary advantages and disadvantages of normal voiding are listed in Table 6-1.

Voided samples are satisfactory for routine urinalysis conducted to screen patients for abnormalities of the urinary tract and other body systems. Depending on specific circumstances, however, it may be necessary to repeat analysis of a urine sample collected by cystocentesis. Voided samples are also satisfactory for serial evaluation of various chemical tests (glucose, ketones, bilirubin, etc.). Comparison of abnormal results in voided urine samples to urinalysis results in samples collected by cystocentesis or catheterization may aid in localization of the underlying cause(s) of the abnormal results (e.g., whether the disorder is proximal and/or distal to the urinary bladder). Unless disease of the urethra or genital tract is suspected, the

TABLE 6-2

MANUAL COMPRESSION OF THE URINARY BLADDER: ADVANTAGES AND DISADVANTAGES

ADVANTAGES
- The risk of iatrogenic lower UTI and iatrogenic trauma is minimal.
- Urine samples may be collected from patients with distended urinary bladders at the convenience of the clinician.

DISADVANTAGES
- The urinary bladder may be traumatized if excessive digital pressure is used. Not only is this detrimental to the patient, but the associated hematuria may interfere with the interpretation of results.
- The urinary bladder may not contain a sufficient volume of urine to facilitate this technique.
- Samples are frequently contaminated with cells, bacteria, and other debris located in the genital tract or on the skin and hair. Therefore they are unsatisfactory for bacterial culture (see section describing urine collection by voluntary voiding).
- Micturition may be difficult to induce in some patients, especially male cats.
- Bladder urine contaminated or infected with bacteria may be forced into the prostate gland, ureters, renal pelves, and kidneys. Unlike normal micturition, where detrusor contraction is associated with a coordinated relaxation of voluntary and involuntary urethral sphincters, manual compression of the bladder increases intravesical pressure but may not be associated with simultaneous relaxation of the urethral sphincters. Application of digital pressure to the urinary bladder for a prolonged period to initiate voiding is associated with a greater risk of reflux into these structures than application of digital pressure for a transient period.
- This technique is unsatisfactory for use during the immediate postoperative phase of cystotomies.

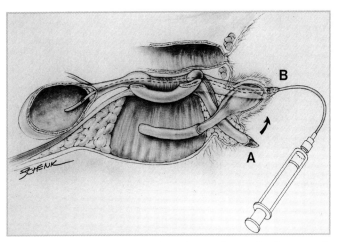

FIGURE 6-4 *Catheterization of a male cat. The penis has been extended from the preputial sheath by pulling it in a caudal position (A). The natural curvature of the caudal portion of the urethra is then minimized by displacing the extended penis in a dorsal direction iwth the objective of aligning the long axis of the urethra with the long axis of the vertebral column (B). (Reprinted with permission of the American Animal Hospital Association. From Osborne CA, Schenk MP: Techniques of urine collection. Forty-Fourth Annual Proceedings of the AAHA, 1977.)*

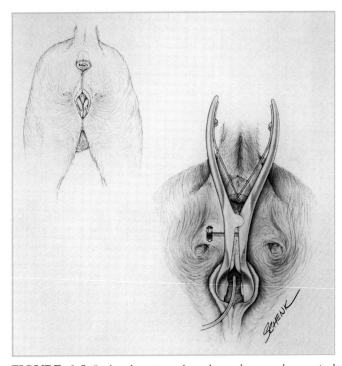

FIGURE 6-5 *Preferred position of nasal speculum, used as vaginal endoscope to permit visualization of the external urethral orifice of female dogs. (From Osborne CA, Stevens JB: Handbook of Canine and Feline Urinalysis. St. Louis, Ralston Purina Co., 1981.)*

first portion of the urine stream should be excluded from the sample submitted for screening analysis because it is often contaminated during contact with the genital tract, skin, and hair.

MANUAL COMPRESSION OF THE URINARY BLADDER

Induction of micturition by application of digital pressure to the urinary bladder through the bladder wall may be used to collect urine samples from dogs and cats. The primary advantages and disadvantages of this procedure are listed in Table 6-2.

TRANSURETHRAL CATHETERIZATION
(Figures 6-2 to 6-8)

Unnecessary catheterization should be avoided, especially in patients with increased risk for bacterial UTI and its sequelae. These include patients with:

- Urinary disease, especially of the lower urinary tract, and renal failure
- Hyperadrenocorticism
- Diabetes mellitus
- Polyuria

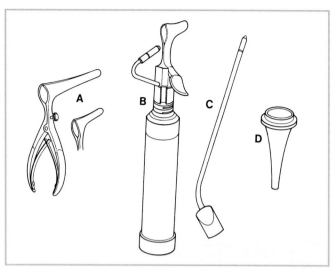

FIGURE 6-6 *Instruments which may be used as vaginal endoscopes. A = nasal specula with blades of different lengths; B = nasal specula with attached light source; C = transilluminator (without handle containing power source); D = otoscope head. (From Osborne CA, Stevens JB: Handbook of Canine and Feline Urinalysis. St. Louis, Ralston Purina Co., 1981.)*

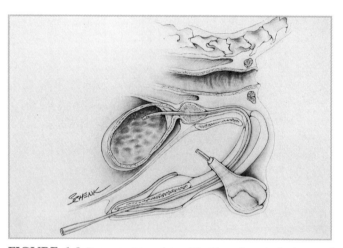

FIGURE 6-8 *Proper position of tip of flexible catheter in the lumen of the urinary bladder of a male dog. Rigid plastic catheters are often unsatisfactory because they may cause trauma and pain during passage through the curved portion of the perineal urethra. (Reprinted with permission of the American Animal Hospital Association. From Osborne CA, Schenk MP: Techniques of urine collection. Forty-Fourth Annual Proceedings of the AAHA, 1977.)*

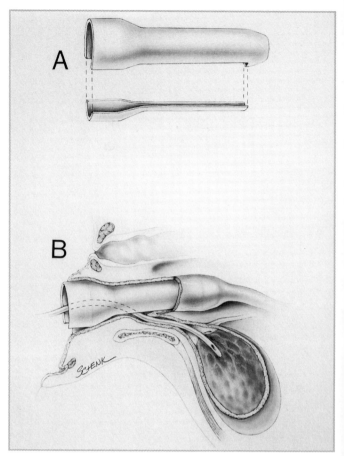

FIGURE 6-7 *Catheterization of a female dog with the aid of an endoscope made from a Monoject disposable syringe container (Sherwood Medical Industries). The endoscope was made by removing a rectangular section from the side of the syringe case (A). Following insertion of the endoscope into the vagina with the open side positioned ventrally, a catheter can readily be directed into the external urethral orifice (B). (Reprinted with permission of the American Animal Hospital Association. From Osborne CA, Schenk MP: Techniques of urine collection. Forty-Fourth Annual Proceedings of the AAHA, 1977.)*

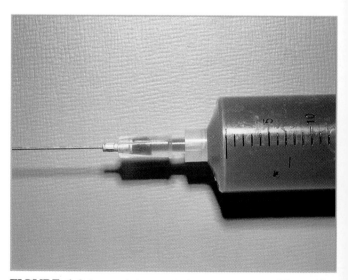

FIGURE 6-9 *Iatrogenic hematuria during cystocentesis. This problem was caused by allowing the tip of the hypodermic needle to contact the mucosal surface of the bladder lumen.*

Catheterization should be performed in an atraumatic and aseptic fashion by persons familiar with correct procedure. Because of the risks of trauma and bacterial UTI, this technique should not be delegated to inadequately trained personnel unaware of the possible consequences.

Only sterilized catheters that are in excellent condition should be used. Nonsterilized catheters should never be used because they may cause iatrogenic infection of the urinary system or they may contaminate urine that is collected for bacterial culture.

Chemical sterilizing solutions containing quaternary ammonia compounds may be used but are less effective than steriliza-

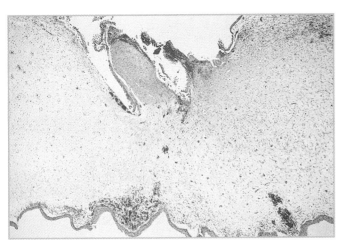

FIGURE 6-10 *Photomicrograph of a section of urinary bladder of a 6-year-old domestic shorthair cat illustrating marked vascular congestion, especially of the submucosa. Transection of these vessels by a 22-gauge needle during cystocentesis would likely be associated with considerable hemorrhage into the bladder lumen. CHBE stain; 4× = original magnification.)*

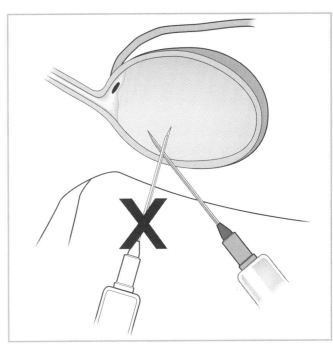

FIGURE 6-12 *Schematic drawing illustrating the correct and incorrect site and angle of penetration of a 22-gauge needle through the bladder wall. Strive to direct the needle through the bladder wall at approximately a 45 degree angle so that an oblique tract will be created. The idea is to create an oblique needle tract to minimize escape of urine into the peritoneal cavity. By inserting the needle in the ventral or ventrolateral baldder wall, iatrogenic trauma to the ureters and major abdominal vessels is minimized. (Adapted from Osborne CA et al: Cystocentesis: Indications, contraindications, technique, and complications. Minn Vet 17:9–14, 1977.)*

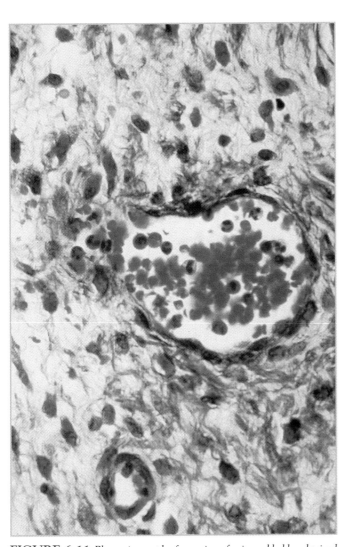

FIGURE 6-11 *Photomicrograph of a section of urinary bladder obtained from a dog with cystitis. Note escape of red blood cells and white cells from the lumen of a congested vessel. (Frazier-Landrum stain; high power magnification.)*

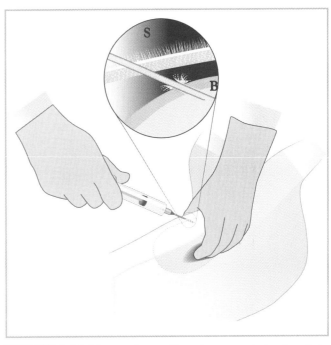

FIGURE 6-13 *Schematic drawing illustrating escape of urine through the bladder wall adjacent to the needle tract as a result of excessive digital pressure used to localize and immobilize the bladder. S = skin; B = wall of urinary bladder. (Adapted from Osborne CA et al: Cystocentesis, in Kirk RW (ed): Current Veterinary Therapy VII. Philadelphia, WB Saunders, 1980, pp 1150–1153.)*

TABLE 6-3

CYSTOCENTESIS: ADVANTAGES AND DISADVANTAGES

ADVANTAGES
- Less risk of iatrogenic infection than with catheterization
- Prevents contamination of urine samples
- Aids in localization of hematuria, pyuria, and bacteriuria

DISADVANTAGES
- Must be sufficient urine in bladder
- May cause microscopic hematuria
- Must be performed with caution in patients with recent cystotomy incisions

tion by autoclaving or ethylene oxide gas. In addition, if residual antiseptic solutions are not thoroughly rinsed from catheters, they may irritate the mucosa of the urethra or urinary bladder, interfere with growth of bacteria, or alter the chemical and enzyme tests.

CYSTOCENTESIS (Figures 6-9 to 6-13)

Cystocentesis (Table 6-3) is a form of paracentesis consisting of needle puncture of the urinary bladder for the purpose of removing a variable quantity of urine by aspiration. Extensive clinical experience has revealed that properly performed cystocentesis is of great diagnostic value. This technique is usually associated with a smaller risk of iatrogenic infection than catheterization and is often better tolerated by patients (especially cats and female dogs) than catheterization.

Diagnostic cystocentesis may be indicated to:

- Prevent contamination of urine samples with bacteria, cells, and debris from the lower urogenital tract
- Aid in localization of hematuria, pyuria, and bacteriuria
- Minimize iatrogenic UTI caused by catheterization, espe-

cially in patients with diseases that predispose them to bacterial UTI

The main contraindications to cystocentesis are an insufficient volume of urine in the urinary bladder and patient resistance to restraint and abdominal palpation. Blind cystocentesis performed without digital localization and immobilization of the urinary bladder is usually unsuccessful and may be associated with damage to the bladder or adjacent structures. Cystocentesis of patients with recent cystotomy incisions should be performed with appropriate caution.

The major diagnostic limitation of cystocentesis is that it is frequently associated with varying degrees of microscopic hematuria. In patients with cystitis, microscopic hematuria should be expected as a result of needle-induced damage to inflamed bladder wall tissue containing an increased number and size of dilated vessels (Figures 6-10 and 6-11). To make the point, consider this illustration. If you scratch normal skin on your forearm, isn't it unlikely that scratching will cause detectable hemorrhage? Alternatively, if you scratch a recently abraded scab-covered lesion on your forearm, isn't bleeding likely to occur?

Please note that bleeding associated with inflammation does not necessarily mean that the bladder is not healing. However, urine samples collected by cystocentesis are not recommended to monitor remission of disease-induced hematuria, because cystocentesis-induced hematuria cannot be readily distinguished from disease-induced hematuria. What is the solution to this dilemma? Evaluation of naturally voided urine samples will not be confounded by the possibility of cystocentesis-induced iatrogenic hematuria.

There are instances when collection of urine samples by cystocentesis is recommended to follow a patient's response to therapy. A notable example is monitoring response to antibacterial treatment of bacterial urinary tract infection. The urinary bladders of patients with irritative cystitis may be too small to safely collect urine by cystocentesis. In this circumstance, inducing diuresis with parenteral fluids or furosemide is acceptable to facilitate diagnostic culture of urine collected by cystocentesis. However, diuresis will reduce quantitative culture counts. Urine formation enhanced with parenteral fluids or furosemide is not suitable for diagnostic urinalysis.

aNebco Distributing, Plymouth, MN.

Chapter 7

Compassion shows others that you care, and compassionate doctors not only care for their patients, they care about their patients.

C.A.O.

"Prophet"-ing More From Urinalysis: Maximizing Reproducible Test Results

A profession consists of an occupation that (1) regulates itself through systematic required education, (2) has a base in technical, specialized knowledge, and (3) has a service rather than a profit orientation, enshrined in an ethical code. With this perspective in mind, it is readily apparent that the primary reason for those of us in the veterinary profession to perform urinalyses should be to assist in the diagnosis, prognosis, treatment, and prevention of diseases. In a symbolic way, results of urinalysis help us to become better medical prophets (or forecasters) of the underlying causes of illnesses and better prophets of the course of the illness (prognosis) with and without treatment. Although monetary income may be derived from performing and evaluating results of urinalysis, this type of "profit" should not be our primary motive for performing urinalyses.

IMPROVING DIAGNOSTIC ACCURACY BY MINIMIZING ERRONEOUS TEST RESULTS

Analysis of urine is a comparatively rapid and inexpensive diagnostic procedure. When properly performed and interpreted, urinalyses provide a fountain of information that assists us in our roles as diagnostic prophets.

In contrast, use of incorrect techniques or outdated reagents and overinterpretation or underinterpretation of test results may seriously hinder our diagnostic prophecies. Incorrect diagnostic information is often a greater stumbling block than lack of diagnostic information because it has a tendency to eliminate the search for correct information. The unfortunate outcome may be misdiagnosis, erroneous prognosis, and administration of ineffective or contraindicated therapy. This outcome is the antithesis of our professional responsibility to ensure that no patient will be worse for having seen the doctor.

Because of the complex nature of normal and abnormal urine, and because of rapid and unpredictable changes in urine composition that may occur following collection, "routine" analysis of this golden liquid should not be regarded as an easy, "routine" task to be delegated to unskilled personnel who have little perspective on the importance of standardization and precision in technique and quality assurance concepts. Caution must also be used not to place a low priority on the techniques of urinalysis when staff are overloaded with work.

As with all diagnostic tests, the value of urinalysis is directly proportional to our diagnostic skills in observation and interpretation. Because results of urinalyses are significantly influenced by biologic as well as technical factors, results should be interpreted in combination with relevant findings from the history and physical examination and radiographic, ultrasonographic, biopsy, and other diagnostic studies.

QUALITY ASSURANCE
Quality Assurance Principles

Quality assurance (QA) encompasses but is not synonymous with the principle of quality control. Quality control involves control of the processes involved in the testing of samples such as urine. Quality assurance is broader in scope than quality control in that it also encompasses validation and verification of the following:

- Proper sample collection
- Correct sample processing (including preservation)
- Proper selection of test methods and testing equipment
- Use of correct terminology when reporting and recording results
- Proper interpretation of results

Thus QA refers to the entire diagnostic process, from collection and identification of urine samples to the technical expertise of staff in interpreting urinalysis results.[2]

Numerous personnel- and technique-related variables may influence the results of urinalysis. The objective of QA is to standardize these variables so that accurate and repeatable results will be produced on every specimen regardless of who does it and which batch of reagent tablets, solutions, or dipsticks were used. When specific errors are identified, corrective steps should be immediately taken to correct the problem(s).

Communication

Confusion and misunderstanding often occur when two people attempt to communicate using two different languages. More commonly, confusion arises between individuals using the same language, each of whom attaches a different meaning or different definition to what appears to be a universally accepted term. If differences in training or personal preference lead to the same type of laboratory test result being reported in different terms, serious misunderstandings may result. Likewise, if different test results are reported using the same terminology, diagnostic chaos is inevitable. Therefore there should be uniform agreement about the terms to be used in reporting, quantifying, and recording urinalysis test results.

Test Standards and Controls

A "standard" solution is one that contains a known amount of an analyte and is used to calibrate a test method. In contrast, "control" reagents or solutions are used to monitor the precision and accuracy of a test method once it has been calibrated with the standard. Control systems should mimic the characteristics of the urine samples being tested.

Accuracy and Precision

The terms accuracy and precision have specific meanings when used in the context of quality assurance:

- **Accuracy** is defined as the ability to obtain the established or true value of an analyte in a sample. Accuracy verifies the correctness of a test result.
- **Precision** is the ability to obtain the same value for repeated measurements of the same analyte in a sample. Precision in measurement verifies the ability of the method to remain accurate upon repeated measures over time.

> As with all diagnostic tests, the value of urinalysis is directly proportional to our diagnostic skills in observation and interpretation.

Accuracy and precision are not synonyms. For example, an inaccurate method may be precise in that it reproduces the same inaccurate measurement over time.

Diagnostic Sensitivity and Specificity of Tests

A laboratory test used to detect disease can have one of four possible outcomes:

- It can yield a positive result for patients that have the disease (true positives).
- It can yield a negative result for patients that do not have the disease (true negatives).
- It can yield a positive result for patients that do not have the disease (false positives).
- It can yield a negative result for patients that have the disease (false negatives).

Sensitivity and specificity are terms used to quantify the ability of diagnostic tests to identify diseased or healthy individuals:

- **Diagnostic sensitivity**—Sensitivity is the probability that a test result will be positive when the patient has a manifestation of the disease the test is designed to detect. It represents the percentage of individuals with the disease that have a positive test result. Sensitivity is calculated by comparing the number of true-positive test results with all patients that should yield positive results with the test.

$$\text{Sensitivity} = \frac{\text{True Positives}}{\text{True Positives} + \text{False Negatives}}$$

Those with the disease that test negative are referred to as false negatives. Highly sensitive tests are likely to identify all patients with disease but may also incorrectly classify healthy patients as having disease.

Practical sensitivity limit is defined in this manual as the concentration of the substance being sought that gives a positive result in 90 out of 100 different samples.

Screening tests for urinalysis must be sensitive enough to detect the lowest level of abnormal concentrations of various substances (glucose, protein, etc.) in urine, but not so sensitive that detection of normal concentrations of these substances gives a false-positive result.

- **Diagnostic specificity**—Specificity is the probability that a test result will be negative when the manifestation of disease the test is designed to detect is not present. It represents the percentage of individuals without the disease that have a negative test. Specificity may be calculated by comparing the number of true negatives with all patients whose test results should have been negative.

$$\text{Specificity} = \frac{\text{True Negatives}}{\text{True Negatives} + \text{False Positives}}$$

Those without the disease that test positive are referred

> There should be uniform agreement about the terms to be used in reporting, quantifying, and recording urinalysis test results.

to as false positives. Highly specific tests are used to confirm a diagnosis suggested by previous diagnostic test results.

- **Sensitivity versus specificity**—A sensitive test is most appropriate for use as a screening test to identify all those that are positive for more definitive testing. A sensitive test will minimize the false-negative rate so that the diagnosis (and therefore treatment) will be missed in as few diseased individuals as possible. When ruling out a disease, sensitivity is more important than specificity because a negative result is relied on more heavily at this point in the diagnostic evaluation.

When it is important to confirm a diagnosis or to "rule-in" a disease, a more specific test should be used to minimize the false-positive rate. Otherwise, a management strategy could be used that is based on a result that incorrectly indicates disease in a healthy patient.

Written Laboratory Protocols

To reduce the subjectivity of urinalysis tests, every step of the procedures used by each laboratory should be defined. Once there is agreement on the procedures to be followed, they should be clearly outlined in written form (Table 7-1). Time and experience have validated the axiom that the strongest memory is weaker than the palest ink. Just as the experienced commercial airline pilot is unable to infallibly recall all the necessary operating procedures at the busy times of takeoff and landing, it is virtually impossible for busy veterinary staff to recall the specific items of each laboratory procedure in proper sequence in the setting of a busy hospital. There are often too many distractions to permit the precision in thinking that is required. As is the situation with poor financial records, poorly defined laboratory procedures are invariably associated with inefficient and erroneous test results. We cannot rely solely on our memories to provide us with the right information about the right test at the right time.

The next critical point is to consistently follow the steps defined in the written protocol. Sample handling and preservation, if used, must be uniform among technical staff. Record keeping, including abbreviations and semiquantitative test reporting, must also be standardized. In addition, record keeping should include documentation of steps taken to ensure that quality assurance procedures are being followed. All laboratory personnel should have ready access to standard operating procedure manuals that have been validated. Inability to find written standard operating procedures is no better than not having them.

Normal Values

Each laboratory should try to develop and record its own normal test reference values as patient populations may vary from hospital to hospital.

In many situations it is impractical for hospitals to establish their own reference ranges. In this situation they must rely on published reference ranges. Limitations associated with many published reference values developed in the past is that they

TABLE 7-1

PROCEDURES FOR ROUTINE SCREENING URINALYSIS

1. To prevent mix-ups in samples from more than one patient, accurately identify the urine specimen by marking the collection container (not just the lid).
2. Record the method of urine collection on the laboratory request/report form (Figure 1-1).
3. Record the time of collection on the laboratory request/report form (Figure 1-1).
4. Record any diagnostic or therapeutic agents given to the patient prior to sample collection on the laboratory request/report form (Figure 1-1).
5. Record the time urinalysis was performed on the laboratory request/report form (Figure 1-1).
6. Strive to use fresh uncentrifuged urine at room temperature.
7. Thoroughly mix the urine sample.
8. Transfer a 5 ml aliquot to a conical tip centrifugal tube. The remainder of the urine sample should be saved until all procedures are completed so that any of the tests can be repeated, if necessary, or other special tests can be performed.
9. Evaluate urine color and turbidity in the transparent centrifuge tube.
10. Completely immerse test portions of the reagent strip into the urine sample and rapidly remove it. With the reagent strip in a horizontal position, gently touch its edge to the edge of collection container and pull it across the container to remove excess urine.
11. Wait for the specified amount of time for the reaction to occur and then compare the color of various reagent pads to the color scale provided by the manufacturer.
    a. Ignore the nitrate test if present.
    b. Ignore the leukocyte test if evaluating feline urine samples.
    c. Ignore the specific gravity test if present.
    d. If the test pad indicates proteinuria, verify its presence by repeating the procedure on urine supernatant. Reagent strip results may be verified with the sulfosalicylic acid test for proteinuria. A urine/protein creatinine ratio may be obtained by utilizing results from the protein and creatinine test pads (Petstix™ 8[a]).
    e. If the test pad indicates glucosuria, test results may be semiquantitated with the copper reduction method for glucosuria.
    f. Evaluate the test for ketonuria.
    g. Use care when interpreting the test for urobilinogen. Do not rely on urobilinogen test pads to screen patients for hemolytic disorders, hepatic disorders, or patency of bile ducts.
    h. Evaluate the test for bilirubinuria.
    i. If the test pad is positive for blood without a pattern of individual spots, repeating the test on urine supernatant may aid in differentiating hematuria from hemoglobinuria and myoglobinuria.
    j. Precautions:
        (1) Allowing the strip to remain in urine for an extended period may result in leaching of reagents from the pad.
        (2) Allowing excess urine to remain on the strip after immersion in the urine sample can result in mixture of reagents between adjacent pads and subsequent distortion of colors. This can be minimized by holding the strip horizontally when it is drawn across the collection container and keeping it horizontal when comparing it to the color chart.
12. Determine urine specific gravity.
    a. Ignore the specific gravity pad on the reagent strip if present.
    b. If a urinometer is used, the temperature of the urine ideally should correspond to the reference temperature of the urinometer.
    c. If a refractometer is used, evaluate uncentrifuged urine if it is clear. If it is turbid, centrifuge (as described below) and use supernatant.
13. Centrifuge 5 ml of urine in a conical tip centrifuge tube for 5 minutes at 1500 to 2000 rpm (or at a relative centrifugation force of 450).
    a. Remove the supernatant by decanting or using a disposable transfer pipette and save for potential chemical analysis. Allow a standard volume (approximately ½ ml) of supernatant to remain in the test tube.
    b. Thoroughly resuspend the urine sediment in the remaining supernatant by agitation of the tube or by "finger flipping" of the tube.
    c. Transfer a drop of reconstituted sediment to a microscope slide with a rubber-topped disposable pipette or an automatic pipette, and place a coverslip over it. Alternatively, use a commercially manufactured sediment system such as the Kova Glasstic Slide[b] system.
    d. Subdue the intensity of the microscope light by lowering the condenser and closing the iris diaphragm (or use a phase microscope).
    e. Systematically examine the entire specimen under the coverslip with the low power objective, assessing the quality and type (casts, cells, crystals, etc.) of sediment.
    f. Examine the sediment with the high power objective to identify the morphology of elements and to detect bacteria.
    g. If the uncentrifuged urine specimen was visibly bloody or very turbid, repeat the dipstick analysis on the supernatant.
    h. If results are questionable, repeat the test and/or confirm the results by another test method.
    i. Record the results.

[a]In the United States, manufactured for IDEXX by Bayer. Petstix is a trademark of Bayer Corporation; used under license by IDEXX Laboratories, Inc. Available in Canada from Bayer, Inc.
[b]Hycor Biomedical, Garden Grove, CA.

have not been modified based on contemporary knowledge and technology. Some include extrapolations of data generated in other species. In addition, reference ranges may have been obtained under a variety of different circumstances using a variety of different techniques. For example, urine concentrations of metabolites are influenced by the amount and composition of diet consumed and also whether urine was collected during conditions of fasting or food consumption.[8,9] Therefore different diets may result in different reference ranges for urine analytes. Until recently, however, little attention has been given to the types of diets that were being consumed at the time normal reference values were being developed.

Following food deprivation, aldosterone secretion increases. Increased aldosterone secretion promotes renal tubular sodium reabsorption and potassium excretion. As a consequence, plasma potassium concentration decreases, urinary potassium excretion increases, and urinary sodium and chloride excretion decrease.[8] During fasting, urinary calcium, magnesium, and uric acid excretions are reduced. However, urinary excretion of phosphorus, oxalate, and citrate are apparently not affected by fasting.[8] When food is withheld from dogs, urinary ammonia, titratable acid, and hydrogen ion excretions decrease and urine pH values rise.[7,8] Therefore measurement of 24 hour urinary solute excretions may be different following food consumption compared to periods when food is withheld.

Consumption of food stimulates gastric secretion of hydrochloric acid. As a result, a decrease in plasma chloride concentration and an increase in bicarbonate concentration occurs in venous blood draining the stomach. Serum total carbon dioxide concentration increases. The resulting metabolic alkalosis is commonly called the postprandial alkaline tide. Urine pH will increase unless acidifying substances are contained in the diet. In a study of healthy beagles, eating was associated with increased urinary excretion of hydrogen ions, ammonia, sodium, potassium, calcium, magnesium, and uric acid.[8]

Laboratory results may be substantially affected by changes in diets fed in a home environment compared to different diets fed in a hospital environment. Urinary excretion of potentially calculogenic metabolites while animals are consuming diets fed in the hospital may be different from calculogenic metabolites excreted by animals eating at home. To determine the influence of home-fed diets on laboratory test results, consider asking clients to bring home-fed diets for use during periods of diagnostic hospitalization.[10]

Positive and Negative Test Control Systems

Because many of the reagents used for analysis of urine are labile, evaluation of dipsticks, solutions, and tablets may be required to ensure proper performance.

Questions about the reliability of a specific manufacturer's lot of reagent strips or tablets may sometimes be answered by repeating the test(s) with new reagents from a different lot number. In addition, positive and negative control samples of urine may be purchased to evaluate some test procedures of routine urinalyses. Test control systems may be either lyophilized pooled human urine or an aqueous solution with various ingredients adjusted to desired concentrations. The manufacturers provide assayed values for each product.

Manufactured products usually have long-term stability in lyophilized form. However, the products usually have limited stability following reconstitution.

Control reagents can be utilized as blind samples (unknown) or as control specimens (known). Control procedures should be performed at regular intervals and every time a new bottle or package of reagents is opened.

> **Techniques used for routine examination of urine sediment for cells, casts, crystals, and so on are more imprecise than most members of the veterinary staff realize.**

Chek-Stix[a] is a positive and negative control strip for urinalysis and is compatible with Bayer reagent strips and tablets.[a] Positive control systems are supplied as a plastic strip with seven pads. Each pad contains one or more natural or synthetic compounds that dissolve into a carefully measured 12 ml volume of distilled or deionized water. Negative control systems are similar in design and use to the positive control systems; however, they have only six reagent pads. Negative or defined results are expected. The strips contain glucose, bilirubin, sodium methylacetoacetate, bovine hemoglobin, bovine albumin, 5-(4-sulfobutoxy)-2-methylindole sodium salt, sodium nitrite, and protease of fungal origin. The reagents are also labile.

Closely follow the manufacturer's directions. The Chek-Stix control solution is made by adding 12 ml of distilled or deionized water to the test tube provided. After adding the strip to water, the system is mixed for 2 minutes and allowed to stand for 30 minutes at room temperature. The tube containing Chek-Stix reagents dissolved in water should then be inverted one more time before removing and discarding the reagent strip. The resulting solutions should be handled and analyzed in a manner identical to an unknown urine specimen.

Kova-Trol,[b] Count-10 Trol,[c] Urine Dipstick Control,[d] and Lyphocheck[e] are control systems that are compatible with Chemstrip urine test[f] strips. Kova-Trol and Count-10 Trol is provided in three levels of control, and Urine Dipstick Control and Lyphocheck are provided in two levels of control. Kova-Trol and Count-10 Trol are reported by the manufacturer to support microscopic values. Tests for microalbuminuria are supported only by Lyphocheck.

Urine Dipstick Control is provided in a ready to use form, but the others require reconstitution. An adequate supply of distilled or deionized water should be available to reconstitute these reagents.

QA also requires proper training in identification and semiquantitation of formed elements found in urine sediments. Kova-Trol contains stabilized red cells and mulberry spores to simulate white cells. QuanTscopics[d] contains stabilized red and white human blood cells and crystals. Materials for total simulation of epithelial cells, casts, and the like are apparently not commercially available.

Techniques used for routine examination of urine sediment for cells, casts, crystals, and so on are more imprecise than most members of the veterinary staff realize. Therefore confirmation of results of urine sediment findings by clinical laboratory supervisors or clinical pathologists is recommended and can be facilitated by use of preserved sediments. Interesting or questionable structures in urine sediment may be preserved by mixing them with an equal volume of Mucolexx[g] preservative and then refrigerating them. Samples may be preserved for several weeks and may be reevaluated by semiquantitative techniques for identification of casts, white and red blood cells, and other formed elements. Struvite crystals tend to dissolve, but most other crystals are preserved. An unidentified crystal may form in some urine samples preserved with Mucolexx (see Chapter 11).

Development of expertise in recognition of red cells and white cells in urine sediments may also be facilitated by adding blood to normal urine and examining the sediment. Similarly, transitional epithelium may be harvested from blood donors with the aid of a catheter or at necropsy and added to normal urine prior to preparation of sediment.

Instruments such as refractometers, urinometers, or centrifuges should be evaluated to ensure that they are properly calibrated. Urinometers and refractometers should be periodically checked for accuracy with solutions of known specific gravity. Preventative maintenance should be regularly scheduled for all laboratory equipment.

Confirmation Tests

Drugs, food, and various endogenous substances can confound urinalysis tests. When interference is suspected, confirmatory tests should be considered. Confirmatory tests should have at least the same sensitivity and specificity as the "routine" test, and, when feasible, should be based on a different biochemical principle. Confirmatory tests for specific reagent strip chemistry tests include but are not limited to Ictotest (to confirm bilirubin dipstick tests), Clinitest (to confirm glucose dipstick tests), Acetest (to confirm ketone dipstick tests), and sulfosalicylic acid (to confirm protein dipstick tests; see Chapter 10).

INFLUENCE OF SAMPLE COLLECTION TIMING ON TEST RESULTS
Randomly Obtained Urine Samples

Urine obtained randomly at any time may be satisfactory for screening analysis; however, the composition of urine may vary considerably throughout the day. Urine samples collected at random could be limited to what has accumulated in the bladder lumen for only a few minutes or it could be a composite of urine formed over several hours.

Early Morning (Fasting) Urine Samples

Early morning samples are preferred to evaluate tubular function because urine from healthy companion animals that have not been drinking while asleep is most likely to be concentrated. Objective evidence of urine concentration provides important insight into the functional status of the kidneys. Also, early morning urine is also more likely to be acid and acid urine pH tends to prevent dissolution of proteinaceous structures.

Since consumption of water is likely to be greatest during the daytime, urine is more likely to be less concentrated at that time. Dilute urine (i.e., specific gravity below approximately 1.008) will lyse formed elements such as red and white cells. In addition, formation of large volumes of unconcentrated or dilute urine tends to reduce the concentration of all substances present in the sample.

Early morning samples are less likely to reveal hyperglycemic glucosuria than a 3 to 4 hour postprandial sample.

> The composition of urine may vary considerably throughout the day.

Also, the morphology of cells is likely to be altered by prolonged exposure to wide variations in pH, osmolality, and waste products. This may cause difficulty in differentiating normal from abnormal cells.

Recently Formed Urine Samples

Cytologic detail in recently formed urine samples is often superior to samples stored in the bladder for several hours. In addition, fastidious bacteria inhibited by urine may be easier to detect.

Recently formed samples may not be sufficiently concentrated to permit evaluation of renal tubular concentrating capacity. Dilute urine may cause lysis or distortion of cells (especially RBC and white cells).

Postprandial Urine Samples

Three to six hour postprandial samples may be utilized to evaluate the effect of various diets on urine pH, crystalluria, glucosuria, and mineral excretion.

Fractional Urine Samples

Water deprivation and vasopressin concentration tests usually require collection of fractions of urine until a desired end point is attained. When interpreting results of these provocative urine concentration tests, care must be used to distinguish events in composite urine samples that have been accumulating in the bladder lumen over time from those in samples collected immediately after all urine has been removed from the bladder lumen.

Timed Urine Samples

Timed (20 minute, 60 minute, and 2, 12, and 24 hour) urine samples are used to determine specific quantities of various analytes (see Chapters 1 and 10). Evaluation of timed urine samples may provide information about:

- Altered renal function (e.g., by measuring glomerular filtration rate, or urine volume)
- Excretion of excessive amounts of metabolites as a consequence of a disorder in a nonurinary system (e.g., excessive excretion of cortisol associated with adrenal disorders)
- The desired and undesired effects of therapy

Collection of timed samples from animals is usually time consuming. In addition, when metabolism cages are used to collect 12 to 24 hour urine samples, some urine voided in the collection pan often evaporates. Voided urine may also be contaminated with feces, hair, and/or food.

Because urine may undergo considerable in vitro change following collection, a preservative is usually added to urine samples collected over 2 or more hours.

If catheterization is required to collect timed urine samples, there is a risk of causing trauma to the urethra and bladder or urinary tract infection.

Detection of the underlying causes of specific types of diseases is often linked to evaluation of the biochemical composition of urine. For best results, at least one and preferably two consecutive

24 hour urine samples should be collected, since determination of fractional excretion of many metabolites in "spot" urine samples does not accurately reflect 24 hour metabolite excretion.

Water consumption and hydration status must be considered when interpreting laboratory results. Decreased water consumption and dehydration are associated with several alterations, including decreased renal clearance of metabolites as well as increased urine specific gravity and urine solute concentrations. Caution must be used in interpreting 24 hour excretion of solutes in the diagnosis and therapy of various diseases if hospitalized animals consume less water than in the home environment.

INFLUENCE OF SAMPLE COLLECTION METHODS ON TEST RESULTS
Overview

In addition to techniques of analysis and interpretation of results, collection of urine is an integral part of urinalysis. The method of collection may influence test results and their interpretation.[11] Therefore this information should be recorded on the urinalysis report form.

Midstream Voided Urine Samples

Midstream voided samples are satisfactory for routine urinalyses obtained to screen patients for abnormalities of the urinary tract and other body systems. Voided samples are frequently contaminated with cells, bacteria, and other debris located in the genital tract or on the skin and hair. Samples may also be contaminated by substances in the external environment or collection container. If difficulty is encountered in distinguishing contaminants from abnormal findings, it may be necessary to repeat analysis of a midstream voided urine sample or a sample collected by cystocentesis.

When possible, the first portion of voided samples should be excluded from the sample submitted for analysis. To facilitate this, two cups may be used to collect the sample. The portion of the sample collected in the second cup, when available, represents a midstream sample; the beginning portion of the sample in the first cup may be discarded or used to localize hemorrhage or inflammatory disease to the urethra or genital tract. If technical difficulties prevent collection of the sample in two cups, the sample in the first cup is still available for analysis.

Voided samples are also satisfactory for serial evaluation of various chemical tests (glucose, ketones, bilirubin, etc.). They are usually unsatisfactory for culture of urine for bacteria.

Manually Induced Voided Urine Samples

Samples collected during induced voiding are also frequently contaminated with cells, bacteria, and other debris located in the genital tract or on the skin and hair. Therefore they are unsatisfactory for the bacterial culture (see the previous section describing urine collection of midstream voided samples).

Catheterized Urine Samples

Urine collected through a transurethral catheter is often altered by catheter-induced hemorrhage. If urine is aspirated from the bladder with the aid of a syringe,

aspiration must be gentle to prevent trauma to the mucosa as a result of sucking it into the "eyes" of the catheter. Unless desired for specific study, the first several milliliters of urine obtained via the catheter should be discarded since it may be contaminated with bacteria, debris, and cells from the genital tract and urethra.

Cystocentesis Urine Samples

The major diagnostic limitation of cystocentesis is that it is frequently associated with varying degrees of microscopic hematuria. The magnitude of hematuria induced by cystocentesis is greatest in patients with inflammation and/or congestion of the urinary bladder. Therefore cystocentesis is not recommended to monitor remission of microscopic hematuria following diagnosis.

SAMPLE PRESERVATION
In Vitro Changes in Urine Composition

Urine is an unpredictably unstable mixture, especially at high temperatures and in an alkaline environment. In vitro changes that may occur in urine samples following collection include those caused by oxidation, photolytic reactions, and/or the effects of bacterial growth and metabolism (Table 7-2). For this reason it is recommended that urine samples (especially those that are alkaline when collected) be examined as soon as possible following collection to eliminate unknown and unpredictable variables. The objective is to analyze samples whose in vitro characteristics are similar to their in vivo characteristics.

In general, the longer the delay between the time of urine collection and the time of analysis, the less reliable are the results. Exactly how long samples can be maintained at room temperature without significantly affecting their composition is unpredictable. However, the yield of red blood cells, white cells, and casts in unrefrigerated samples (especially if alkaline and/or dilute) will be inaccurate within a few hours of collection.

One of the most detrimental alterations that occurs when urine is allowed to remain at room temperature following collection is a variable increase in pH secondary to escape of CO_2 from urine into the atmosphere and secondary to proliferation of urease-producing bacterial contaminants. Alkaline urine promotes false-positive dipstick protein tests as well as lysis of red blood cells, casts, and especially white cells within a few hours. In addition, in vitro alkalinization may alter crystal composition.

Contamination of Urine with Bacteria

Microorganisms are normal inhabitants of distal portions of the urethra. Bacteria also normally inhabit the vaginal vault and labia of females and prepuce of males. Urine may be a good culture medium for some of these microorganisms (Figure 7-1). Proliferating microorganisms may in turn alter the chemical characteristics of urine. For example, bacteria may:

- Catabolize glucose
- Change urine pH
- Cause urine to become cloudy if they multiply to large numbers
- Create an ammoniacal odor

The method of collection may influence test results and their interpretation.

TABLE 7-2

IN VITRO CHANGES THAT MAY OCCUR IN UNPRESERVED URINE

Property	Change
Physical Properties	
Color	■ Colorless urobilogen to orange-brown urobilin ■ Yellow bilirubin to green biliverdin ■ Red hemoglobin to brown methemoglobin
Transparency	■ Increased turbidity due to formation of crystals or proliferation of bacteria
Odor	■ Ammoniacal (strong smelling) due to degradation of urea to ammonia by urease-producing bacteria
Chemical Properties	
pH	■ Increased due to bacterial degradation of urea and/or escape of CO_2 ■ Decreased if microbes metabolize glucose to form acids
Glucose	■ Decreased if metabolized by cells or microbes
Ketones	■ Decreased if microbes metabolize acetoacetate to less reactive acetone
Bilirubin	■ Decreased if exposure to light results in formation of nonreactive biliverdin and/or free bilirubin
Urobilinogen	■ Decreased due to oxidation to urobilin
Nitrite	■ Increased if bacteria convert nitrate to nitrite
Sediment Characteristics	
Red blood cells, white cells, casts	■ Decreased due to disintegration in dilute or alkaline urine
Crystals	■ Increased or decreased depending on crystal solubility in alkaline urine
Bacteria	■ Increased due to in vitro growth

In addition, certain microorganisms produce peroxidase activity that leads to false-positive tests for blood, myoglobin, and hemoglobin. Therefore some form of preservation is indicated if urinalysis cannot be performed within 1 to 2 hours after collection. Proper preservation is especially important for urine to be cultured for bacteria and for 24 hour urine collections.

Fresh Urine Samples

Most agree that urine samples submitted for "routine" analysis should be analyzed within 1 to 2 hours of the time of collection. Otherwise, refrigeration should be considered. If a delay in culturing urine for bacteria is unavoidable, urine specimens designated for culture should be refrigerated immediately following collection. To aid in meaningful interpretation of results, the time of collection, the type of preservation, and the time of analysis should be recorded independently on the urinalysis form (Figure 1-1).

Freshly Formed versus Freshly Voided or Collected Urine

A fresh urine sample is the most desirable for analysis. However, freshly formed urine is not necessarily synonymous with freshly voided urine or freshly collected urine. Urine stored in the urinary bladder for several hours may change in composition. From a diagnostic standpoint, this generality is especially applicable to casts, cells, bacteria, and perhaps pH and crystals. Growth of bacteria may be enhanced or inhibited, depending on the species of bacteria and composition of urine. Bacteria themselves may alter the concentration of metabolites such as glucose and nitrate (consult preceding section, Timing of Analysis, for additional considerations).

In Vitro Preservation of Urine
Objective of Preservation

The objective of all preservation procedures is to prevent in vitro alterations from occurring in the physical and chemical properties of urine, and to prevent in vitro degenerative changes in cellular elements and casts. Preservatives are used in an attempt to provide samples whose in vitro characteristics are similar to their in vivo characteristics.

Basic Actions of Urine Preservatives

Because there is no universal preservative that is satisfactory for all aspects of urinalysis procedures, many different types of chemical preservations are available. Each alters different characteristics of urine. Therefore their general use for routine urinalysis is discouraged. A fresh urine sample is most desirable for analysis.

Two general categories of preservatives exist. One group prevents microbial growth, while the other prevents chemical changes.

Basis for Choice of Preservatives

Choice of the proper urine preservative should be based on:

■ The method of sample collection
■ The test to be performed (i.e., knowledge of the analyte[s] to be measured)
■ The biochemical method to be used to measure the analyte(s)
■ The time delay between urine collection and analysis

It is also helpful to know the type of deterioration that is like-

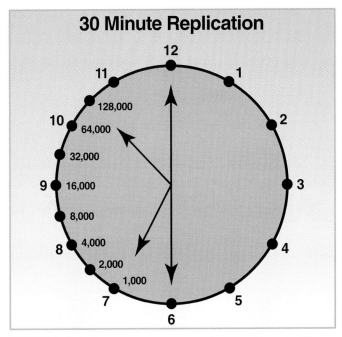

30 Minute Replication

FIGURE 7-1 *Illustration of in vitro proliferation of bacteria following collection of a contaminated urine sample. If a urine sample containing 1000 bacteria per milliliter was collected at 7 AM and allowed to remain at room temperature before being cultured, the numbers of bacteria could increase to 128,000 per ml in 3.5 hours.*

ly to affect the analytes. When requesting measurement of special analytes in urine, consult the laboratory that is to perform the test for specific instructions on which preservative to use (if any).

Adverse Influence of Urine Preservatives on Test Results

Examples of detrimental effects of preservatives are:

■ Interference with one or more chemical tests by bacteriostatic or bactericidal agents
■ Alteration of cellular and crystalline elements and interference with test responses of reagent sticks by acid preservatives
■ Destruction of cellular elements as a consequence of freezing
■ Interference with semiquantitation of results caused by dilution following addition of a significant volume of preservative in proportion to the volume of the urine sample
■ Interference caused by addition of excess ascorbic acid; whereas ascorbic acid in concentrations of approximately 100 mg/dl prevents oxidation of bilirubin, ascorbic acid in concentrations greater than 20 mg/dl interferes with methods utilizing glucose oxidase to detect glucose

If preservatives designed for urine sediment are used that interfere with chemical tests, consider dividing the urine sample into two aliquots of appropriate size. Add an appropriate quantity of preservative to the portion saved for sediment examination. Do not add the preservative to the aliquot saved for chemical analysis.

Refrigeration

Refrigeration is used to preserve urine for routine urinalysis

since it is unlikely to interfere with reagent strip chemical tests. If it is known that routine analysis of a urine specimen will not be performed within 1 to 2 hours of the time of its collection, the sample should be immediately refrigerated (2° to 8°C).

The length of time that various components of canine and feline urine samples will remain unaltered or will undergo minimal alteration during refrigeration has not been determined under controlled conditions. Uncontrolled clinical impressions have been interpreted by most investigators to indicate that the sample may be preserved for several hours and probably overnight. Consider the results of studies performed in refrigerated urine:

■ Red blood cells remain stable in refrigerated *acid* urine for several days.
■ White cells remained stable for about 3 days in refrigerated urine and for more than 10 days in refrigerated urine.

Some perspective on the alterations that occur during refrigeration may be obtained by comparing results of the pH and chemical composition of the sample determined with diagnostic reagent strips   refrigeration and again   refrigeration. Until more refined data become available, we cautiously suggest that refrigerated urine is suitable for examination after 6 to 8 hours. If no alternative exists, it may be used for examination up to 12 hours. After that time the value of examining an unpreserved sample must be considered in light of availability of additional suitable pretreatment urine samples from the patient and the purpose of the urinalysis.

Refrigerated urine samples should be stored in containers with tight-fitting lids to minimize evaporation. Specimens should be stored in amber or opaque containers to protect them from prolonged exposure to light, especially sunlight. Bilirubin, as detected by diazo tests, will become undetectable within 1 hour of exposure to sunlight.

Containers used to collect urine voided by patients in metabolism cages can be surrounded by ice packs and then insulated. Immediately following collection of all urine the composite sample is thoroughly mixed. As needed for various tests, different preservatives may be added to separate aliquots prior to storage.

Refrigerated urine samples should be warmed to room temperature prior to analysis to enhance the proper temperature for enzyme-based tests such as glucose oxidase. Rewarming samples may also help to redissolve substances that precipitated at colder temperatures. In addition, the specific gravity of cold urine is higher than warm urine because cold urine is more dense (consult the discussion on urinometers in Chapter 9).

Freezing

Freezing is a satisfactory method of preserving urine for most chemical reactions (including bilirubin) since it inhibits bacterial growth and retards decomposition of most metabolites. Freezing is a satisfactory method of preserving calcium, sodium, potassium, chloride, magnesium, and phosphate for at least 10 weeks. Reliable measurements of canine uric acid in frozen urine requires dilution of the sample (1 part urine to 20 parts deionized water) at the time of collection and prior to freezing. Xanthine in urine may also be measured by high pressure liquid chromatography. In one study xanthine concentrations in urine obtained from beagles could be reproducibly measured in undiluted or diluted samples preserved by freezing for up to 12 weeks.

Freezing is not a satisfactory method of preserving samples for sediment examination since it will cause varying degrees of cellular disruption. Also, freezing may result in significant losses of the following metabolites: antidiuretic hormone, creatinine, epinephrine, hydroxyproline, norepinephrine, and urea nitrogen.

Samples to be preserved by freezing should be stored in tightly closed containers to minimize evaporation. Depending on the laboratory test to be performed, it may be important to rewarm the sample to room temperature to promote solution of precipitated substances and/or to facilitate the reaction of enzyme-based tests.

Acidification

Cells, casts, and some chemical constituents may be preserved for a short time by acidifying urine, especially if the sample is alkaline when collected from the patient. Concentrated hydrochloric acid and glacial acetic acid will damage cells in sediment. To use acidification to preserve urine sediment, determine the pH of the urine sample. Add boric acid dropwise while mixing until the pH becomes acid. Crystals normally found in alkaline urine will tend to dissolve after acidification, while crystals found in acid urine will tend to form.

Urine preserved with glacial acetic acid may be used for calcium, oxalic acid, phosphorus, delta-aminolevulinic acid, catecholamines, estradiol, estrogens, estrone, and hydroxyproline.

Addition of hydrochloric acid (5 to 10 ml of 10% HCl per liter to reduce the urine pH to 3 or less) is commonly used to preserve urine specimens collected for analysis of calcium and oxalic acid. However, acidified urine is unsuitable for preservation of samples for uric acid determinations since uric acid and its salts will precipitate in an acid environment (see the section on freezing).

For preservation of urine for amino acid analysis, add drops of boric acid until a pH of 3 is reached. The sample should then be frozen.

Mucolexx

Morphologic details of cells and casts and some crystals can also be preserved by the addition of Mucolexx. Mucolexx contains polyethylene glycol, isotonic metallic salts, formaldehyde, and pH buffers. A quantity of Mucolexx approximately equal to the quantity of sediment is added to the test tube, and then the tube is capped.

Formaldehyde

Formaldehyde prevents microbial growth and therefore aids in preservation of casts and cells in urine sediment. One drop of

> **When requesting measurement of special analytes in urine, consult the laboratory that is to perform the test for specific instructions on which preservative to use (if any).**

40% formalin per 30 ml of urine is adequate. Mixing 20 ml of urine with 40 ml of 4% formaldehyde in water has also been reported to provide good results.

Formaldehyde interferes with the determination of glucose by techniques utilizing glucose oxidase. Since it is a reducing agent, if present in sufficient concentration, it may give false-positive results for glucose measured by copper reduction tests.

Thymol

Thymol is usually selected as an antimicrobial preservative. It may be used to preserve glucose and urine sediment. It will induce false-positive reactions for protein if sulfosalicylic acid or Exton's reagent is used. It does not interfere with the reagent strip test for protein. Thymol is added to urine as a 10% (w/v) solution in isopropanol. Between 5 to 10 ml is sufficient to preserve a 24 hour urine collection from an average-sized dog.

Boric Acid

Boric acid at a concentration of 0.8% (1/4 saturation) has been reported to be superior to formaldehyde, chloroform, and toluene in inhibiting bacterial growth. However, some bacterial growth may occur. One gram of boric acid is adequate to preserve a 24 hour sample. Urine preserved with boric acid may be used for protein and sediment analysis. With the exception of pH, it does not interfere with routine dipstick tests.

Urine preserved with boric acid may be used for analysis of androsterone, chorionic gonadotropin, dehydroepiandrosterone, 17-ketogenic steroids, pituitary gonadotropins, pregnanediol, pregnanetriol 5-hydroxyindole acetic acid, and vanillylmandelic acid.

Boric acid in lower concentrations combined with sodium formate is also used in commercially manufactured systems (Cul-Tect™,[h] B-D Urine C & S Transport Kit[i]) to stabilize the number of bacteria for culture, quantification, and identification.[1] These systems are designed to stabilize urine specimens for up to 72 hours at room temperature without altering microbiologic testing procedures. However, refrigeration combined with these systems appears to be more effective.[1] They are used to preserve samples sent to laboratories by mail.

Toluene

Toluene floats on the surface of the specimen. When added in sufficient quantities to cover the surface of urine in the collection container, toluene will minimize surface contamination with airborne microbes. However, it may not prevent growth of bacteria within the sample. The portion of the urine specimen to be examined should be collected from beneath the surface layer of toluene.

Toluene will help prevent loss of acetone but will alter the quantity of acetone detected since acetone is half as soluble in toluene as in water. Toluene is a solvent and may dissolve cups

TABLE 7-3

DOs AND DON'Ts IN TECHNIQUE AND INTERPRETATION

DOs

- Try to collect and analyze a urine specimen whose in vitro characteristics are similar to its in vivo characteristics. If routine analysis can't be performed within 1 to 2 hours of the time of collection, refrigerate the sample. If a delay in culturing urine for bacteria is unavoidable, urine specimens designated for culture should be refrigerated immediately following collection.
- Measure urine pH at the time of urine collection and again at the time of urinalysis when more then one half hour is expected to elapse between the times of collection and analysis. Differences between the two pH values suggest that in vitro changes have occurred and should be considered when interpreting the significance of test results. This step is especially applicable when mailing urine samples to diagnostic laboratories.
- Consider alternatives before discarding unpreserved urine samples. The value of results obtained from such samples must be considered in light of availability of additional suitable pretreatment urine samples, the status of the patient, and the purpose of the urinalysis.
- Use a clean collection container that does not contain cleaning compound residues that could alter the sample.
- Properly identify the sample to prevent mixups in the laboratory.
- Minimize variations in laboratory results by consistently performing all steps in analysis of urine in a standard fashion.
- Rewarm refrigerated urine to room temperature before analysis.
- Store commercial reagents in a cool dry place (not a refrigerator).
- Keep reagents in a tightly capped original container away from moisture, direct sunlight, heat, acids, alkalis, and volatile fumes.
- Immerse all reagent pads of the strip briefly but completely in urine.
- Remove excess urine from the reagent strip by drawing the strip across the top of the container or by pressing the edge against absorbent paper.
- Minimize contamination of reagents from one test pad with reagents from an adjacent test pad by keeping reagent strips horizontal after they are exposed to urine.
- Read reagent strip color changes against a white background in a properly lighted room.
- Evaluate test results at times specified by the manufacturer.

- Use a pH meter to confirm results of questionable pH values detected by reagent strip tests.
- Use a reliable pH meter when there is need for accurate urine pH values.
- Standardize the method of urine sediment preparation.
- Record test results in an orderly fashion immediately after they are obtained.
- Consider the method of urine collection and urine specific gravity before interpreting the significance of test results.
- Use caution in interpretation of results. With the exception of Petstix™ 8,[a] the reliability and specificity of most commercially manufactured tests for humans have not necessarily been evaluated in animals under controlled conditions.
- Evaluate test reagents against positive and negative control reagent systems.
- Repeat urinalysis when unexpected or questionable results are obtained to verify whether abnormalities are transient or pesistent and to monitor the patient's response to treatment.

DON'Ts

- **Don't** rely on urine samples collected and submitted by clients for diagnostic evaluation.
- **Don't** administer diagnostic or therapeutic agents prior to collection of urine for screening diagnostic tests.
- **Don't** rely on a contaminated sample.
- **Don't** remove the desiccant from the reagent strip container.
- **Don't** use outdated or deteriorated reagents.
- **Don't** touch test pads on reagent strips.
- **Don't** rely on color changes in reagents that develop after times specified by the manufacturer.
- **Don't** rely on reagent strip tests to evaluate urine specific gravity.
- **Don't** prepare urine sediment by centrifugation at excessive speeds.
- **Don't** rely on samples preserved by refrigeration for evaluation of in vivo crystalluria.
- **Don't** rely on light microscopic evaluation of urine sediment to detect bacteria.
- **Don't** use "always or never" or "all or none" interpretations about normal or abnormal test results.

[a]In the United States, manufactured for IDEXX by Bayer. Petstix is a trademark of Bayer Corporation; used under license by IDEXX Laboratories, Inc. Available in Canada from Bayer, Inc.

and other collection containers composed of synthetic material. It is also flammable.

Chloroform

Chloroform is an antimicrobial agent when added in sufficient quantities to saturate urine. It is heavier than urine and thus sinks to the bottom of the container, where it may interfere with sediment evaluation. Five milliliters of chloroform is adequate to preserve a 24-hour urine sample obtained from an average-sized dog.

> We cautiously suggest that refrigerated urine is suitable for examination after 6 to 8 hours.

Sodium Fluoride

Sodium fluoride may be used to preserve glucose in urine because it prevents certain enzymes from degrading glucose. Sodium fluoride will inhibit enzymatic tests for glucose and occult blood, including those in commonly used dipsticks. Therefore it is unsatisfactory as a "routine" preservative. Because sodium fluoride is not a good antibacterial agent, thymol is usually also added (10 mg sodium fluoride + 1 mg thymol per 1 ml urine). The sample is suitable for hexokinase analysis of glucose.

Metaphosphoric Acid

Metaphosphoric acid (HPO_3) may be used to preserve vitamin C. An aqueous solution of 10% metaphosphoric acid is used. One volume of acid is added to five volumes of urine.

Commercially Manufactured Preservative

According to the manufacturer, Sedi-Tect consists of urine preservative tablets that maintain structures in urine sediment (red and white cells, casts, crystals, ova, bacteria) for up to 5 days at room temperature.

DRUG-INDUCED ERRORS OF ROUTINE URINALYSIS
Value of Pretreatment Samples

Because drugs may alter laboratory test values by a variety of pharmacologic, physical, and/or chemical mechanisms, diagnostic urine samples should be collected prior to administration of diagnostic and therapeutic agents. Even though test results may not be available until after therapy has been initiated, they still provide accurate baseline information for:

- Assessing the suitability of symptomatic and supportive therapy
- Comparing serial laboratory data obtained to monitor the efficacy and safety of therapy
- Monitoring the rate of progression or remission of the problem

If therapy has been given prior to sample collection, the time and sequence of therapy and sampling should be recorded on the report form to facilitate proper interpretation of results. In some situations it may be advisable to repeat the test after therapy is discontinued.

Acidifiers and Alkalinizers

Administration of acidifiers or alkalinizers may alter crystal composition in addition to altering urine pH. Highly alkaline urine samples may induce false-positive reactions for protein detected by commonly used reagent strips and false-negative reactions for protein tested for with sulfosalicylic acid.

Methionine and other drugs that contain free sulfhydryl groups such as captopril, d-penicillamine, and 2-MPG may cause a false-positive reaction for ketones detected by reagent strips.

Ascorbic acid may cause a false-positive reaction for glucose detected by copper reduction methods and a false-negative reaction for glucose detected by glucose oxidase methods. Ascorbic acid may also inhibit reduction of nitrate to nitrite, tests for bilirubinuria, and chemical tests for red cells, hemoglobin, and myoglobin.

Analgesics

Phenazopyridine may cause false-positive reactions for protein detected by dipsticks. It may also cause false-positive reactions for tests to detect ketones, bilirubin, urobilinogen, and nitrite.

> Formaldehyde prevents microbial growth and therefore aids in preservation of casts and cells in urine sediment.

Anticystinuria Drugs

d-Penicillamine, 2-MPG (Thiola™ʲ), and captopril (which are drugs containing free sulfhydryl groups and used to increase the solubility of cystine in urine) may cause a false-positive reaction for ketones detected by reagent strips.

Antihypertensive Drugs

Captopril, an angiotensin-converting enzyme inhibitor that contains free sulfhydryl groups, may cause a false-positive reaction for ketones detected by reagent strips.

Antimicrobial Drugs

Urine for diagnostic culture should be collected 3 to 5 days prior to administration of antimicrobial drugs. In instances where diagnostic culture is needed following initiation of antimicrobial therapy, we suggest that therapy be withdrawn for 3 to 5 days before samples for culture are collected.

High doses of carbenicillin and benzylpenicillin have caused an increase in urine specific gravity in humans.[12]

Release of formaldehyde from methenamine may inhibit glucose oxidase and peroxidase systems utilized in some glucose and occult blood, hemoglobin, and myoglobin determinations. Formaldehyde may also interfere with tests for urobilinogen.

Large doses of penicillins may precipitate following addition of sulfosalicylic acid, giving a false-positive appearance of protein. Large doses of cephaloridine, aminoglycosides, and sulfisoxazole have also been reported to give a false-positive reaction for protein when precipitated by sulfosalicylic acid.[4]

Corticosteroids

Corticosteroids may reduce urine specific gravity and osmolality by interfering with normal concentrating mechanisms, especially in dogs. As a result of the dilutional effect of increased urine volume, all other components of urinalysis may also be affected.

Fluids and Diuretics

Oral or parenteral administration of fluids or diuretics may alter urine specific gravity and osmolality. Increased urine volumes may suppress positive test results by dilution of analytes, cells, casts, crystals, and so on. Dilute urine (urine specific gravity <1.008) may also cause varying degrees of cell lysis.

Administration of parenteral solutions containing glucose may cause varying degrees of glucosuria and diuresis. Therapeutic dosages of furosemide may cause urine to become acid. Acetazolamide may increase urine pH and falsely elevate dipstick readings for protein.

Radiopaque Contrast Agents

Commonly used triiodinated radiopaque contrast agents may alter urine specific gravity and osmolality.[5,6] With respect to triiodinated contrast agents given intravenously, if the preadministration urine sample has a specific gravity below approximately 1.040, the specific gravity will typically rise following urinary excretion of radiopaque contrast agents. If the preadministration urine sample has a specific gravity above approximately 1.040, the specific gravity will typically fall following urinary excretion of radiopaque contrast agents (possibly as a result of osmotic diuresis). If triiodinated radiopaque contrast agents are directly injected into the urinary tract via a catheter, urine specific gravity will increase.

Triiodinated radiopaque contrast agents may precipitate in an acid medium to induce false-positive reactions for protein detected by sulfosalicylic acid. Evaluation of the precipitates by light microscopy will reveal that the radiopaque contrast agents form crystalline precipitates, whereas protein forms amorphous (noncrystalline) precipitates.

Radiopaque contrast agents may cause crystalluria, although in our experience this phenomenon is uncommonly detected. See the section on crystalluria in Chapter 11 for additional details. Radiopaque contrast agents may also alter the morphology of cells in urine sediment, and they may alter survival rates of some bacterial pathogens.

Radiopaque contrast agents may cause false-positive reactions (often black or greenish black) for glucose detected by the copper reduction method.

Other Drugs

Consult discussions of specific tests of routine urinalyses for additional information about drug-induced errors of results.

---

[a]Available from Bayer Corporation, Elkhart, IN.

[b]Available from Hycor Biomedical, Garden Grove, CA.

[c]Available from V-Tech, Inc., Pomona, CA.

[d]Available from Quantimetrix, Hawthorne, CA.

[e]Available from Biorad Laboratories, Anaheim, CA.

[f]Available from Boehringer Mannheim Corp., Indianapolis, IN.

[g]Available from Lerner Laboratories, Pittsburgh, PA.

[h]Globe Scientific, Paramus, NJ.

[i]Becton Dickinson and Company, Franklin Lakes, NJ.

[j]Mission Pharmacal, San Antonio, TX.

REFERENCES AND SUGGESTED READINGS

1. Allen TA, Jones RL, Purvance J: Microbiologic evaluation of canine urine: Direct microscopic examination and preservation of specimen quality for culture. *JAVMA* 190:1289–1291, 1987.
2. Bakes-Martin RC: Quality assurance, in Anderson SC, Cockayne S (eds): *Clinical Chemistry. Concepts and Application*. Philadelphia, WB Saunders, 1993, pp 39–71.
3. Bartges JW, Osborne CA, Felice LJ, et al: Effects of time and dilution on concentration of xanthine in frozen urine and plasma in dogs. *Am J Vet Res* 58:118–120, 1997.
4. Bradley M, Schumann GB, Ward PCJ: Examination of urine, in Henry JB (ed): *Clinical Diagnosis and Management by Laboratory Methods*, ed 17. vol 1. Philadelphia, WB Saunders, 1979, pp 559–634.
5. Feeney DA, Osborne CA, Jessen CR: Effects of radiographic contrast media on the results of urinalysis. *JAVMA* 176:1378–1781, 1980.
6. Feeney DA, Walter PA, Johnston GR: The effect of radiopaque contrast media on the urinalysis, in Kirk RW (ed): *Current Veterinary Therapy*, vol 9. Philadelphia, WB Saunders, 1986, pp 1115–1117.
7. Lemieux G, Plante GE: The effect of starvation in the normal dog including the Dalmatian coach hound. *Metabolism* 17:620, 1968.
8. Lulich JP, Osborne CA, Parker ML, et al: Urine chemistry values in non-fasted and fasted normal Beagle dogs. *J Am Vet Res* 52:1573–1578, 1991.
9. Lulich JP, Osborne CA, Smith CL: Canine calcium oxalate urolithiasis: Risk factor management, in Bonagura JD, Kirk RW (eds): *Kirk's Current Veterinary Therapy*, vol 11. Philadelphia, WB Saunders, 1992, pp 892–899.
10. Osborne CA, Lulich JP, Bartges JW, et al: Medical dissolution and prevention of canine and feline uroliths: Diagnostic and therapeutic caveats. *Vet Rec* 127:369–373, 1990.
11. Osborne CA, Stevens JB: A clinician's analysis of urinalysis, in Osborne CA, Finco DR (eds): *Canine and Feline Nephrology and Urology*. Baltimore, Williams & Wilkins, 1995, pp 136–205.
12. Swelling LA, Balow JE: Hypersthenuria in high doses of carbenicillin therapy. *Ann Intern Med* 89:225–226, 1978.

Chapter 8

Compassion is an acquired quality. By example, compassionate doctors teach others to be compassionate.

C.A.O.

Macroscopic Urinalysis: Volume, Color, Clarity, and Odor

URINE VOLUME

Indications

Indications for determination of urine volume include the following:

■ For verification of an observation of polyuria or oliguria
■ For quantitation of substances excreted in urine (such as protein, amino acids, hormones, and minerals)
■ For evaluation of renal perfusion in patients with shock
■ For evaluation of fluid deficits and excesses during parenteral fluid therapy

Methodology

Guesstimation of urine volume by observation during the voiding phase of micturition is unreliable. Use of metabolism cages provides more accurate data (Table 8-1; consult the section in Chapter 1 entitled Qualitative, Semiquantitative, and Quantitative Urinalyses for additional information).[7]

Measurements of urinary excretion of hormones, electrolytes, minerals, and other metabolites have the advantage of reflecting average plasma concentrations and therefore average production rates over the 24 hour collection period. However, this method of collection does not reflect circadian rhythms of plasma or urine concentrations of metabolites or variations due to postprandial and fasting states.[1,7]

TABLE 8-1

PROTOCOL FOR MEASUREMENT OF 24 HOUR VOLUME AND URINARY EXCRETION OF VARIOUS METABOLITES

TECHNIQUE

- If the objective of the collection of a 24 hour urine sample is to measure urinary excretion of electrolytes as influenced by diet, consider acclimating the patient to the diet. For approximately 10 to 14 days in the home environment, provide either the diet being consumed just prior to detection of the illness in question or a standard diet of known composition. We commonly use Prescription Diet k/d[a] as our standard diet.
- If possible, for at least 1 day prior to urine collection, hospitalize and feed the dog in the metabolism unit to be used for urine collection. As patients become acclimated to this environment, they are more likely to consume quantities of food and water similar to those consumed in their home environment.
- If analytes are to be measured in the composite 24 hour urine sample, consult the laboratory for recommendations about proper methods of urine preservation (see the section on urine preservation in Chapter 7) before starting collection of urine. The method of preservation may vary depending on the substances being measured and the tests used to measure them. Urine removed by intermittent catheterization can usually be stored in the refrigerator in clean containers with screwtop lids. Containers used for continuous collection beneath metabolism cages can be surrounded by ice packs and then insulated. *Caution:* Refrigeration may cause some minerals to precipitate out of solution.
- Administration of a broad-spectrum antibiotic that achieves high concentrations in urine is initiated approximately 8 hours prior to initial transurethral catheterization to prevent catheter-induced urinary tract infection. The dosage, dosing interval, and route should be based on recommendations provided by the manufacturer. We recommend that antimicrobial administration be continued for 3 to 5 days following urine collection. This represents the time required for normal urothelial repair and replacement (see Appendix C, Table 17).
- Begin each 24 hour urine collection by removing urine from the urinary bladder by transurethral catheterization. This urine is discarded. Record the exact time that urine collection is initiated.
- Weigh the patient after emptying the urinary bladder. This information is necessary to convert final values to a kilogram of body weight basis.
- Feed patients the chosen diet as if they were in their home environment. Drinking water should be available continuously.

- To avoid loss of urine, keep the patient in the collection cage. When using metabolism cages designed for urine collection, catheterization of the urinary tract is not needed except at the end of the 24 hours. House-trained dogs may not voluntarily void in their cage. In this situation urinary catheterization may be used to obtain urine. Dogs may be catheterized as often as necessary to keep them comfortable (usually every 6 to 8 hours). Save all urine removed during the 24 hour collection period.
- If performing renal clearance tests, collect and process a blood sample at approximately the halfway point during the 24 hour collection.
- At the end of each 24 hour collection period, use a transurethral catheter to atraumatically remove all urine. This urine is saved.
- The exact time that the 24 hour collection is completed is recorded.
- All urine collected during the 24 hour period is pooled in a single container, and its volume is measured.
- Pooled urine is thoroughly mixed prior to removing representative aliquots for analysis. Save urine aliquots of sufficient volume in appropriate containers that will prevent contamination and evaporation. We recommend saving samples in triplicate in anticipation of handling and laboratory accidents.

STANDARDIZING FINAL CALCULATIONS OF 24 HOUR URINE VOLUME

- Collecting perfectly timed 24 hour urine samples is often difficult. To adjust the volume of urine collected during a timed period to a 24 hour period, use the following formula:

$$\frac{\text{Actual time interval (minutes)} \times \text{Urine volume}}{1440 \text{ minutes per 24 hours}}$$

- *Example:* A 24 hour urine collection was started at 8:30 AM and ended the following day at 9:00 AM. During this period, 400 ml of urine were collected.

$$\text{Urine volume adjusted} = 1440 \text{ min}/1470 \text{ min} \times 400 \text{ ml}$$
$$= 392 \text{ ml for 24 hours}$$

[a]Hill's Pet Nutrition, Topeka, KS.

Urine volume may be inferred from urine specific gravity. If the urine specific gravity of nonglucosuric urine samples is greater than 1.030 (dog) or 1.035 (cat), it is unlikely that polyuria exists. A specific gravity of this magnitude indicates that water is being reabsorbed from glomerular filtrate in excess of solute. If the urine specific gravity is below 1.030 (dog) or 1.035 (cat), the patient might have any of the following:

- Physiologic polyuria

- Pathologic polyuria
- Pathologic oliguria

Observations and Interpretations
Normal Urine Volume

Normal urine volume is influenced by several variables (Table 8-2). It has been estimated that normal adult dogs in a normal environment will produce approximately 20 to 40 ml of urine per kilogram of body weight per 24 hours (1.0 to 2.0

TABLE 8-2

FACTORS THAT MAY AFFECT NORMAL DAILY URINE VOLUME

- Species
- Body weight and size
- Dietary metabolites and ingredients (water, minerals, and other nutrients) that affect urine volume and renal concentrating capacity
- Fluid intake
- Fluid loss from nonrenal sources such as the gastrointestinal tract
- Physical activity
- Environmental factors such as temperature and humidity
- Urinary solute excretion

TABLE 8-3

CHARACTERISTIC URINE VOLUMES AND URINE SPECIFIC GRAVITY (U_{SG}) VALUES ASSOCIATED WITH DIFFERENT TYPES OF AZOTEMIA IN DOGS AND CATS[a]

Prerenal Azotemia
Physiologic oliguria
    Dogs: $U_{SG} \geq 1.030$
    Cats: $U_{SG} \geq 1.035–1.040$[a]

Primary Acute Ischemic or Nephrotoxic Azotemia
Initial oliguric or nonoliguric phase
    Dogs: $U_{SG} = 1.006$ to ~1.029
    Cats: $U_{SG} = 1.006$ to ~1.034 to 1.039[a]

Subsequent Polyuric Phase
    Dogs: $U_{SG} = 1.006$ to ~1.029
    Cats: $U_{SG} = 1.006$ to ~1.034 to 1.039[a]

Obstructive Postrenal Azotemia
Initial oliguria or anuria
    Dogs: $U_{SG} = 1.006$ to ~1.029
    Cats: $U_{SG} = 1.006$ to ~1.034 to 1.039[a]
Diuresis and polyuria following relief of obstruction
    Dogs: $U_{SG} = 1.006$ to ~1.029
    Cats: $U_{SG} = 1.006$ to ~1.034 to 1.039[a]

Primary Chronic Azotemia
Polyuria
    Dogs: $U_{SG} = 1.006$ to ~1.029[b]
    Cats: $U_{SG} = 1.006$ to ~1.034 to 1.039[a,b]

Terminal nonpolyuric phase
    $U_{SG} = 1.007$ to ~1.013

Reversible oliguria may be caused by onset of nonrenal disorder that induces prerenal azotemia
    Dogs: $U_{SG} = 1.006$ to ~1.029
    Cats: $U_{SG} = 1.006$ to ~1.034 to 1.039[a]

[a]Some cats with primary renal azotemia may concentrate urine to 1.045 or greater.
[b]Urine specific gravity may become fixed between approximately 1.007 and 1.013 if sufficient nephron function is altered. The specific gravity of glomerular filtrate is approximately 1.008 to 1.012.

---

ml/kg/hour). In one study normal adult cats produced an average of 28 ml of urine per kilogram of body weight per 24 hours.[10]

Normal 24 hour urine volume for kittens has been estimated to range between 5 and 60 ml per kilogram of body weight.[3] Newborn puppies have a comparatively limited ability to concentrate or dilute urine in response to changes in extracellular fluid volume. Puppies and kittens are predisposed to rapid dehydration as a result of their higher water requirements, their comparatively greater insensible water losses, and their decreased ability to maximally concentrate urine.

Polyuria and Polydipsia (Tables 1-4, 1-5, and 8-3; Figures 1-4 and 8-1)[8]

Polyuria is defined as the formation and elimination of large quantities of urine. The term diuresis is also defined as formation of abnormally large volumes of urine. Urine volume in excess of 45 ml/kg/day in dogs and 40 ml/kg/day in cats is consistent with polyuria. Depending on the body's need to conserve or eliminate water and/or solutes, polyuria may be normal (physiologic or compensatory) or abnormal (pathologic). For example, polyuria is an appropriate response to water consumption in excess of need. However, polyuria is inappropriate when dehydration is present. The clinical significance of polyuria without knowledge of additional information obtained from the history, physical examination, results of urinalysis, and so on cannot be reliably determined.

Polydipsia is defined as increased thirst or greater than normal water consumption. Daily maintenance water requirements may be calculated as follows:

For dogs—$140 \times$ (Body weight in kg)$^{0.75}$
For cats—$80 \times$ (Body weight in kg)$^{0.75}$

Normal water consumption should not exceed 90 ml/kg/day in dogs or 45 ml/kg/day in cats. Water consumption greater than this is evidence of polydipsia.

Physiologic Polyuria

The most common cause of polyuria is physiologic polyuria. It usually occurs as a compensatory response to increased fluid intake. Verification that a patient has physiologic polyuria may require a provocative water deprivation or vasopressin response test.[6]

Pharmacologic Polyuria

Pharmacologic polyuria may occur under a number of different circumstances:

- Following ingestion of sufficient quantities of salt to increase thirst

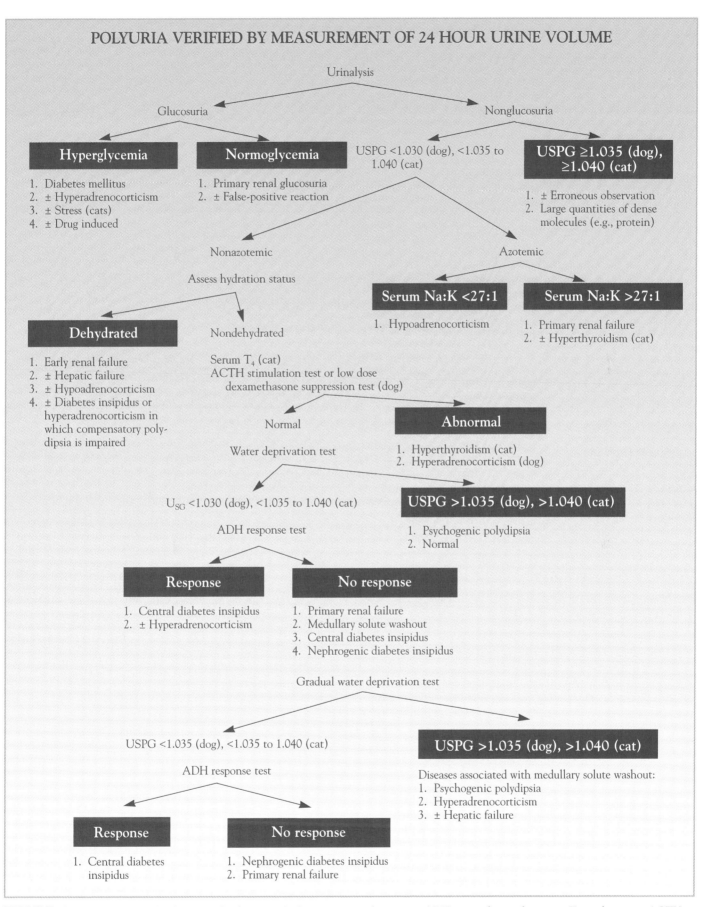

POLYURIA VERIFIED BY MEASUREMENT OF 24 HOUR URINE VOLUME

Urinalysis

Glucosuria — Nonglucosuria

Hyperglycemia
1. Diabetes mellitus
2. ± Hyperadrenocorticism
3. ± Stress (cats)
4. ± Drug induced

Normoglycemia
1. Primary renal glucosuria
2. ± False-positive reaction

USPG <1.030 (dog), <1.035 to 1.040 (cat)

USPG ≥1.035 (dog), ≥1.040 (cat)
1. ± Erroneous observation
2. Large quantities of dense molecules (e.g., protein)

Nonazotemic

Assess hydration status

Azotemic

Serum Na:K <27:1
1. Hypoadrenocorticism

Serum Na:K >27:1
1. Primary renal failure
2. ± Hyperthyroidism (cat)

Dehydrated
1. Early renal failure
2. ± Hepatic failure
3. ± Hypoadrenocorticism
4. ± Diabetes insipidus or hyperadrenocorticism in which compensatory polydipsia is impaired

Nondehydrated

Serum T_4 (cat)
ACTH stimulation test or low dose dexamethasone suppression test (dog)

Normal

Abnormal
1. Hyperthyroidism (cat)
2. Hyperadrenocorticism (dog)

Water deprivation test

U_{SG} <1.030 (dog), <1.035 to 1.040 (cat)

USPG >1.035 (dog), >1.040 (cat)
1. Psychogenic polydipsia
2. Normal

ADH response test

Response
1. Central diabetes insipidus
2. ± Hyperadrenocorticism

No response
1. Primary renal failure
2. Medullary solute washout
3. Central diabetes insipidus
4. Nephrogenic diabetes insipidus

Gradual water deprivation test

USPG <1.035 (dog), <1.035 to 1.040 (cat)

ADH response test

USPG >1.035 (dog), >1.040 (cat)
Diseases associated with medullary solute washout:
1. Psychogenic polydipsia
2. Hyperadrenocorticism
3. ± Hepatic failure

Response
1. Central diabetes insipidus

No response
1. Nephrogenic diabetes insipidus
2. Primary renal failure

FIGURE 8-1 *Algorithm for the diagnosis of polyuria. USPG = urine specific gravity; ADH = antidiuretic hormone; T_4 = thyroxine; ACTH = adrenocorticotropic hormone. (Modified from Osborne CA: Clinical algorithms: Tools that foster quality patient care, in Kirk RW (ed): Current Veterinary Therapy IX. Philadelphia, WB Saunders, 1989.)*

■ Following administration of diuretic agents
■ Following administration of glucocorticoids, especially in dogs
■ Following parenteral administration of fluids
■ Following administration of phenytoin (antidiuretic hormone [ADH] inhibition)
■ Following administration of synthetic thyroid hormone supplements

Pathologic Polyuria

On the basis of different pathophysiologic mechanisms, polyuria may be classified as water diuresis or solute diuresis.

In general, water diuresis is characterized by a urine specific gravity (SG = 1.001 to 1.006) and osmolality (Osm = 50 to ± 150 mOsm/kg H_2O) below that of glomerular filtrate (SG = 1.008 to 1.012; Osm = ± 300 mOsm/kg H_2O). Water diuresis commonly results from insufficient ADH (central diabetes insipidus), decreased renal response to adequate concentrations of ADH (renal diabetes insipidus), or excessive water consumption (pathologic thirst including psychogenic polydipsia).

In general, solute diuresis is characterized by a urine specific gravity and osmolality equal to or greater than that of glomerular filtrate. Solute diuresis results from excretion of solute in excess of tubular capacity to absorb it (i.e., glucose in diabetes mellitus), impaired tubular reabsorption of one or more solutes (i.e., urea, creatinine, phosphorus, and other solutes in primary renal failure), and/or abnormal reduction in medullary solute concentration that impairs the countercurrent system (i.e., decreased renal medullary urea in patients with portovascular shunts and decreased renal medullary sodium in patients with hypoadrenocorticism). Disorders associated with pathologic polyuria and solute diuresis include chronic primary renal failure, the diuretic phase of acute renal failure, postobstructive diuresis, hyperadrenocorticism, and some hepatic disorders (Table 8-2; Figures 1-4 and 8-1).

Polyuria that occurs in association with clinical dehydration (caused by vomiting, diarrhea, etc.) indicates that the kidneys are unable to conserve water when the body needs water. If renal function were normal, physiologic oliguria would be expected to occur as a compensatory response of the kidneys to restore fluid balance. Diseases that commonly, but not invariably, are associated with polyuria, vomiting, and clinical dehydration include primary renal failure (regardless of cause), diabetic ketoacidosis, some cases of pyometra, and some cases of liver disorders. Although polyuria, polydipsia, and dehydration may be associated with central diabetes insipidus, nephrogenic diabetes insipidus, hyperadrenocorticism, and primary polydipsia, these diseases are not typically associated with severe vomiting.

Oliguria (Table 8-2)

The term oliguria has been used to describe either of the following:

■ Decreased urine formation by kidneys
■ Decreased elimination of urine from the body

> Polyuria that occurs in association with clinical dehydration indicates that the kidneys are unable to conserve water when the body needs water.

Oliguria associated with formation of a reduced quantity of urine is related to renal function and may be physiologic or pathologic in nature.

Physiologic Oliguria

Physiologic compensatory oliguria occurs when normal kidneys conserve water in excess of solute to maintain or restore normal body fluid balance. Physiologic oliguria is characterized by formation of a small volume of urine of high specific gravity and high osmolality. The production of a decreased volume of highly concentrated urine in patients with prerenal azotemia is an example of physiologic compensatory oliguria. Prerenal azotemia is often caused by abnormalities that reduce renal function by reducing renal perfusion with blood (i.e., dehydration, shock, cardiac dysfunction). Since blood pressure provides the force necessary for glomerular filtration, a marked decrease in blood pressure will result in reduction of glomerular filtrate. A variable degree of retention of substances normally filtered by glomeruli (urea, creatinine, phosphorus, etc.) results. To combat low perfusion pressure and reduced blood volume, the body secretes ADH to promote conservation of water filtered through glomeruli. Production of urine of high specific gravity, high osmolality, and low volume is the normal response. Prerenal azotemia provides evidence that the kidneys are structurally adequate to maintain homeostasis and are initially capable of quantitatively adequate function provided the prerenal cause is rapidly removed. If the prerenal cause is allowed to persist, however, primary ischemic renal disease leading to renal failure may develop.

Pathologic Oliguria

Formation of inappropriately concentrated urine in quantities of less than 0.5 to 1.0 ml/kg/hour is evidence of pathologic oliguria in dogs and cats.

Pathologic oliguria may occur during the early phase of acute primary renal failure due to generalized ischemic or nephrotoxic tubular disease (Table 8-3). The exact pathophysiology involved in the production of oliguria in patients with acute renal failure is attributable to several mechanisms. Depending on the inciting cause(s), any one or a combination of the following mechanisms may be involved:

■ Marked renal vasoconstriction
■ Decreased glomerular permeability
■ Obstruction of tubular lumens
■ Abnormal reabsorption of filtrate through damaged tubular walls

Pathologic oliguria associated with acute renal failure may persist for hours, days, or weeks. In some instances its duration is so transient that it is not detected.

In some patients, particularly those with drug-induced nephrotoxicity, the term "nonoliguric" is used to reflect a relatively constant, but still inappropriate, volume of urine that is intermediate between oliguria and polyuria. Generally, patients with acute nonoliguric renal failure have a more favorable prognosis for recovery than those with acute oliguric renal failure. However, prognosis is dependent on many factors including specific initiating cause, magnitude and severity of intrinsic damage to renal tissues, and the experience of those providing specific, supportive, and symptomatic therapy.

The specific gravity and osmolality of urine (regardless of volume) formed by patients with acute renal failure will reflect impaired concentrating capacity if a sufficient quantity of nephrons have been damaged. The damage may be reversible or irreversible. Irreversible damage may be nonprogressive or progressive.

A state of pathologic oliguria may develop in patients with primary polyuric renal failure if some prerenal abnormality (vomiting, decreased water consumption, cardiac decompensation, etc.) develops. The oliguria is related to reduced renal perfusion resulting in reduction in the amount of glomerular filtrate that is formed. If this prerenal cause(s) is reversible and/or if adequate renal perfusion is restored, polyuria will resume.

Oliguria or a nonpolyuric state may develop as a terminal event in patients with chronic progressive generalized renal disease.

Oliguria in the context of reduction in the volume of urine expelled from the urinary bladder during the voiding phase of micturition is associated with diseases of the lower urinary system (ureters, urinary bladder, urethra) that impair flow of urine through the excretory pathway. Examples of such diseases include:

- Neoplasms, strictures, or uroliths that partially occlude the urethral lumen
- Herniation of the urinary bladder that partially obstructs urine outflow through the urethra or urine inflow from the ureters
- Rupture of the urinary bladder

Anuria

The term anuria has been used to indicate the absence of urine formation by the kidneys and absence of elimination of urine from the body. Although it is possible that anuria could occur as a result of complete shutdown of renal function due to lack of renal perfusion caused by thromboembolic disease or severe bilateral renal medullary papillary necrosis, anuria is usually associated with total obstruction of urine outflow or rents in the lower urinary tract.

URINE COLOR
Indications for Evaluation

Changes in urine color are sometimes the primary reason clients seek veterinary advice. However, evaluation of urine color per se is of limited diagnostic value. Because of ease and lack of expense, determination of urine color is included in the routine complete urinalysis.

Methodology

Care should be taken to evaluate urine color under a good light source that is consistently used. A standardized volume of urine in a standardized clear plastic or glass container should be used to view urine color against a white background. It is important to differentiate color from transparency.

Interpretation

The color of urine is a composite of all the colored substances it contains. The intensity of urine color may be affected by several variables including:

- The quantity of the colored substance in urine
- Urine pH
- The biochemical structure of the substance, which can change in vitro and in vivo

Because the intensity of colors is dependent on the quantity of water in which associated pigments are excreted, the significance of color should be interpreted in light of urine specific gravity.

Urine color may be altered by in vivo changes associated with a number of factors (Table 8-4),[2,5] including:

- Urine concentration and dilution
- A variety of diseases
- Some pharmacologic agents
- Some ingested substances

Most foods and drugs lose their colors during digestion and metabolism and therefore do not have any recognizable effect on urine color. The color, turbidity, and odor will change in vitro in urine allowed to stand at room temperature.

Caution: Do not overinterpret the significance of urine color. Remember that significant disease may exist when urine is normal in color (i.e., glucosuria) and unusual colors are not always indicative of disease.

Normal Urine Color

Normal urine is typically transparent, light yellow, yellow, or amber. The intensity of the yellow color in normal urine varies with the degree of urine concentration or dilution. The yellow color is imparted primarily by renal excretion of urochrome in plasma. Urochrome is a yellow, lipid-soluble, sulfur-containing oxidation product of a colorless urochromogen. Because the 24 hour urinary excretion of urochrome is relatively constant, urine color provides a crude index of the degree of urine concentration and dilution. Highly concentrated urine will be amber in color, while dilute urine may be almost colorless or light yellow. The quantity of urochrome may also increase in urine kept at room temperature.[9]

> The production of a decreased volume of highly concentrated urine in patients with prerenal azotemia is an example of physiologic compensatory oliguria.

TABLE 8-4

SOME CAUSES OF DIFFERENT URINE COLORS

Pale Yellow, Yellow, or Amber
- Normal urochromes
- Urobilin

Deep Yellow
- Highly concentrated urine
- Bilirubinuria
- Quinacrine (Atabrine); following acidification (H)
- Nitrofurantoin (H)
- Phenacetin (H)
- Riboflavin (large quantities; H)
- Phenolsulfonphthalein (acid urine)

Blue
- Methylene blue
- Indigo carmine and indigo blue dye (H)
- Indicans (H)
- *Pseudomonas* infections (H)

Green (mixture of blue plus yellow)
- Methylene blue
- Dithiazanine iodine
- Indigo blue (H)
- Evans blue (H)
- Biliverdin
- Riboflavin (H)
- Thymol (H)
- Amitriptyline (H)

Orange-Yellow
- Highly concentrated urine
- Excess urobilin
- Bilirubin (yellow foam when shaken)
- Phenazopyridine
- Salicylazosulfapyridine (H)
- Fluorescein sodium (H)

Red, Pink, Red-Brown, Red-Orange, Orange
- Hematuria
- Hemoglobinuria
- Myoglobinuria (red-brown)
- Porphyrinuria
- Congo red
- Phenolsulfonphthalein (following alkalinization)
- Neoprontosil
- Metronidazole (H)
- Warfarin (orange; H)
- Rhubarb (H)
- Carbon tetrachloride (H)

- Phenazopyridine
- Phenothiazines (H)
- Diphenylhydantoin (H)
- Bromsulphalein (following alkalinization)
- Sulfasalazine (following alkalinization)

Brownish
- Methemoglobin
- Melanin
- Salicylazosulfapyridine (H)
- Nitrofurantoin (H)
- Phenacetin (H)
- Naphthalene (H)
- Sulfonamides (H)
- Bismuth (H)
- Mercury (H)

Yellow-Brown, Green-Brown
- Bile pigments

Brown to Black (Brown or Reddish Brown When Viewed in Bright Light or in Thin Layer)
- Melanin
- Methemoglobin
- Myoglobin
- Bile pigments
- Thymol (H)
- Phenolic compounds (ingested or from decomposed protein) (H)
- Nitrofurantoins (H)
- Nitrites (H)
- Naphthalene (H)
- Chlorinated hydrocarbons (H)
- Aniline dyes (H)
- Homogentisic acid (H)

Colorless
- Overhydration (water diuresis)
- Diuretics
- Diabetes insipidus

Milky White
- Chyle
- Pus
- Phosphate crystals
- Fat (surface layer)

H = Reported in humans.

Urochrome may darken when exposed to light.[4] Increased quantities of urochrome may be excreted as a result of fever or starvation.

Urobilin, an orange-brown degradation product of the colorless urobilinogen, may also contribute to the yellow color of urine.

Abnormal Urine Color (Table 8-4)

Detection of abnormal urine color should prompt questions related to diet, administration of medications, and environment. Abnormal colors of the same type are caused by several endogenous or exogenous pigments. Although they indicate an abnormality, they provide relatively nonspecific information in terms of localizing cause(s). Causes of abnormal colors should be substantiated with appropriate laboratory tests and examination of urine sediment.

The color associated with hematuria may vary from red to black, depending on the quantity of blood in urine, the degree of urine acidity, and the time interval that blood has been in contact with urine. As red cells disintegrate, they release hemoglobin, which, when oxidized to methemoglobin, becomes brown or black. Hemoglobinuria resulting from hemoglobinemia may also cause freshly voided urine to appear brown or black in color if hemoglobin has been oxidized to methemoglobin. Myoglobinuria may also cause urine to appear brown.

Bilirubin or its degradation products may result in a yellow color that is darker than normal. Green urine may be associated with oxidation of large quantities of bilirubin to biliverdin (see Figure 10-6).

Urine color may interfere with colorimetric test results to a variable degree.

URINE CLARITY/TRANSPARENCY
Terminology
Turbidity is derived from the Latin word "turbidus," meaning troubled or disturbed. In context of urine it is commonly used to connote cloudiness of the sample.

Nephloid is a term derived from the Greek term "nephele," meaning cloudy. Nephology (not nephrology, as nephro is the Greek root word for kidney) is a branch of meteorology related to clouds. Nephloid urine means cloudy urine. The degree of cloudiness or turbidity can be measured with an instrument called a nephlometer.

Indications for Evaluation
Freshly voided urine should be transparent. If it is turbid or cloudy, this is cause for further evaluation.

Methodology
The degree of clarity (transparency) or cloudiness (turbidity) is determined at the time of assessment of urine color using the same standardized methodology. The transparency or turbidity of urine is commonly estimated by reading newspaper print through the clear container. The degree of turbidity may be reported as clear, slightly turbid, moderately turbid, or extremely turbid:

- A clear sample contains no visible particulate matter.
- A slightly turbid sample is characterized by visible precipitates that do not obscure newsprint viewed through the specimen.
- A moderately turbid sample is characterized by visible precipitates that obscure newsprint viewed through the specimen.
- An extremely turbid sample is characterized by inability to read newsprint viewed through the specimen.

Interpretation
Turbidity of urine is caused by precipitates that scatter light.

> **Urine color provides a crude index of the degree of urine concentration and dilution.**

The causes of urine turbidity may be associated with normalcy, contamination of the sample, or an underlying abnormality. These causes are usually best investigated by light microscopic evaluation of urine.

Normal
In most species freshly voided midstream urine is transparent or clear. Lipiduria, which is often present in urine samples obtained from healthy cats, is often characterized by visible turbidity at the surface of the specimen.

Caution: Clear urine is not always normal as it may contain abnormal amounts of glucose, protein, and ketones. Clear urine may also contain abnormal numbers of casts, cells, and crystals that are not present in sufficient quantity to alter the clarity of the sample.

Turbidity
Concentrated urine is more likely to be turbid than dilute urine.

Artifactual Turbidity
In vitro alterations, especially changes in temperature and pH, may cause varying degrees of loss of transparency that are not associated with any in vivo abnormalities.

In vitro formation of crystals in urine is a common cause of urine turbidity. The solubility of most crystals is influenced by temperature. Hence crystals may form as urine as body temperature cools to room or refrigeration temperature. If crystals interfere with microscopic examination of sediment, crystal dissolution may be promoted by warming the sample in a 37°C water bath. Precipitation of crystals may also be influenced by pH. Consult the discussion about crystals in Chapter 11 for further information.

Other in vitro causes of turbidity include contaminants from the collection container, contamination with semen, and contamination with feces.

Abnormal Turbidity
Causes of abnormal urine turbidity include:

- Crystals
- Red blood cells, white cells, and/or epithelial cells
- Bacteria, yeasts, and the like
- Lipid droplets

Macroscopic hematuria typically results in brownish to red (occasionally black) turbid urine. Hemoglobinuria (and myoglobinuria) results in brownish to red (occasionally black) transparent urine.

URINE ODOR
Indications for Evaluation
Detection of abnormal urine odors is rarely of specific diagnostic significance. However, detection of abnormal urine odors indicates the need for further evaluation.

Improperly stored urine samples typically have a very strong odor. Therefore it is useful to determine whether urine samples with strong odors have been properly preserved before proceeding with urinalysis and interpreting the results.

Methodology

Urine odor is evaluated by our sense of smell. Odor may be described as normal (urinoid), ammoniacal, putrid, disagreeable, or with slang terms. An abnormally strong odor should be noted on the urinalysis report form.

The cause of abnormal urine odor is best determined by evaluation of a complete urinalysis. Depending on the cause, additional laboratory tests and/or clinical investigation may be required.

Interpretation
Normal Odor

Normal urine has a characteristic odor that varies among species and between genders within species. Urine obtained from uncastrated male cats is particularly pungent. Urine from horses also has a characteristic aromatic odor.

Abnormal Odor

In humans abnormal urine odors in newborn infants are sometimes associated with metabolic defects. Urinary tract infections and excretion of drugs, such as ampicillin, may be associated with abnormal and sometimes characteristic odors.

Urine with an ammoniacal odor is a common abnormality. NH_3 (ammonia) imparts the characteristic odor; NH_4^+ (ammonium) and urea are odorless. Fresh normal urine at room temperature does not have an ammoniacal odor because it contains an insignificant quantity of NH_3. It contains large quantities of urea, however, and may contain a large quantity of NH_4^+.

Potential causes of ammoniacal odor include transformation of NH_4^+ to NH_3 by endogenous or exogenous heat and degra-

> The cause of abnormal urine odor is best determined by evaluation of a complete urinalysis.

dation of urea to NH_3 by urease-producing bacteria. Urease-producing bacteria may be pathogens or contaminants. Freshly voided urine with an ammoniacal odor suggests (but does not prove) infection of the urinary tract with urease-producing bacteria.

A putrid odor also indicates bacterial degradation of a large quantity of protein and is abnormal.

Ketonuria has been reported to impart a characteristic sweet or fruity odor to urine. Many individuals are unable to detect this odor. Laboratory tests are more reliable in detecting ketonuria.

Sometimes urine will have the odor characteristic of the container in which it was collected. Examples include odors from detergents used to clean containers and odors from cosmetic and perfume containers.

REFERENCES AND SUGGESTED READINGS

1. Bartges JW, Osborne CA: Influence of fasting and eating on laboratory values, in Bonagura JD (ed): *Current Veterinary Therapy XII*. Philadelphia, WB Saunders, 1995, pp 20–23.
2. Brunzel NA: *Fundamentals of Body Fluid Analysis*. Philadelphia, WB Saunders, 1994.
3. Crawford MA: The urinary system, in Hoskins JD (ed): *Veterinary Pediatrics*. Philadelphia, WB Saunders, 1990, pp 271–292.
4. deWardner HE: *The Kidney*, ed 5. New York, Churchill Livingstone, 1985, p 205.
5. Free A, Free H: *Urinalysis in Clinical Laboratory Practice*. Cleveland, CRC Press, 1975.
6. Hardy RM, Osborne CA: Water deprivation and vasopressin concentration tests, in Kirk RW (ed): *Current Veterinary Therapy VII*. Philadelphia, WB Saunders, 1980, p 1081.
7. Lulich JP, Osborne CA, Polzin JP, et al: Urine metabolite values in fed and nonfed clinically normal beagles. *Am J Vet Res* 52:1573–1578, 1991.
8. Osborne CA, Stevens JB: *Handbook of Canine and Feline Urinalysis*. St. Louis, Ralston Purina Co, 1981.
9. Oslow M, Philo S: The chief urinary pigment: The relationship between the rate of excretion of the yellow pigment and the metabolic rate. *Am J Med Sci* 207:507–512, 1944.
10. Worden AN, Waterhouse CE, Sellwood EHB: Studies of the composition of normal cat urine. *J Small Anim Pract* 1:11–29, 1960.

Chapter 9

To the extent we learn to put ourselves in another's shoes, paws, hooves, or claws, we will be able to be compassionate.

C.A.O.

Urine Specific Gravity, Refractive Index, or Osmolality: Which One Would You Choose?

CASE SCENARIO

Suppose you are evaluating a persistently polyuric golden retriever. The serum biochemical profile is normal. Evaluation of urine reveals 3+ proteinuria (determined by reagent strip), with no abnormalities in urine sediment. Which of the following test results obtained from a refrigerated urine sample (40°F) most accurately reflects urine concentrating capacity: (1) urine osmolality = 1400 mOsm/kg, (2) urine specific gravity = 1.025 by urinometer, (3) urine specific gravity = 1.014 by dipstick test, or (4) urine specific gravity = 1.017 by refractometer. What is the basis for your choice?

TABLE 9-1

DIFFERENTIATION OF DIFFERENT FORMS OF AZOTEMIA

Factor	Prerenal Azotemia	Primary Intrarenal Azotemia	Postrenal Azotemia	Primary Renal Azotemia with Functional Glumerulotubular Imbalance
Serum urea nitrogen concentration	Increased	Increased	Increased	Increased
Serum creatinine concentration	Increased	Increased	Increased	Increased
Urine specific gravity	≥1.035 (Dog) ≥1.040 (Cat[a])	±1.007–1.029 (Dog) ±1.007–1.039 Cat[a])	Variable	±1.020–1.030 (Dog) ±1.035–1.040 (Cat)
Proteinuria with normal sediment	Usually negative	Variable depending on cause	Usually negative	Positive
Proteinuria with red cells and/or white cells	Usually negative	Variable depending on cause	Often positive	Positive
Prerenal cause	Present	Absent	Absent	Usually negative
Postrenal cause	Absent	Absent	Present	Absent
Response to correction of postrenal cause	Not applicable	Not applicable	Within hours to a few days	Absent
Response to correction of renal perfusion with fluids	Within 1–3 days	Minimal if normally hydrated Some response if dehydrated	Minimal	Minimal

[a]Some cats with primary renal azotemia may concentrate urine to 1.045 or greater.

WHAT ARE THE INDICATIONS FOR MEASUREMENT OF URINE SPECIFIC GRAVITY AND OSMOLALITY?

The kidneys excrete unwanted solute (metabolic garbage) in a volume of water that is not required to maintain homeostasis. Elimination of unwanted solutes and water is the result of carefully regulated glomerular filtration, tubular reabsorption, and tubular secretion. Measurement of urine osmolality, either directly by osmometry or indirectly by evaluation of urine specific gravity, is the primary method used to evaluate the kidney's "response ability" to concentrate (remove water in excess of solute) or dilute (remove solute in excess of water) urine according to varying needs. Thus evaluation of urine osmolality or specific gravity is an index of tubular reabsorption. Consult Chapter 1 for additional details. Knowledge of urine osmolality or specific gravity is also extremely helpful when attempting to differentiate the underlying cause(s) of polyuria and when localizing the pathophysiologic mechanisms of azotemia (Tables 1-2, 2-1, and 9-1). Consult Chapters 1, 2, and 8 for additional details.

Another major indication for routine evaluation of urine specific gravity involves interpretation of tests that are part of the complete urinalysis. Interpretation of other test results of the urinalysis are dependent on knowledge of specific gravity (or osmolality) since these data provide information regarding the ratio of solutes to solvent (water). Tests of routine urinalyses are typically performed on a relatively small sample of urine without regard to the rate of formation of urine or total urine volume. Semiquantitative interpretation of results is unfeasible in such samples without knowledge of specific gravity. Consider proteinuria as an example. Does 2+ proteinuria at a specific gravity of 1.010 reflect an equal or greater loss of protein than a 2+ proteinuria at 1.050? The answer is obvious—there is more protein in the less concentrated sample. The same concept is applicable to interpretation of positive test results for glucose, ketones, bilirubin, occult blood, and constituents in urine sediment.

Another indication for evaluation of urine specific gravity and/or osmolality is as an aid for monitoring the patient's fluid balance, especially during therapy with parenteral fluids.

METHODOLOGY
What Is Urine Osmolality?
Application of Basic Concepts

The clinical unit of osmotic concentration is the *osmole*. An osmole is defined as the quantity of a substance that dissociates to produce 1 mole of particles in solution. Consider the effects of relatively large albumin molecules (molecular weight = 68,000), much smaller glucose molecules (molecular weight = 180), and tiny sodium chloride molecules (molecular weight = 58) on the osmolality of urine (Table 1-3). Does albumin, glucose, or NaCl have the greater effect on osmolality? One mole of albumin provides 1 osmole of solute because albumin does not dissociate in urine to form an increased quantity of solute. Likewise, 1 mole of glucose provides 1 osmole of solute because glucose does not dissociate in urine to form an increased quantity of solute. However, 1 g of glucose per deciliter has a greater effect on osmolality than 1 g of albumin per deciliter because the number of molecules in 1 g/dl is much larger for glucose than the number of particles of albumin in 1 g/dl. What about NaCl? In urine, 1 mole of NaCl will dissociate to form 2 osmoles (one sodium ion and one chloride ion) in solution. Thus a 1 g/dl solution of NaCl has many hundred times the osmotic activity of a 1 g/dl solution of albumin because undissociated and dissociated salt molecules contribute many small molecules in large numbers while the same weight of protein contributes fewer large molecules. However, because of their high molecular weight, proteins could substantially affect specific gravity measurements. When urine contains 1 g of protein per deciliter, 0.003 must be subtracted from the observed specific gravity. In contrast, the effect of 1 g of protein per deciliter on urine osmolality is negligible (less than 1 milliosmole per kilogram).

Since the *osmole* represents a large mass of solute, the *milliosmole* has been developed for clinical use (1 milliosmole [mOsm] = 0.001 osmole). Use of milliosmoles eliminates the necessity of using fractions when evaluating osmolality of biological fluids.

For osmolality the unit of solvent measurement is mass (kilograms), and therefore osmolality is expressed as mOsm/kg of solution. For osmolarity the unit of solvent measurement is volume (liter), and therefore osmolality is expressed as mOsm/L of solution. Unlike osmolality, osmolarity measurements are temperature dependent. However, the numerical difference between osmolality and osmolarity values of biological fluids is usually small, and therefore the values are commonly used interchangeably.

Osmometers

Conceptual understanding of how osmolality is measured in plasma and urine is linked to the following characteristics of colligative properties of solutions. What are colligative properties? Colligative properties are physical rather than chemical in nature. In context of urine, colligative properties are physical characteristics that are dependent only on the number of particles of dissolved solute that it contains. Dissolution of one or more substances (or solutes) in a solvent (water) changes four

> In context of urine, colligative properties are physical characteristics that are dependent only on the number of particles of dissolved solute that it contains.

mathematically interrelated physical characteristics: (1) osmotic pressure, (2) freezing point, (3) vapor pressure, and (4) boiling point. What are colligative properties? They are not dependent on the specific chemical nature, size, shape, weight, or electrical charge of solutes. Now, consider this fact. As solute is added to urine (1) osmotic pressure increases, (2) boiling point increases, (3) vapor pressure (the pressure at which rate of evaporation is equal to the rate of condensation) decreases, and (4) freezing point decreases. One osmole of an ideal solution in 1 kg of water will have a freezing point of $-1.86\,°C$ compared to pure water.

Commercial osmometers determine osmolality by measuring relative changes in freezing point or vapor pressure of unknown solutions, utilizing standard solutions as reference points. Currently available equipment utilizes microprocessors to provide rapid digital readout of data on samples as small as 0.2 ml. Unfortunately, osmometers are relatively expensive.

Although osmometers provide a measurement of the number (or concentration) of osmotically active particles in solution, they do not indicate the type(s) of solute present. In addition, different types of osmometers have different advantages and limitations. For example, unlike vapor pressure osmometers, freezing point osmometers measure the effect of volatile solutes (such as ethylene glycol) on osmolality. However, vapor pressure osmometers have been superior to freezing point osmometers for measurement of extremely high solute concentrations of urine samples. In studies of concentrated feline urine performed at the University of Minnesota, freezing point osmometers were not capable of accurately measuring the osmotic concentration of samples whose specific gravity (SG) was greater than 1050.[17] Although osmometers provide a measurement of the number (or concentration) of osmotically active particles in solution, they do not indicate the type(s) of solute present.

What Is Urine Specific Gravity?
Application of Basic Concepts

The density of a substance is the ratio of its mass (weight) to its volume. Density of urine reflects the total mass (which is related to weight and thus to gravity) of all solutes per unit volume of solution. Stated in another way, urine specific gravity is the ratio of the density (or weight) of urine to the density (or weight) of an equal volume of distilled water, both measured at the same temperature:

$$\text{Specific Gravity} = \frac{\text{Density (weight) of urine}}{\text{Density (weight) of water}}$$

The SG of water is 1.000 under conditions of standard temperature and pressure. If the density of urine were equal to the density of water, the specific gravity value would be 1. However, it is physiologically impossible for the kidneys to excrete pure water. Urine is more dense than water because it is composed of water and various solutes of different densities and therefore always has a specific gravity greater than 1.

Because specific gravity is a measurement of density, it is affected by the number of particles of solute present. Unfortunately, it is also affected by the molecular weight of each solute present. Therefore there is only an approximate relationship between specific gravity and total solute concentration.[17] For example, we observed a urine specific gravity value of 1.048 in three different dogs. The urine osmolality values of the same urine samples from these three dogs were 1734, 1820, and 1978 mOsm/kg.

Each species of solute has its own characteristic effect on the SG of urine. Urine samples having equivalent numbers of solute molecules per unit volume may have different SG values if different mixtures of solutes are present. For example, equal numbers of molecules of urea, sodium chloride, albumin, globulin, fibrinogen, and glucose all have a different quantitative effect on specific gravity. Looking at this illustration in a slightly different context, addition of either (1) 0.147 g of sodium chloride, (2) 0.36 g of urea, (3) 0.27 g of glucose, or (4) 0.4 g of albumin to 100 ml of urine will increase SG by 0.001.

Urinometers

Hydrometers are devices for measurement of the density of liquids by the buoyancy of a plummet with a calibrated stem. There are hydrometers for alcoholic solutions (alcoholometer), sugar (saccharometer), milk (lactometer), and urine (urinometer).

A urinometer consists of a weighted glass bulb attached to a cylindrical stem designed to measure the specific gravity of urine. A scale calibrated in specific gravity units is etched on the surface or placed inside the cylindrical stem. When placed in a solution such as urine with a spinning motion to be sure that it is floating freely, the urinometer displaces a volume of urine equal to its weight. The more solute that urine contains, the less volume the urinometer displaces. The fluid level is read at the bottom of the meniscus where urine intersects with the urinometer scale.

Although the weight of urine remains constant regardless of its temperature, the density of urine decreases with an increase in temperature. Conversely, the density of urine increases with a decrease in temperature. Therefore, urinometers are calibrated at a reference temperature (usually close to room temperature). The reference temperature is usually identified on the stem (Figure 9-1). For precise work, measurements should be corrected by adding 0.001 for each 3°C that urine temperature is above the reference temperature of the urinometer or by subtracting 0.001 for each 3°C that urine temperature is below the reference temperature. For screening evaluation this calculation is unnecessary, although the concept should be considered when interpreting the results.

Compared to refractometry and osmolality, the precision of urinometers is not great. One reason already mentioned is that measurements vary with temperature. In addition, there may be difficulty in reading the meniscus. Froth or bubbles on the surface of urine should be broken (touch with a piece of filter paper), and the reading taken at the

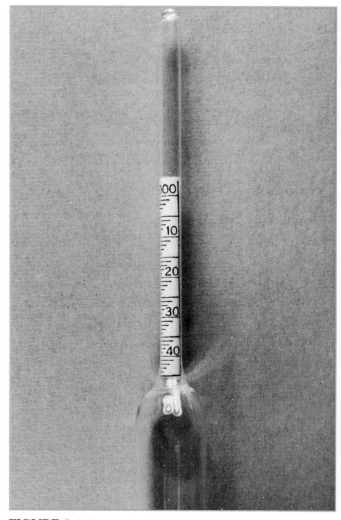

FIGURE 9-1 *Photograph of a urinometer. The specific gravity scale is printed on a piece of paper located in the stem. Movement of this paper could erroneously alter test results.*

level of the bottom of the meniscus. Another disadvantage is that there is a tendency for urinometers to "drag" against the side of narrow deep cylinders containing the urine sample. This may result in erroneous specific gravity values.

The specific gravity scales of urinometers are often inaccurate. Therefore each urinometer should be checked for accuracy after purchase and periodically thereafter. To validate the reliability of urinometers, distilled water, which has an SG = 1.000, may be used. An 0.58% NaCl solution has a specific gravity of 1.003; a 3% NaCl solution has a specific gravity of 1.020. Further, 75 ml of xylene and 28 ml of bromobenzene have an SG = 1.030.

Yet another disadvantage of urinometers is that a relatively large volume of urine (i.e., 5 to 15 ml or more depending on the size of the urinometer and the size of the container) is required in which to float this instrument. Specific gravity may be determined with urinometers on smaller samples of urine by addition of a known volume of water and by correcting the observed measurement for the dilution. To

> There is only an approximate relationship between specific gravity and total solute concentration.

obtain the actual specific gravity of a diluted urine sample, to the value 1.000 add the product obtained when the observed value minus 1.000 is multiplied by the dilution factor. For example, if the dilution is one part urine to two parts water and the observed specific gravity is 1.007, the corrected specific gravity is 1.021:

$$1.007 - 1.000 = 0.007$$
$$0.007 \times 3 = 0.021$$
$$1 + 0.021 = 1.021$$

Values obtained by the dilution method are less accurate than undiluted values because errors introduced by measurement are multiplied by the dilution factor.

Specific Gravity Reagent Strips

The reagent strip specific gravity test is an indirect colorimetric method of assessment of "ionic" urine specific gravity. Indirectly measuring urine specific gravity with test strips is based on the change in pK (dissociation constant) of a polyelectrolyte in the test pad in relation to the concentration of ionic solutes in urine.[5] The test pad is impregnated with a polyelectrolyte (polymethylvinyl ether/maleic acid in Multistix®,[a] and ethyleneglycol-bis tetraacetic acid in Chemstrip®[b]) and a pH indicator (bromthymol blue) that are maintained at an alkaline pH. When the test pad is immersed in urine, the polyelectrolyte reagent ionizes and releases protons in proportion to the concentration of urine ionic analytes. The protons released from the polyelectrolyte decrease the pH of the test pad, causing a color change in the indicator dye from dark blue-green (SG = 1.000) to yellow-green (SG = 1.030). The greater the number of ionic solutes in urine, the greater the release of hydrogen ions from the test pad, and the greater the color change in the test pad indicator dye.

This method is not influenced by nonionic urine analytes, such as urea or glucose. Therefore specific gravity values determined by this method do not need to be corrected for significant quantities of urine glucose. However, the total specific gravity of urine is dependent on both ionic and nonionic solutes. In addition, urine pH values of 6.5 or greater could influence test results because the indicator dye bromthymol blue is active in this range.

Because the highest value that these reagent strips can detect is approximately 1.025 to 1.030, they are unsatisfactory for detection of adequate renal concentrating capacity in dogs or cats. We have also found them to be unreliable in less concentrated urine samples.

What Is Urine Refractive Index?
Application of Basic Concepts

Aqueous solutions such as urine contain substances that absorb various wavelengths of light. This may be measured by determining the refractive index of the light. The refractive index of light is defined as the ratio (or comparison) of the velocities of light in two different media.

In context of urine, refractive index is the unitless ratio of refraction of light in air compared to the refraction of light in

> Ideally, refractometers should be calibrated for the species being studied by using urine samples of known specific gravity.

urine. As the solute concentration of urine increases, the velocity of light passing from air through urine decreases and the light beam is refracted. As a consequence, the light rays "bend" (that is, the angle of light refraction changes). The index of refraction may be measured by an instrument called a refractometer. Refractometry provides an indirect assessment of osmolality and specific gravity.

Refractometers

Small hand-held refractometers calibrated to determine urine specific gravity are commonly used. The design of refractometers is beyond the scope of this discussion but has been described in detail.[21] The basic components of clinical laboratory refractometers consist of a prism, a liquid compensator, and a chamber cover designed to direct a specific wavelength of light (usually 589 nm) onto a calibrated scale.

Measurement of the refractive index of urine is affected by the concentration of all solutes (ionic and nonionic) in urine. In addition to urine solute concentration, temperature affects the density (or specific gravity) of urine. Therefore refractometers are calibrated at a reference temperature. Some refractometers have a built-in compensating mechanism for temperatures between 60°C and 100°C (Leica Vet360[c]). In addition, within the limits of their design, all refractometers permit temperature compensation by the following mechanism. Because the temperature of the small drop of urine required to obtain a measurement with refractometers rapidly equilibrates with temperature of the instrument, a temperature-corrected result may be obtained provided the instrument's temperature is near the reference temperature. Caution should be used to prevent significant alterations in the temperature of the instruments as a result of holding it for prolonged periods, storing it adjacent to heating vents, etc.

There is considerable variability in the quality and cost of refractometers. Ideally, refractometers should be calibrated for the species being studied by using urine samples of known specific gravity. Therefore dog and cat urine require different scales (Figure 9-2). Those designed for physicians are calibrated for human urine.

High quality refractometers typically provide reproducible results. They have an adjustable scale and contain a built-in mechanism for temperature correction (from 60° to 100°C). However, many refractometers acquire an increasing error with increasing amounts of solids.[21]

Summary

In summary, measurements made by osmometers, refractometers, urinometers, and reagent strips are related but not interchangeable. Measurement of urine osmolality provides information that is more closely related to renal concentrating capacity than does specific gravity or refractive index. Osmometers provide a more accurate assessment of osmolality of individual urine samples than refractometers or urinometers.

Urine specific gravity is a direct, but not proportional, function of the number of solute particles in urine. Urine SG varies with the kind of solute present, whereas urine osmolality is independent of the types of solute present. Therefore, urine specific gravity provides only an estimation of osmolality. Indirect measurement of urine specific gravity by refractometry is a very useful screening test of renal function. However, osmolality measured with osmometers should be used for patients with undiagnosed persistent polyuria when errors in assessment of renal function are of significant consequence (i.e., in conjunction with provocative water deprivation and vasopressin response tests). Vapor pressure osmometers are preferable to freezing point osmometers when assessing urine samples with high osmolality.

Evaluation of specific gravity is essential when interpreting test results of the complete urinalysis. Refractometry is entirely satisfactory for routine screening by urinalysis. Refractometers are recommended over urinometers for determination of urine specific gravity because:

- They provide more reproducible results.
- They require a small sample size.
- They are temperature compensated.
- They are technically easy to use.

INTERPRETATION
Terminology

The root word "sthen" is Latin for the English word "*strength*." Hypersthenuria, isosthenuria, and hyposthenuria are terms that depict the solute concentration (or strength) in urine compared with the concentration of solute in glomerular filtrate (Table 1-5). Hypersthenuria (also called baruria) depicts urine of high specific gravity and osmolality compared with glomerular filtrate. Hyposthenuria depicts formation of dilute urine with a specific gravity and osmolality that are significantly lower than those of plasma and glomerular filtrate. Isosthenuria depicts urine with a specific gravity and osmolality similar to those of (or with the same strength as) plasma and glomerular filtrate. Complete loss of ability to concentrate or dilute glomerular filtrate according to body need is sometimes referred to as "fixed" specific gravity.

In context of quantifying urine concentration, terms that are more useful than hypersthenuria are (1) maximum urine concentration, (2) functionally adequate urine concentration, and (3) inappropriate urine concentration (Table 9-2). There is significant species variability in maximum and functionally adequate urine concentrating capacities. Refer to the sections in this chapter entitled "Normal Urine Specific Gravity Values," "Significance of Urine Specific Gravity of 1.025 in Humans, Dogs, and Cats," and "Abnormal Urine Specific Gravity Values" for further explanations.

Osmotic Activity in Extracellular Fluid and Urine

Sodium, chloride, and bicarbonate account for approximately 90% of the osmotic activity of extracellular fluid. Nonelectrolytes such as urea, proteins, and glucose account for the remainder of the osmotic activity. Sodium, chloride, and urea account for the majority of osmotic activity in urine.

There is usually no significant difference between the osmo-

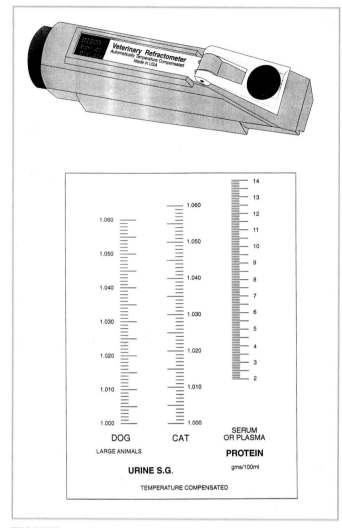

FIGURE 9-2 *Temperature-compensated veterinary refractometer, model 10436. (Misco Products Division, Cleveland, OH.)*

lality (or specific gravity) of uncentrifuged urine and the supernatant of centrifuged urine because cells, casts, etc. do not contribute significantly to osmotic pressure. There is no significant difference between serum and plasma osmolality since fibrinogen does not exert a significant osmotic effect. However, the quantity and type of anticoagulant used to obtain plasma may be of significance. For example, EDTA may contribute 5 to 20 mOsm/kg to plasma osmolality, depending on the amount of blood in a 2 ml Vacutainer[Bd] tube.[19] Heparin is usually utilized as the anticoagulant for plasma osmolality determinations.

Normally the osmotic concentration of urine is variable, being dependent on the fluid and electrolyte balance of the body and the nitrogen content of the diet. Species differences in the ability to concentrate urine are also significant (Table 9-2).

Interpretation of urine osmolality is usually enhanced when the values of serum or plasma osmolality are also available. The osmotic concentration of plasma, serum, interstitial fluid, transcellular fluid, and intracellular fluid is approximately 280 to 310 mOsm/kg of water. The osmotic concentration of glomerular filtrate is about 300 mOsm/kg of water. The ratio of urine osmolality (U_{osm}) to plasma osmolality (U/P_{osm}) is a good clinical index of the ability of the kidneys to concentrate or dilute glomerular filtrate.[4]

- A U/P_{osm} ratio above 1 indicates that the kidneys are concentrating urine above plasma and glomerular filtrate. Following water deprivation the U/P_{osm} of normal dogs may be 7 or higher.[13]
- A U/P_{osm} ratio of approximately 1 indicates that water and solute are being excreted in a state that is isoosmotic with plasma.
- A U/P_{osm} ratio significantly below 1 indicates that the tubules are capable of absorbing solute in excess of water (i.e., they are diluting glomerular filtrate).

Normal Urine Specific Gravity Values (Tables 1-1, 9-2, and 9-3)

Overview

The SG of urine of normal animals is variable, being dependent on the fluid and electrolyte balance of the body, the protein, mineral, and water composition of the diet, and other variables related to species and individuals. Refer to the section on urine volume in Chapter 8 for additional information about these factors. The urine SG typically fluctuates widely from day to day and within the same day.

Urine specific gravity may range from 1.001 to 1.070 or greater in normal adult dogs and from 1.001 to 1080 or greater in normal adult cats. Depending on the requirements of the body for water and/or solutes, any specific gravity value within these ranges may be normal. *Therefore the concept of an average normal specific gravity is misleading because it implies that values above or below the average may not be normal!*

Randomly collected urine samples from normal adult dogs and cats often have a specific gravity that encompasses a narrower range than those just mentioned, but an individual urine sample with a specific gravity outside these values is not reliable evidence of renal dysfunction (Tables 1-1 and 9-3).[2,4,13]

A urine specific gravity that is similar to that of glomerular filtrate (1.008 to 1.012) may be observed in individuals with normal renal function that have no need to concentrate urine. Although values in this range may be normal in hydrated nonazotemic patients, they should be viewed as a presumptive evidence of an abnormality, especially if this pattern is repeated in multiple random samples. Further tests will be required, however, to prove or disprove this presumption.

Urine Concentration

The ability of patients to excrete urine with a specific gravity significantly above that of glomerular filtrate (1008 to 1.012) is dependent on a functional system for production and release of antidiuretic hormone, a sufficient population of functional nephrons to generate and maintain a high solute concentration in the renal medulla, and a sufficient population of functional tubules to respond to antidiuretic hormone. See Chapter 1 for additional information.

Data obtained from partially nephrectomized dogs with remnant kidneys suggest that only about one-third of the nephrons of both kidneys is required to concentrate urine to 1.025 or greater.[15] Results of these studies are the primary basis for the clinical axiom that significant impairment of the canine kidney's ability to concentrate (or dilute) urine is usually not detected until at least two-thirds of the total renal functional parenchyma has been impaired. Although some variation from this value may be expected in canine patients with naturally occurring renal diseases, in general, dogs in which at least one-third of the total nephron population is functional have adequate renal function to prevent polysystemic clinical signs of primary renal failure. Please note that the aforementioned clinical axiom does not apply to cats as they have greater urine concentrating capacity than dogs (Tables 9-2 and 9-3).

Urine Dilution

Since metabolic work is required to dilute glomerular filtrate (SG = 1.008 to 1.012) by removing solute in excess of water, a urine SG significantly below 1.008 indicates that a sufficient number of functional nephrons (commonly estimated to be at least one-third of the total population) are present to

TABLE 9-2

SPECIES VARIATION IN MAXIMUM, FUNCTIONALLY ADEQUATE, QUESTIONABLE, AND INAPPROPRIATE URINE CONCENTRATION OF ADULT ANIMALS AS EVALUATED BY SPECIFIC GRAVITY

Species	Specific Gravity Values			
	Maximum	Functionally Adequate	Questionable[a]	Inappropriate[a]
Canine	1.060–1.065	>1.040	1.030–1.040	≤1.029
Feline	1.080–1.085	>1.045[b]	1.040–1.045	≤1.039
Human	1.035–1.040	>1.025		≤1.025

[a]Specific gravity values in azotemic or dehydrated patients prior to any form of therapy that could affect urine concentrating capacity.
[b]Some cats with primary renal failure can concentrate urine to 1.045 or greater.

TABLE 9-3

OSMOLALITY AND SPECIFIC GRAVITY VALUES FOR ADULT DOG, CAT, AND HUMAN URINE

Factor	Species		
	Dog	Cat	Human
Specific gravity—maximum range	1.001 to ±1.070	1.001 to ±1.085	1.001 to ±1.035+
Osmolality—maximum range (mOsm/kg)	50 to 2800	50 to 3200	50 to 1400
Specific gravity—typical range when normally hydrated	1.015 to 1.050	1.035 to 1.060	1.015 to 1.025
Osmolality—typical range when normally hydrated	450 to 2000	1500 to 2500	450 to 800
Specific gravity—expected value if dehydrated	1.050 to 1.070	1.050 to 1.085	1.025 to 1.040
Osmolality—expected range if dehydrated	1800 to 2800	1600 to 3200+	800 to 1400

Data compiled from references 2, 4, 7, 13, 17, 19, 23, 24.

dilute urine and therefore to prevent clinical signs associated with primary renal failure. Dilution of urine is an appropriate and expected compensatory response to overhydration. However, formation of dilute urine when the patient is in negative water balance is abnormal.

Although the minimum number of nephrons required to dilute canine or feline urine to a specific gravity of 1.005 or lower has apparently not been determined, it has been assumed to be similar to that required for urine concentration (i.e., about one-third of the total nephron population). However, normal dilution ability apparently can be maintained with fewer functional nephrons than normal concentration ability.[20]

Immature Dogs and Cats

Appropriate caution must be used when interpreting the significance of urine specific gravity and osmolality values in immature animals since they apparently have different average and minimum and maximum values than those of mature animals. The kidneys of newborn human infants can concentrate urine only to a maximum of 700 to 800 mOsm/kg at the time of birth but can dilute urine to values as low as 40 mOsm/kg.[8,10,12] Maximum and minimum specific gravity values for infant and immature dogs and cats have apparently not been evaluated. Likewise, the time of maturation of various renal functions in immature dogs and cats is unknown. In one study of kittens consuming a maintenance dry cat food, urine osmolality ranged from 618 to 2680 ($\bar{x}$ = 1424) in those 4 to 6 weeks old, 1214 to 3474 ($\bar{x}$ = 2432) in those 7 to 12 weeks old, 1408 to 3814 ($\bar{x}$ = 2797) in those 13 to 19 weeks old, and 918 to 3384 ($\bar{x}$ = 2383) in those 20 to 24 weeks old.[6,16] In one study measurement of urine specific gravity values of canine fetuses prior to birth revealed values that ranged from 1.008 to –1.025.[22] Randomly collected urine samples from dogs that were 2 days old had an osmolality approximately twice that of plasma, but the ratio was

approximately seven times that of plasma when the pups were 77 days old. These observations suggest that kidneys of newborn puppies can concentrate urine to some degree, and that concentration capacity improves with age.

Studies of human infants suggest that refractometry may be less reliable for measurement of urine concentrating capacity compared to measurement of osmolality.[3] This observation raises questions about the reliability of refractometer measurements of urine specific gravity in animal infants.

Significance of Urine SG Values of 1.025 in Humans, Dogs, and Cats

The ability of dogs to concentrate urine to a specific gravity of 1.025 was at one time generally accepted as evidence of "adequate" renal concentrating capacity (i.e., at least one-third of the total nephron population functional) to maintain homeostasis. The urine specific gravity end point of 1.025 was extrapolated from human data. Since humans can concentrate their urine to a maximum of 1.035 to 1.040 whereas values for dogs may reach 1.060 or more and values for cats may reach 1.080 or more, concentration of urine to 1.025 implies better renal tubular function in humans than in cats or dogs. A significant degree of impaired urine concentrating capacity exists in dehydrated or azotemic dogs unable to concentrate their urine to a specific gravity more than 1.025. In one study the maximal urine specific gravities of three partially nephrectomized dogs (two-thirds of total nephrons removed) subjected to 48 hours of water deprivation were 1.023, 1.018, and 1.027.[15]

Clinical observations in dogs indicate that detection of a urine specific gravity of 1.040 indicates a functionally adequate population of nephrons to prevent clinical signs associated with primary renal failure (Table 9-2). Likewise, urine specific gravity values between 1.030 and 1.040 in normally hydrated nonazotemic dogs are considered indicative of adequate renal function. However, urine specific gravity values between 1.030 and 1.040 in dehydrated or azotemic dogs should raise suspicion of some impairment of urine concentrating capacity and warrant further investigation.

Although we commonly have used a specific gravity value of 1.035 to 1.040 to indicate adequate urine concentrating capacity for cats, further studies are required to determine the urine SG value that best indicates an adequate population of functional nephrons to prevent clinical signs associated with primary renal failure. Studies of partially nephrectomized cats with remnant kidneys have revealed that animals with less than 25% functional nephrons could concentrate their urine significantly higher than SG = 1.040.[1,18,23] Pending results of further studies, urine specific gravity values of 1.035 to 1.040 in dehydrated or azotemic cats should be viewed as questionable in terms of urine concentrating capacity and indicate the need for further evaluation. Values of 1.045 or higher usually suggest adequate urine concentrating capacity to prevent intrarenal azotemia.

Abnormal Urine Specific Gravity Values
Impaired Urine Concentration

Interpretation of urine SG values of randomly obtained samples is dependent on knowledge of the patient's hydration status, diet history, the plasma or serum concentration of urea nitrogen or creatinine, and knowledge of drugs or fluids that have been administered to the patient. Knowledge of urine volume and water consumption may also be helpful. In some instances, interpretation may require knowledge of serially performed evaluation of urine specific gravity on multiple samples. In others, evaluation of urine and plasma osmolality is needed.

If sufficient clinical evidence is present to warrant examination of the patient's renal function by determining the serum concentration of creatinine or blood urea nitrogen, the urine specific gravity (or osmolality) should be evaluated a the same time. Why? Because an adequately concentrated urine sample associated with an abnormal elevation in serum creatinine or urea nitrogen concentration suggests the probability of *prerenal azotemia* whereas *intrarenal azotemia* is probable in patients with elevated serum urea nitrogen and creatinine concentrations and less concentrated urine (Tables 1-2, 2-1, and 9-1).

Varying degrees of impaired ability to concentrate or dilute glomerular filtrate are a consistent finding in all forms of primary renal failure but not all forms of renal disease. Because the kidneys have substantial functional reserve capacity, impairment of their ability to concentrate or dilute urine may not be detected until at least two-thirds (dogs) or more (cats) of the total population of nephrons has been damaged.

Complete inability of the nephrons to modify glomerular filtrate typically results in formation of urine with a specific gravity

that is similar to that of glomerular filtrate (1.008 to 1.012). This phenomenon has been commonly called "fixation of specific gravity." Once the ability to concentrate or dilute urine has been permanently destroyed, repeated evaluation of specific gravity will not be of aid in evaluation of progressive deterioration of renal function. Therefore serial evaluation of urine specific gravity is of greatest aid in detecting functional changes earlier during the course of progressive primary renal failure or in monitoring functional recovery associated with reversible renal diseases.

Total loss of the ability to concentrate and dilute urine (SG = 1.008 to 1.012) often does not occur as a sudden event but may develop gradually. For this reason urine specific gravity values between approximately 1.007 to 1.029 in dogs and 1.007 to 1.039 in cats associated with azotemia are highly suggestive of primary renal failure, although on occasion hypoadrenocorticism may induce similar findings (Tables 1-2, 2-1, and 9-1). Likewise, urine specific gravity values between approximately 1.007 to 1.029 in dogs and 1.007 to 1.039 in cats that are clinically dehydrated but not azotemic are highly suggestive of primary renal failure or other disorders that impair urine concentrating capacity.

If nonazotemic patients have impaired ability to concentrate urine, causes of pathologic polyuria should be investigated. Determination of urine specific gravity or osmolality may allow one to determine whether a polyuric disorder characterized by water (1.001 ± 1.006) or solute (±1.008 or greater) diuresis is probable. Consult the section on urine volume in Chapter 8 for additional information related to physiologic and pathologic polyuria and physiologic and pathologic oliguria.

If a *nondehydrated, nonazotemic* patient suspected of having pathologic polyuria does not have a urine specific gravity that indicates that the kidneys can definitely concentrate urine, further "provocative" tests are required before conclusions are established about the kidneys' capacity to concentrate urine. By depriving the nonazotemic, nondehydrated patient of water consumption for an appropriate period of time, antidiuretic hormone will normally be released from the posterior pituitary gland as a compensatory response to hydropenia.[9,11,13,14] Antidiuretic hormone enhances fluid reabsorption from the distal tubules and collecting ducts by increasing tubular epithelial cell permeability to water.

Clinical experience has revealed that the results of water deprivation tests are often difficult to reproduce. Boundary values have been established above which renal function is assumed to be adequate and below which it is assumed to be impaired. A zone of doubt exists in between. Uncontrolled clinical observations indicate that dogs with "adequate" renal function will excrete urine with a high specific gravity (1.030), high osmolality, and relatively small volume (physiologic oliguria). Studies of dogs with completely normal renal func-

> In cats, further studies are required to determine the urine SG value that best indicates an adequate population of functional nephrons to prevent clinical signs associated with primary renal failure.

tion were interpreted to indicate that 95% of normal dogs subjected to water deprivation sufficient to produce a slight degree of dehydration should have a urine specific gravity of at least 1.048, a urine osmolality of at least 1,787 mOsm/kg, and a U/P_{osm} ratio of at least 5.7 to 1.[13,14] If such values are not obtained, nephron dysfunction may exist. The degree of dysfunction, however, may not be severe enough to be associated with clinical signs. Patients unable to concentrate urine following appropriately conducted water deprivation tests should be evaluated for diseases that cause medullary solute depletion, central diabetes insipidus, and/or renal diabetes insipidus.

Mechanisms of Polyuria in Primary Renal Failure

When urine specific gravity reflects impaired ability to concentrate (or dilute) urine, it is more an index of nephron function than of distal tubular and collecting duct function. Why? In addition to generalized tubular lesions that impair the function of the countercurrent system, this abnormality may be intensified as a result of factors not specifically related to tubular damage. These factors include:

- Compensatory increase in glomerular filtration (so-called hyperfiltration) that occurs as a result of a decrease in the quantity of functional nephrons. Increased production of glomerular filtrate floods the distal tubules and collecting ducts with solute and water. It is associated with decreased fractional tubular reabsorption of sodium and phosphorus by viable nephrons.
- Decrease in the number of functioning nephrons. The latter is associated with impaired ability of the countercurrent mechanism to maintain the high osmotic gradient normally present in renal medulla.
- Osmotic diuresis in remaining functional nephrons as a result of increased filtration of solutes (azotemia, hyperphosphatemia, etc.) in them secondary to reduced glomerular filtration (Figure 9-3). This accentuates the degree of obligatory polyuria.

Once the ability to concentrate or dilute urine has been permanently destroyed, repeated evaluation of specific gravity will not be of aid in evaluation of progressive deterioration of renal function. Therefore serial evaluation of urine specific gravity is of greatest aid in detecting functional changes earlier in the course of progressive primary renal failure or in monitoring functional recovery associated with reversible renal diseases.

Diseases Associated With Urine Dilution

Formation of dilute urine (SG < 1.007; especially in patients that need to conserve water) may represent an abnormality associated with several diseases including:

- Central or renal diabetes insipidus
- Hyperadrenocorticism
- Hypercalcemia

- Pyometra
- Liver disorders
- Psychogenic water consumption

Urine Specific Gravity Values and Localization of Azotemia
Overview

Although the following generalities apply to dogs and cats, it is emphasized that some azotemic cats with primary renal failure retain comparably greater urine concentrating capacity than dogs. In dogs with progressive disease resulting in primary renal failure, azotemia usually follows loss of the ability to concentrate urine to at least SG of 1.030. In some cats with primary renal failure, azotemia may precede loss of the ability to concentrate urine to values of 1.040 to 1.045.[1,18,23]

Prerenal Azotemia
Causes and Pathogenesis

Extraurinary diseases may cause varying degrees of alteration in glomerular filtration as a result of reduction of renal blood flow. Inadequate perfusion of normal glomeruli with blood, regardless of cause (dehydration, cardiac disease, shock, hypoadrenocorticism, decreased plasma colloidal osmotic pressure), may cause prerenal azotemia (Tables 1-2, 2-1, and 9-1).

Prerenal azotemia is initially associated with structurally normal kidneys that are capable of quantitatively normal renal function, provided compromised renal perfusion is corrected prior to the onset of ischemic nephron damage. Progression of prerenal azotemia to intrarenal (primary) renal failure due to persistent ischemia prolongs and reduces the likelihood of complete recovery.

A diagnosis of prerenal azotemia should be considered if

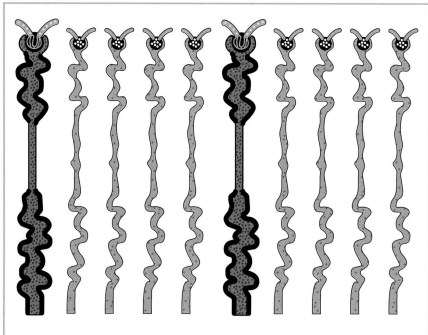

FIGURE 9-3 *Schematic illustration of mechanism of solute-enhanced polyuria in patients with azotemic renal failure. Because of elevated concentrations of urea, creatinine, phosphorus, and other solutes in plasma, the quantity of these solutes in glomerular filtrate are higher than normal. As a result, they exceed the absorptive capacity of remaining functional nephrons and induce solute diuresis.*

abnormal elevation in the serum or plasma concentration of urea nitrogen and creatinine is associated with adequately concentrated urine (specific gravity 1.035 in dogs; specific gravity 1.040 in cats) in patients with no specific evidence of generalized glomerular disease. Detection of adequately concentrated urine in association with azotemia indicates that a sufficient quantity of functional nephrons are present to prevent primary renal azotemia. Significant elevations in the serum or plasma concentration of urea nitrogen or creatinine due to primary renal failure cannot be detected in dogs until approximately 70% to 75% of the nephron population is nonfunctional. Elevation in urine specific gravity associated with prerenal azotemia probably reflects a compensatory response by the body to combat low perfusion pressure and blood volume by secreting antidiuretic hormone (and possibly other substances) to conserve water filtered through glomeruli. Restoration of renal perfusion by appropriate volume replacement therapy is typically followed by a dramatic drop in the concentration of serum urea and creatinine to normal in approximately 1 to 3 days.

Another form of potentially reversible prerenal azotemia associated with primary renal disease may develop in patients with glomerulonephropathy and severe hypoalbuminemia. At the level of the glomerulus, hypoalbuminemia enhances glomerular filtration rate due to a reduction in colloidal osmotic pressure. However, decreased renal blood flow and glomerular filtration that occur in association with marked reduction in vascular volume secondary to a reduction in colloidal osmotic pressure result in a proportionate degree of retention of substances normally cleared by the kidneys (creatinine, urea, etc.). These two mechanisms have opposite effects on glomerular filtration. Therefore the significance of an abnormal increase in the serum concentration of urea nitrogen or creatinine (or a reduction in creatinine clearance) must be carefully interpreted in hypoproteinemic nephrotic patients. Azotemia cannot be accepted as indisputable evidence of severe primary glomerular lesions since a component of the azotemia may be associated with a potentially reversible decrease in renal perfusion caused by hypoalbuminemia.

Diagnosis

Diagnosis of prerenal azotemia is based on the following (Table 9-1):

- Elevation of serum urea nitrogen or creatinine concentration
- Oliguria
- High specific gravity (1.035 in dogs; 1.040 in cats) or osmolality
- Detection of underlying cause
- Rapid correction of azotemia following administration of appropriate therapy to restore renal perfusion

Prognosis

The prognosis of prerenal azotemia is dependent on reversibility of the primary cause. The prognosis is favorable for renal function if perfusion is rapidly restored. However, *complete* loss of renal perfusion in excess of 2 to 4 hours may result in general-

ized ischemic renal disease. With the exception of shock, this degree of reduced renal perfusion is uncommon. Thus the onset of generalized renal disease would be expected to require a longer period of altered renal perfusion.

Postrenal Azotemia
Pathogenesis

Diseases that prevent excretion of urine from the body may cause postrenal azotemia. The kidneys are structurally normal initially and capable of quantitatively normal function provided the underlying cause is corrected. However, if the underlying cause is allowed to persist, death from alterations in water, electrolyte and acid-base, and endocrine balance, in addition to accumulation of metabolic waste products, will occur within a few days. If there is only partial obstruction of urine outflow, allowing the patient to survive for a longer time, varying degrees of hydronephrosis may subsequently occur.

Causes

Complete obstruction of urine outflow (i.e., obstruction in urethra, bladder, or both ureters) that persists for more than 24 hours usually results in postrenal azotemia. Unilateral ureteral occlusion (an example of renal disease) is not associated with azotemia unless generalized disease of the nonobstructed kidney is also present. Azotemia that occurs as a sequela to rupture of the excretory pathway (most commonly the bladder) is primarily related to absorption of urine from the peritoneal cavity. Unless damaged as a result of hypovolemic shock or trauma secondary to the underlying cause of rupture of the excretory pathway, the kidneys are structurally and functionally normal.

Diagnosis

A diagnosis of postrenal azotemia is based on the integration of clinical findings. Lesions causing urine outflow obstruction are commonly associated with:

- Elevation in serum urea nitrogen and creatinine concentration
- Oliguria or anuria, dysuria, and tenesmus
- Detection of obstructive lesion(s) by physical examination (urethral plug, herniated bladder, etc.), radiography, ultrasonography, etc
- Variable urine specific gravity values

Rupture of the excretory pathway is commonly associated with:

- Progressive elevation in serum urea nitrogen or creatinine concentration
- Progressive depression; painful abdomen; ascites
- A history of trauma and associated physical examination findings
- Inability to palpate the urinary bladder
- Detection of a modified transudate or exudate by abdominocentesis
- Abnormalities detected by ultrasonography or retrograde contrast (positive or negative) cystography or urethrocystography

> Complete obstruction of urine outflow that persists for more than 24 hours usually results in postrenal azotemia.

Because of variability, the urine specific gravity of patients with postrenal azotemia is not relied on to the same degree for assessment of renal function as it is in patients with primary renal and prerenal azotemia.

Prognosis Associated With Obstructive Lesions

If the patient has total obstruction to urine outflow for a period of 3 to 6 days, death from uremia will occur. Death usually occurs before significant hydronephrosis has time to develop. Death is caused by alteration of fluid, acid-base, electrolyte, nutrient, and endocrine balance, as well as accumulation of metabolic waste products.

The prognosis is favorable for renal function if the obstructive lesion(s) is rapidly removed. The long-term prognosis is dependent on the reversibility of the underlying cause.

Prognosis Associated With
Rupture of the Excretory Pathway

If a persistent rent in the excretory pathway is of sufficient magnitude to result in progressive azotemia, it is likely that the patient will die if it is not repaired. The prognosis for recovery of adequate renal function is favorable if the rent is repaired or heals. The long-term prognosis is dependent on the reversibility of the underlying cause.

Primary Intrarenal Azotemia
Pathogenesis

Intrarenal azotemic renal failure may be caused by a large number of disease processes (glomerular, tubular, interstitial, and/or vascular) that have in common destruction of approximately three-fourths or more of the parenchyma of both kidneys. Depending on the biologic behavior of the disease in question, primary renal failure associated with intrarenal azotemia may be reversible or irreversible, acute or chronic. Chronic irreversible azotemic renal failure is usually slowly progressive.

Diagnosis

In dogs impairment of at least two-thirds of the nephron mass is indicated if a dehydrated patient (that has not received fluid, diuretic, or glucocorticoid therapy) has impaired ability to concentrate urine. Total loss of ability to concentrate and dilute urine does not always occur as a sudden event but often develops gradually. For this reason a urine specific gravity between approximately 1.007 to 1.029 for dogs or 1.007 to 1.039 for cats associated with clinical dehydration or azotemia is indicative of intrarenal azotemia (Tables 1-2 and 9-1). Total inability of the nephrons to concentrate or dilute urine (so-called fixation of specific gravity or isosthenuria) results in the formation of urine that is similar to that of glomerular filtrate (approximately 1.008 to 1.012).

If a hydrated patient has an elevation in

> **If a hydrated patient has an elevation in the serum or plasma concentration of urea nitrogen and creatinine and impaired ability to concentrate or dilute urine, it is likely that impairment of at least three-fourths of the functional capacity of the nephron mass has occurred.**

TABLE 9-4

CHECKLIST OF CLINICAL FINDINGS THAT SUGGEST THAT PRERENAL AZOTEMIA EXISTS IN PATIENTS WITH INTRARENAL AZOTEMIA

- Clinical dehydration
- Laboratory evidence of hemoconcentration
  - Elevated packed cell volume
  - Elevated serum concentration of proteins
- Decreased capillary refill time
- Rapid and weak pulse
- Signs of cardiovascular dysfunction
- Rapid reduction in the magnitude of azotemia in response to correction of prerenal component of azotemia

the serum or plasma concentration of urea nitrogen and creatinine and impaired ability to concentrate or dilute urine, it is likely that impairment of at least three-fourths of the functional capacity of the nephron mass has occurred.

More definitive studies (ultrasonography, radiography, biopsy, exploratory surgery, etc.) are required to establish the underlying cause of primary azotemic renal failure. When formulating a prognosis and therapy, recall that the uremic signs are not directly caused by renal lesions but rather are related to varying degrees of fluid, acid-base, electrolyte, and nutrient imbalances, vitamin and endocrine alterations, and retention of waste products of protein catabolism that develop as a result of nephron dysfunction caused by an underlying disease. See Appendix 2 for additional information.

Azotemia Associated With
Glomerulotubular Imbalance

In some patients with primary renal failure caused by generalized glomerular disease, abnormal elevation in the serum concentration of urea nitrogen or creatinine may occur in association with varying degrees of urine concentration (Tables 9-1 and 9-4). Caution should be used not to overinterpret the absolute value of the urine specific gravity in such patients, since it may be slightly elevated by the effect of protein. Addition of 40 mg of protein per 100 ml of urine will increase the urine specific gravity by approximately 0.001.

The renal lesion in such patients must be characterized by glomerular damage that is sufficiently severe to impair renal clearance of urea and creatinine but that has not yet induced a sufficient degree of ischemic atrophy and necrosis or renal tubular cells to prevent varying degrees of urine concentration. Thus glomerular filtrate that is formed may be concentrated to such degree that prerenal azotemia is initially considered. However, this group of patients may be differentiated from patients with prerenal azotemia by failure of a search for one of the extrarenal causes of poor perfusion, by persistent proteinuria, and by persistent azotemia despite restoration of vascular volume and perfusion with appropriate therapy (Table 9-1).

Combinations of Primary Intrarenal Azotemia, Prerenal Azotemia, and Postrenal Azotemia

Pathogenesis

Severely diseased kidneys have impaired ability to compensate for stresses imposed by disease states, dietary indiscretion, and change in environment. In patients with previously compensated primary renal disease, uremic crises are commonly precipitated or complicated by a variety of concomitant extrarenal factors (Table 9-4).

Extrarenal mechanisms that may be associated with uremic crises include the following:

- Factors (anorexia, infection, extensive tissue necrosis, administration of catabolic drugs) that accelerate endogenous protein catabolism increase the quantity of metabolic by-products in the body since the kidneys are incapable of excreting them. Protein by-products contribute significantly to the production of uremic signs in patients with renal failure.
- Stress states (fever, infection, change of environment) are associated with release of glucocorticoids from the adrenal glands. Glucocorticoids stimulate conversion of proteins to carbohydrates (gluconeogenesis) and thus increase the quantity of protein waste products in the body.
- Abnormalities that decrease renal perfusion (i.e., decreased water consumption, vomiting, diarrhea, shock, cardiac decompensation) cause prerenal uremia.
- Administration of nephrotoxic drugs to a patient with chronic renal failure may precipitate an acute uremic crisis by damaging nephrons.

Diagnosis

Combinations of causes of azotemia should be considered on the basis of:

- A previous history of compensated primary renal failure.
- Detection of primary extrarenal disease processes in addition to generalized renal disease.
- Detection of clinical dehydration. Dehydration associated with azotemia and impaired urine concentration is reliable evidence that a portion of the azotemia is prerenal in origin.
- How the patient responds to therapy. Patients with uremic crises precipitated by reversible extrarenal disorders (pancreatitis, hepatic disease, gastroenteritis, etc.) may rapidly respond to supportive and symptomatic therapy, as evidenced by a rapid and significant reduction in the magnitude of azotemia. The therapeutic response of patients with uremic crises caused by progressive irreversible destruction of nephrons is usually slower, as evidenced by only a marginal reduction in the magnitude of azotemia.

Prognosis

Prognosis related to the severity of altered glomerular filtration rate should be withheld until the magnitude of azotemia is reassessed after correction of the prerenal or postrenal components of azotemia.

[a]Bayer Corporation, Elkhart, IN.
[b]Boehringer Mannheim Corporation, Indianapolis, IN.
[c]Leica Microsystems Inc., Buffalo, NY.
[d]Becton Dickinson and Company, Franklin Lakes, NJ.

REFERENCES AND SUGGESTED READINGS

1. Adams LG, Polzin DJ, Osborne CA, O'Brien TD: Effects of dietary protein restriction in clinically normal cats and cats with surgically induced chronic renal failure. *Am J Vet Res* 54:1643–1662, 1993.
2. Barlough JE, Osborne CA, Stevens JB: Canine and feline urinalysis; Value of macroscopic and microscopic examination. *JAVMA* 178:61–63, 1981.
3. Benitz OA, Benitz M, Stijen T, et al: Inaccuracy in neonatal measurement of urine concentration with a refractometer. *Clinical and Laboratory Observations* 108:613–616, 1986.
4. Bovee KC: Urine osmolality as a definitive indicator of renal concentrating ability. *JAVMA* 155:30–35, 1969.
5. Cialla AP, Newsome B, Kaster J: Reagent strip method for specific gravity. An evaluation. *Lab Med* 16:38–40, 1985.
6. Crawford MA: The urinary system, in Hoskins JD (ed): *Veterinary Pediatrics*. Philadelphia, WB Saunders, pp 271–292, 1990.
7. DiBartola SP, Chew DJ, Jacobs G: Quantitative urinalysis including 24-hour protein excretion in the dog. *JAAHA* 16:537–546, 1980.
8. Edelmann CM Jr, Barnett HL, Troupkov V: Renal concentrating mechanism in newborn infants. Effects of dietary protein and water content, role of urea, and responsiveness to antidiuretic hormone. *J Clin Invest* 39:1062–1069, 1960.
9. Feldman EC, Nelson RW: *Canine and Feline Endocrinology and Reproduction*. Philadelphia, WB Saunders, 1987.
10. Fettman MJ, Allen TA: Developmental aspects of fluid and electrolyte metabolism and renal function in neonates. *Compend Contin Educ Pract Vet* 13:392, 1991.
11. Finco DR: Kidney function, in Kaneko JJ (ed): *Clinical Biochemistry of Domestic Animals,* ed 4. New York, Academic Press, 1989, pp 496–542.
12. Guignard P: Renal function in the newborn infant. *Ped Clin North Am* 29:777–790, 1982.
13. Hardy RM, Osborne CA: Water deprivation test in the dog: Maximal normal values. *JAVMA* 174:479–484, 1979.
14. Hardy RM, Osborne CA; Water deprivation and vasopressin concentration tests in the differentiation of polyuric syndromes, in Kirk RW (ed): *Current Veterinary Therapy VII*. Philadelphia, WB Saunders, p 1080, 1980.
15. Hayman JM, Shumway NP, Dunke P, et al: Experimental hyposthenuria. *J Clin Invest* 18:195–211, 1939.
16. Hoskins JD, Turnwald GH, Kearney MT, et al: Quantitative urinalysis in kittens from four to thirty weeks after birth. *Am J Vet Res* 52:1295–1299, 1991.
17. Lees GE, Osborne CA, Stevens JB: Antibacterial properties of urine: Studies of feline urine specific gravity, osmolality, and pH. *JAAHA* 15:135–141, 1979.
18. Lulich JP, Osborne CA, O'Brien TD, Polzin DJ: Feline renal failure: Questions, answers, questions. *Compend Contin Educ Pract Vet* 14:127–152,1992.
19. Osborne CA, Stevens JB: *Handbook of Canine and Feline Urinalysis*. St. Louis, Ralston Purina Co., 1981.
20. Papper S: *Clinical Nephrology*, ed 2. Boston, Little, Brown and Co, 1980.
21. Pradella M, Dorizzi RM, Rigolin F: Relative density of urine: Methods and clinical significance. *CRC Crit Rev Clin Lab Sci* 26:195–242, 1988.
22. Rahill WH, Subramanian S: Use of fetal animals to investigate renal development. *Lab Anim* 23:92–96, 1973.
23. Ross LA, Finco DR: Relationship of selected renal function tests to glomerular filtration rate and renal blood flow in cats. *Am J Vet Res* 42:1704–1710, 1981.
24. Thrall BE, Miller LG: Water turnover in cats fed dry rations. *Feline Pract* 6:10–17, 1976.

Chapter 10

As doctors, let us provide the type of compassionate care for our patients as we would have our doctors provide compassionate care to us.

C.A.O.

Biochemical Analysis of Urine: Indications, Methods, Interpretation

SECTION 1: URINE pH

I. **Indications**
A. Diagnostic
B. Therapeutic

II. **Methodology**
A. pH Meters
B. Reagent Strips
C. Confirmatory Testing

III. **Interpretation**
A. Normal
B. Abnormal (Inappropriate)
C. Renal Tubular Acidosis
D. Artifacts

SECTION 2: GLUCOSE

I. **Indications**
A. Diagnostic
B. Therapeutic

II. **Methodology**
A. Historical Tests
B. Colorimetric Tests Based on Glucose Oxidase Activity
1. Clinistix®
2. Petstix™, Diastix®, and Multistix®
3. Chemstrip® 2GP, 4OB, 6, 7, 8, 9, and 10 with SG
4. Chemstrip® uG and uGK
C. Colorimetric Tests Based on Copper Reduction
1. Clinitest®
D. Confirmatory Testing

III. **Interpretation**
A. Specificity of Methods

1. Glucose Oxidase
a. Glucose Specific Test
b. False-Positive Reactions
c. False-Negative Reactions
2. Copper Reduction
B. Sensitivity of Methods
1. Ascorbic Acid versus Sensitivity
C. Physiologic Glucosuria
D. Pharmacologic Glucosuria
E. Pathologic Glucosuria
F. Consequences of Glucosuria

SECTION 3: KETONES

I. **Indications**

II. **Methodology**
A. Nitroprusside Tests
B. Confirmatory Testing

III. **Interpretation**
A. Specificity
B. Sensitivity
C. Applied Physiology
D. Significance of Ketonuria

SECTION 4: BILIRUBIN

I. **Indications**

II. **Methodology**
A. Ictotest®
B. Petstix™ and Multistix®
C. Chemstrip®
D. Confirmatory Testing

III. **Interpretation**
A. General

B. Specificity
1. Ictotest®
2. Multistix® and Petstix™
3. Chemstrip®
C. Sensitivity
1. Ictotest®
2. Petstix™ and Multistix®
D. Applied Physiology
E. Significance
1. In Dogs
2. In Cats

SECTION 5: OCCULT BLOOD, HEMOGLOBIN, AND MYOGLOBIN

I. Indications

II. Methodology
A. Overview
B. Hematest®
C. Petstix™, Hemastix®, and Multistix®
D. Chemstrip® 4OB, 6, 7, 8, 9, and 10 with SG

III. Interpretation
A. Specificity
1. False-Positive Reactions
2. False-Negative Reactions
B. Sensitivity
C. Applied Physiology
1. Red Blood Cells
2. Hemoglobin
3. Myoglobin

V. Significance
A. Interpretations and Misinterpretations
B. Hematuria
C. Hemoglobinuria
D. Myoglobinuria

SECTION 6: PROTEINURIA

I. Indications
A. Overview
B. Definitions

II. Methodology
A. Generalities
B. Sample Collection
C. Sulfosalicylic Acid Turbidimetric Test
D. Dipstick Colorimetric Test
E. Bence Jones Proteinuria
F. Twenty-Four Hour Urine Protein Determination
G. Urine Protein-Creatinine Ratios

III. Interpretation
A. Overview
B. Specificity of Tests
1. Sulfosalicylic Acid Turbidimetric Test
2. Dipstick Colorimetric Test
C. Sensitivity of Tests
D. Applied Physiology
1. Renal Handling of Protein
2. Tubular Reabsorption and Disposal of Absorbed Protein
3. Proteins Originating from the Urinary Tract
4. Normal Urine Protein Concentration
E. Abnormal Urine Protein Concentration
1. Preglomerular Proteinuria
2. Glomerular Proteinuria
3. Postglomerular Proteinuria
4. Pseudoproteinuria (False-Positive Proteinuria)
5. False-Negative Proteinuria

SECTION 7: UROBILINOGEN

I. Indications

II. Methodology
A. Multistix® SG, 9, 10 SG, N-Multistix®, N-Multistix® SG
B. Chemstrip® 8, 9, 10 SG
C. Confirmatory Testing

III. Interpretation
A. Specificity
1. Multistix®
2. Chemstrip®
B. Sensitivity
1. Multistix®
2. Chemstrip®
C. Applied Physiology

SECTION 8: NITRITURIA

SECTION 9: LEUKOCYTES

I. Indications

II. Methodology

III. Interpretation

SECTION 10: URINE SPECIFIC GRAVITY

I. Indications

II. Methodology

III. Interpretation

Section 1: Urine pH

INDICATIONS
Diagnostic

Urine pH may be used as a crude index of body acid-base balance. The body generally produces an excess of acid metabolites. The lungs regulate acid-base balance by retention or elimination of carbon dioxide (and therefore carbonic acid), while the kidneys regulate acid-base balance primarily via recovery of bicarbonate from the ultrafiltrate and/or the excretion of protons (H^+) in the form of ammonium ions and phosphate ions. In dogs and cats the principal buffer is phosphate, whereas in herbivores it is ammonium.

There may be significant diurnal variation in urine pH. Type of diet and type of disease may also induce considerable variation in urine pH. As was the situation with urine specific gravity, differentiation between normal and abnormal (or inappropriate) urine pH values is not possible without additional information. Both may fall within the same range.

Knowledge of urine pH may aid in determination of the type of uroliths present prior to mineral analysis. Calcium phosphate (apatite) and magnesium ammonium phosphate (struvite) uroliths tend to form in alkaline urine. Cystine and uric acid uroliths tend to form in acid urine. Ammonium urate crystals may be flocculated by hydrogen ion (acid pH) or ammonium ion (alkaline pH). The solubility of calcium oxalate and silica uroliths in urine is apparently not significantly influenced by urine pH per se.

Urinary tract infections caused by urease-producing bacteria (primarily staphylococci and *Proteus* spp.) frequently cause urine to become alkaline. Urinary tract infections are commonly associated with acid urine since most bacterial pathogens do not produce urease.

Knowledge of urine pH trends is of value for a number of reasons:

- It may suggest that certain animals are predisposed to urinary tract infections with urease-producing bacteria.
- It may help in the interpretation of other urine tests. For example, very alkaline urine may result in a positive dipstick test for protein.
- It may be important in interpretation of findings in urine sediment. Red blood cells, white cells, casts, and other proteinaceous structures tend to disintegrate in alkaline urine.
- It may suggest that negative tests for leptospirosis organisms are false because these organisms may not survive in acid urine.

Therapeutic

Urine pH is commonly manipulated to aid in the dissolution or prevention of certain uroliths. Calcium phosphate and magnesium ammonium phosphate crystals are more soluble in acid urine, whereas cystine and uric acid crystals are more soluble in alkaline urine. Ammonium urate crystals are least likely to precipitate in urine without a neutral pH.

Because acid urine may inhibit bacterial growth, urinary acidifiers are sometimes used as ancillary treatment of urinary tract infections (dog and cat) or preventatives (swine). In addition, the therapeutic efficacy of some antimicrobial agents may be enhanced by alteration of urine pH. The solubility of some antimicrobial agents may also be pH dependent. In the past therapeutic manipulation of pH has been recommended for management of myoglobinuria.

METHODOLOGY
pH Meters

Although pH meters provide excellent results, they have not been commonly used for routine urinalysis because of their expense and because of the technical ease provided by reagent strips.

Relatively inexpensive "pocket" pH meters are widely available and are recommended for evaluation of patients with urolithiasis.

Laboratory pH meters are commonly used in conjunction with determination of titratable acidity. Procedures for measurement of titratable acidity include concurrent determination of bicarbonate and ammonium ion concentration.

Hydrogen ions may be excreted in urine in a form (such as HPO_4 or NaH_2PO_4) not detectable by simple pH measurements but detectable by a method called titratable acidity. Urinary excretion of monobasic phosphate results in elimination of hydrogen ions and reabsorption of sodium and bicarbonate. Titration of urine formed during 24 hours with a standard base (or acid) to a pH of 7.4 allows quantitation of the quantity of hydrogen ions excreted in this form. This method is called titratable acidity. Hydrogen ions combined with other salts are not measured. Conceptually, titratable acidity is measured by titrating a representative aliquot of a 24 hour urine sample with a 0.1 N sodium hydroxide or hydrochloric acid to a pH of 7.4 as indicated by a pH meter.

Titratable acidity is usually reported as the number of milliliters of 0.1 "N" NaOH or HCl required to neutralize a 24 hour specimen. It is reported as a negative or positive value depending on the quantity of HCl(−) or NaOH(+) needed to adjust the pH of urine to 7.4. A negative result indicates conservation of hydrogen ion, while a positive result indicates excretion of excess acid.

Titratable acidity is primarily influenced by filtered phosphate, bicarbonate, and ammonia. It can also be affected by diet. Diets rich in sulfur-containing amino acids (methionine and cystine) lead to the production of acid urine, because oxidation of neutral sulfate results in the generation of hydrogen ion and sulfate ion. Diets high in vegetables and fruits usually contain an excess of free anions (such as lactate, citrate, malate, etc.), which fix the hydrogen ion when they are catabolized to carbon dioxide and water; thus they tend to alkalinize urine.

Proteinuria will cause a varying degree of interference with titratable acidity because of the buffering capacity of proteins. Increased production of beta-hydroxybutyric acid and acetoacetic acid in ketotic

> Diet and disease may induce considerable variation in urine pH.

Unless otherwise listed, manufacturer information for all products can be found in Table 10-1 (pp. 90–91).

states may also result in positive values for titratable acidity. The pK of beta-hydroxy-butyric acid is 4.4. Therefore at lower limits of urine acidification a small amount of the beta-hydroxybutyric acid is excreted in dissociated form. The pK of acetoacetic acid is even lower, accounting for the fact that only a small amount will be excreted as free acid.

> Petstix™ 8 is a new urinalysis strip designed for veterinary use.

Reagent Strips

Urine pH can readily be determined by any one of a number of commercially available test strips impregnated with indicator dyes. The most reliable results are obtained by evaluation of fresh specimens.

Litmus paper is too insensitive for diagnostic use. Nitrazine paper is capable of detecting changes in pH from 4.5 to 7.5. The color ranges from yellow to blue and can be matched to standard colors for estimation of urine pH. However, this range is too narrow for diagnostic use. Wide-range hydrogen paper (pH 5.5 to 9) is satisfactory for routine analyses. It is available as LoBuff® pH Paper.[a]

Diagnostic strips (Petstix™, Multistix®, and Chemstrip®; Table 10-1) that measure pH are very similar in chemical composition. Petstix™, Multistix®, and Chemstrip® contain both methyl red (which turns red in acid urine and yellow in neutral and alkaline urine) and bromthymol blue (which turns green and blue in alkaline urine and yellow in acid urine). The range provided on the strips is from pH 5.0 to 9.0 in 0.5 unit increments. pH can be estimated within 1 pH unit with these strips.

Petstix™ and Multistix® reagent strips are capable of monitoring changes in urine pH from 5 to 8.5 visually and 5 to 9 instrumentally. Care must be taken with Petstix™ and Multistix® to prevent buffer in the adjacent protein test from being transported by urine to the pH test pad, since this phenomenon will result in an acid pH change.

Instrumentally read strips (Multistix®, Clinitek® 200) underestimated pH below 6.5 and overestimated pH above 7.5. At pH 7.5 the error compared to a pH meter was about 1.5 pH units. Dog and rat urine were used in the study.[7]

Petstix™ 8 is a new urinalysis strip designed for veterinary use. This product will be commercially available in 1999. The pH zone was tested at the University of Minnesota and at the University of Guelph in 62 dogs, 8 cats, and 4 horses: 92% of the urines were within 0.5 units of the pH meter values.

Confirmatory Testing

pH meters can be used to confirm results, particularly when pigmenturia obscures or alters test pad color. Extremely dilute urine samples may read at a higher pH than indicated by reagent strips.

INTERPRETATION
Normal

The kidneys are capable of adjusting the pH of urine between 4.5 and approximately 8.5, depending on the acid-base status of the body. Therefore the pH of urine provides a reflection of the metabolic state of the body.

Ingestion of animal protein typically results in production of acid urine. However, commercially manufactured animal protein diets may be modified to produce neutral or alkaline urine pH. The pH of dog and cat urine commonly lies between 5.5 and 7.0.[5] In a study of 517 hospitalized cats at the University of Minnesota, the mean pH was 6.7 (range of 5.0 to 9.0).[4]

Urine pH tends to vary throughout the day, in part because of events associated with eating and digestion. Urine of dogs and cats tends to become less acidic shortly following ingestion of food. This is related to the "alkaline tide" and presumably is due to increased secretion of hydrochloric acid in the stomach.[3]

It is logical to assume that the magnitude of change in urine pH following eating will be dependent on the composition of the diet, the frequency of eating, and the quantity of food consumed. Following several hours of sleep, the pH of human urine tends to be more acid, presumably a reflection of respiratory acidosis associated with decreased ventilation during sleep.

Abnormal (Inappropriate)

Abnormal or inappropriate urine pH values are similar to normal values. Meaningful interpretation may require knowledge of blood pH and TCO_2, plasma bicarbonate concentration, and response to controlled administration of acidifying or alkalinizing substances. The infrequency with which urine pH values below 5.5 and above 7.5 occur in dogs should arouse suspicion of an abnormality when they are observed (see Table 10-2).

Renal Tubular Acidosis

Renal tubular acidosis (RTA) may be more appropriately defined as an inability to acidify urine in response to body needs. The urine pH may be 6.5 or higher.

A relatively alkaline urine in an acidotic animal may suggest either proximal or distal RTA. Urine excretion of ammonium is inappropriately low in all forms of distal RTA in humans and presumably in dogs but high in other forms of metabolic acidosis, including proximal RTA (i.e., ammonium ion is not produced and excreted in distal RTA).

The urine anion gap is defined as the sum of sodium concentration and potassium concentration minus chloride concentration and is reported as negative or positive. If the positive ammonium ion is present in significant amounts, the sum of the positive ions will be greater than chloride ion, yielding a positive urine anion gap. Based on one study, a large negative urine anion gap (more chloride) was a reliable index of urine NH_4^+ excretion in dogs with metabolic acidosis other than distal RTA.[7] The urine anion gap is positive in most situations that result in hyperchloremic metabolic acidosis but is negative in distal RTA.

Large amounts of ketone bodies can mask excessive amounts of ammonium in the urine as determined by this method. Therefore determination of ammonium secretion may discriminate between distal RTA and chronic systemic acidosis from other causes.

TABLE 10-1

SUMMARY OF CHEMISTRY TESTS EVALUATED BY REAGENT STRIPS AND TABLETS

Product List	Glucose	Bilirubin	Ketone	Specific Gravity	Blood in Urine
Petstix™[a,b]					
Multistix®[c]					
Multistix® SG[c]					
Multistix® 2[c]					
Multistix® 7[c]					
Multistix® 8SG[c]					
Multistix® 9SG[c]					
Multistix® 9[c]					
Multistix® 10SG[c]					
N-Multistix®[c]					
N-Multistix® SG[c]					
Bili-Labstix®[c]					
Hemacombistix®[c]					
Combistix®[c]					
Uristix®[c]					
Uristix® 4[c]					
Keto-Diastix®[c]					
Labstix®[c]					
Diastix®[c]					
Acetest®[c]			Tablet		
Ictotest®[c]		Tablet			
Clinitest®[c]	Red-Ox				
Hematest®[c]					
Micro-Bumintest™[c]					
Microstix®-3[c]					
Hemastix®[c]					
Albustix®[c]					
Ketostix®[c]					
Clinistix®[c]					
Chek-stix®[c]					
Chemstrip® 2GP[d]					
Chemstrip® 2LN[d]					
Chemstrip® 4OB[d]					
Chemstrip® 6[d]					
Chemstrip® 7[d]					
Chemstrip® 8[d]					
Chemstrip® 9[d]					
Chemstrip® 10 with SG[d]					
Chemstrip® uG[d]					
Chemstrip® uGK[d]					

[a]Also detects creatinine.

[b]In the United States, manufactured for IDEXX by Bayer. Petstix is a trademark of Bayer Corporation; used under license by IDEXX Laboratories, I
Available in Canada from Bayer, Inc.

Test List

Blood in Feces	pH	Protein	Microalbumin	Urobilinogen	Nitrite	Leukocytes
Tablet						

cBayer Corporation, Elkhart, IN.
dBoehringer Mannheim Corporation, Indianapolis, IN.

TABLE 10-2

EXAMPLES OF DISORDERS ASSOCIATED WITH ABNORMAL URINE pH VALUES

Excretion of Acid Urine
- Respiratory and metabolic acidoses
- Diabetic acidosis
- Primary renal failure
- Severe vomiting (so-called paradoxical aciduria of vomiting)
- Severe diarrhea
- Starvation
- Pyrexia
- Catabolism of endogenous or exogenous proteins
- Oxygen debt

Excretion of Alkaline Urine
- Urinary tract infections caused by urease-producing pathogens
- Respiratory or metabolic alkalosis
- Vomiting

TABLE 10-3

DRUGS AND FOOD ADDITIVES THAT AFFECT URINE pH

Acidifying Products
- Phosphate salts (sodium, potassium, or ammonium)
- D,L-Methionine
- Ammonium chloride
- Ascorbic acid (although studies in cats indicate that ascorbic acid was incapable of altering urine pH at commonly recommended therapeutic dosages)[1]
- Citric acid
- Therapeutic doses of furosemide

Alkalinizing Products
- Sodium bicarbonate
- Sodium lactate
- Sodium acetate
- Potassium citrate
- Acetazolamide
- Chlorothiazide

See Table 10-3 for listings of drugs and food additives that affect urine pH.

Artifacts

Contamination of urine with urease-producing bacteria from the distal urethra, genital tract, or environment may result in alkalinization of urine, whereas contamination with other bacteria, particularly urine containing glucose, may cause acidification. This problem may be minimized by using sterilized cups to collect urine that must be stored for several hours before testing. Alkalinization may also occur as a result of storage of samples at room temperature (due to loss of CO_2) and following exposure to detergents and disinfection agents in collection containers.

ªMicroessential Laboratory.

REFERENCES AND SUGGESTED READINGS

1. Chow FHC, Taton GF, Lewis LD, Hamar DW: Effects of dietary ammonium chloride, *dl*-methionine, sodium phosphate and ascorbic acid on urinary pH and electrolyte concentrations in male cats. *Feline Pract* 8:29–34, 1978.
2. Dee SA, Tracy JD, Kin V: Using citric acid to control urinary tract disease in swine. *Vet Med* 89:473–476, 1994.
3. Finco DR, Admas D, Crowell WA, et al: Food and water intake and urine composition in cats: Influence of continuous versus periodic feeding. *Am J Vet Res* 47(7):1986.
4. Lees GE, Osborne CA, Stevens JB: Antibacterial properties of urine: Studies of feline specific gravity, osmolality and pH. *JAAHA* 15:135–141, 1979.
5. Osborne CA, Stevens JB, Polzin DJ, Klausner JS: Clinical significance of urine pH. *Minn Vet* 21:24–27, 1981.
6. Paquignon A, Tran G, Provost JP: Evaluation of the Clinitek 200 urinary test-strip reader in the analysis of dog and rat urine in pre-clinical toxicology studies. *Lab Anim* 27:240–246, 1993.
7. Shaw DH: Relationship between urine ammonium ion excretion and urine anion gap in dogs. *Am J Vet Res* 52(12):1956, 1991.

Section 2: Glucose

INDICATIONS

Diagnostic

Although a small quantity of glucose is normally present in urine (2 to 10 mg/100 ml in humans), the quantity is insufficient to be detected by screening tests commonly used as a part of routine urinalyses. Detection of glucosuria should prompt consideration of hyperglycemic and normoglycemic states, which may be physiologic, pharmacologic, or pathologic (Figure 10-1).

Therapeutic

The dosage of insulin given to patients with diabetes mellitus is commonly adjusted based on semiquantitative measurements of urine glucose, usually taken in the nonstressful home environment.[11] Although the concentration of urine glucose is related to the concentration of blood glucose, the relationship may be influenced by many variables. Periodic evaluation of blood glucose concentration is required to establish insulin dose regimens and to confirm response to therapy based on evaluation of urine glucose concentrations. Detection of urine glucose is commonly used as a qualitative index of response to therapeutic osmotic diuresis induced by parenteral administration of hypertonic dextrose (so-called intensive osmotic diuresis).

METHODOLOGY

Historical Tests

In ancient times, urine was tasted to detect sugars. The

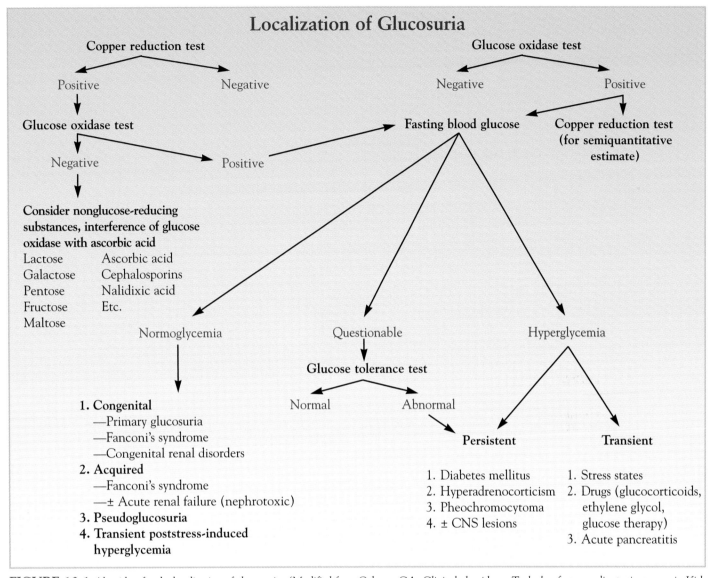

FIGURE 10-1 *Algorithm for the localization of glucosuria. (Modified from Osborne CA: Clinical algorithms: Tools that foster quality patient care, in Kirk RW (ed):* Current Veterinary Therapy IX. *Philadelphia, WB Saunders, 1989.)*

Greek words "mellitus" (meaning honey and implying a sweet taste) and insipidus ("in" is a prefix meaning without and "sapid" means taste) were used to describe different types of diabetes. Diabetes, a term derived from Greek and literally meaning "to pass through," was used to refer to formation of a large volume of urine.

Colorimetric Tests Based on Glucose Oxidase Activity (Table 10-1)

Dipsticks and reagent tapes impregnated with glucose oxidase/peroxidase and several other reagents are available from commercial sources. Although these enzymatic tests for detection of urine glucose are technically easy to perform, they involve interrelated enzymatic reactions that occur in a sequential fashion (Figures 10-2 and 10-3). The reliability of the results depends on adherence to the manufacturers' recommendations for use.

Although different chromogens are present in various tests (potassium iodide in Multistix®; tetramethyl benzidine in

Chemstrip®), the intensity and shade of colors are reported to be roughly proportional to the quantity of glucose in urine. Color scales for comparison are provided by manufacturers.

Glucose oxidase enzyme reacts specifically with glucose; the enzyme will not react with nonglucose-reducing substances (see discussion on colorimetric tests based on copper reduction).[1] However, the tests incorporate colorimetric indicators that may react with nonglucose substances. Conversely, some substances may inhibit the test reaction.

Glucose oxidase and peroxidase are labile proteins. Therefore test strips have a limited shelf-life as indicated by the expiration date on their container.

Test results may be influenced by temperature. Pilot studies performed at the University of Minnesota on canine urine with a known concentration of glucose in water (0, 100, 250, 500, 1000, and 2000 mg/dl) revealed that almost 25% of the samples refrigerated at 6°C and immediately tested at room temperature (21°C) with Clinistix® were falsely negative. These data indicate that refrigerated samples should be warmed to room tem-

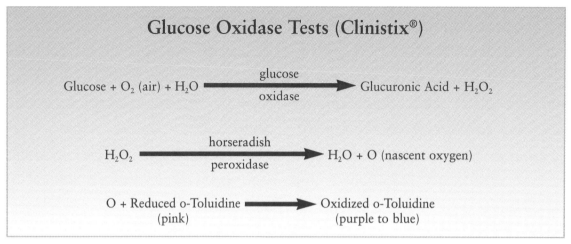

FIGURE 10-2 *Interrelationship of reagents in Clinistix® and their reaction with urine glucose.*

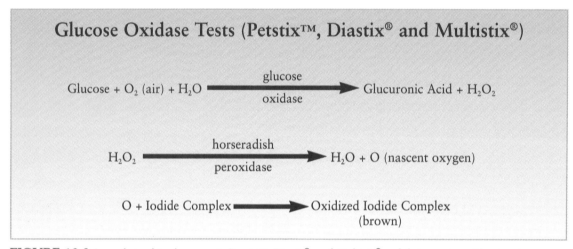

FIGURE 10-3 *Interrelationship of reagents in Petstix™, Diastix®, and Multistix® and their reaction with urine glucose.*

perature before evaluation for glucose with enzyme-dependent tests requiring short reaction times (10 seconds).

Inhibition by ascorbic acid at concentrations ≥ 50 mg/dl is likely to occur only at the lowest detectable glucose concentration (50 mg/dl for Chemstrip® and 100 mg/dl for Multistix®). Reactivity of the Multistix® glucose test decreases as the urine SG increases. Oxidizing cleaning agents may cause false positive results with the Chemstrip® glucose test. As always, strips should be handled as described in the package insert to avoid reagent deterioration.

The sensitivity of glucose oxidase tests may also be influenced by reagent deterioration and possibly other factors. Because many variables have the potential to affect the validity of the test, appropriate caution must be used in interpretation of semiquantitative results.

Clinistix®

Dry, solid-state reagent pads attached to a plastic strip contain glucose oxidase, peroxidase, and a colorimetric indicator (ortho-tolidine). A red background dye is used to provide an easily matched negative color (see Figure 10-2).

Color reactions are matched at 10 seconds. Color changes that occur after 10 seconds are ignored.

Three positive color blocks are light (100 mg/dl), medium (250 mg/dl), and dark (500 mg/dl+) purple (Table 10-4).

Petstix™, Diastix®, and Multistix®

These tests are based on the same principle as Chemstrip®, but potassium iodide is used as the chromogen (see Figure 10-3). A light blue background dye is also incorporated into the system.

Color reactions are matched at 30 seconds, but can be read up to 2 minutes. A blue color is negative, while positive results are indicated by shades of green through brown to represent 100, 250, 500, 1000, and 2000 mg/dl glucose (see Table 10-4).

The manufacturer indicates that Diastix® or Clinitest® provides more reliable semiquantitative results than Clinistix®.

Urine gains access to the glucose test pad on Petstix™ and Multistix® from the side. Therefore, if urine is applied by a dropper or by a syringe, it must be applied to the side and not the top of the test pad.

Chemstrip® 2GP, 4OB, 6, 7, 8, 9, and 10 with SG

The glucose oxidase/peroxidase test principle is used. Glucose oxidase reacts only with glucose. A second enzyme, peroxidase, catalyzes the reaction of hydrogen peroxide with the

TABLE 10-4

SENSITIVITY OF TESTS FOR URINE GLUCOSE

Test	Normal	<50 mg/dl	100 mg/dl	250 mg/dl	500 mg/dl	750 mg/dl	1000 mg/dl	2000 mg/dl	5000 mg/dl
Chemstrip®[a]	Yellow-gold	Yellow-green (trace)	Green (+)	Dark green	Dark green		Green-blue (+++)		
Clinistix®[b]	Red		Light purple	Medium purple	Dark purple				
Multistix®[b]	Pale blue	Light green (trace)	Light green	Darker green	Olive		Light brown	Brown	
Petstix™[c]	Pale blue		Light green	Darker green	Olive		Light brown	Brown	
Diastix®[b]	Pale blue		Light green	Darker green	Olive		Light brown	Brown	
Clinitest®[b] Five drop method	Blue			Blue green	Olive green	Pea green	Brown	Orange	
Two drop method					Green		Olive green	Brown	Orange

[a]Boehringer Mannheim Corp., Indianapolis, IN.
[b]Bayer Corp., Elkhart, IN.
[c]In the United States, manufactured for IDEXX by Bayer. Petstix is a trademark of Bayer Corporation; used under license by IDEXX Laboratories, Inc. Available in Canada from Bayer, Inc.

chromogen tetramethylbenzidine to form a green color. The original test pad color is yellow, and any green is taken as a positive reaction.

Reagent impregnated paper is sandwiched between an iodate scavenger pad and an absorbent pad. The iodate scavenger oxidizes ascorbic acid and allows interaction between the products of the peroxidase enzyme and the chromogen. The absorbent pad prevents reagents from washing into neighboring test pad areas. The complex is held to the plastic dipstick by means of a laminated nylon mesh.

The color can be compared to the color chart provided after 60 seconds. The color is stable for up to 2 minutes. A yellow color is normal. Positive results are indicated by increasing intensity of green. The reagent strips are calibrated as normal, 1/20% (50 mg/dl), 1/10% (100 mg/dl), 1/4% (250 mg/dl), 1/2% (500 mg/dl), and 1% (1000 mg/dl) glucose.

Chemstrip® uG and uGK

The test principle is the same as that previously described using tetramethylbenzidine as the chromogen. Changing concentrations of the chromogen changes test sensitivity. In addition, the reagents are not impregnated on paper but are included in a plastic dispersion.

The Chemstrip® uG has two test zones. The light yellow zone changes from light to dark green with increasing glucose concentrations. The most intense green corresponds to a 2% glucose concentration. A second white zone changes to light blue and then to blue over a glucose concentration range of 0.5% to 5%. These twin test areas with overlapping concentration ranges allow an observer to estimate concentration gradations over a range up to 5% glucose. The Chemstrip® uGK has an additional area for the detection of ketone bodies in urine.

Colorimetric Tests Based on Copper Reduction

Copper reduction methods are based on color changes associated with change of cupric ions (blue) to cuprous oxide (orange-red; by reducing substances Figure 10-4). Blue through green to orange colors are dependent on the concentration of reducing compounds (including glucose) in urine.

Clinitest®

Clinitest® is a commercially prepared tablet test system. Each tablet contains cupric sulfate, citric acid, sodium hydroxide, and sodium carbonate. A tablet is added to 5 drops of urine and 10 drops of water in a test tube. The reaction of citric acid with sodium bicarbonate generates carbon dioxide bubbles, which prevents room air from participating in the chemical reastion. Dissolution of sodium hydroxide and its interaction with water provide the

Copper Reduction Tests (Clinitest®)

Cupric ions (blue) + Glucose $\xrightarrow[\text{alkali}]{\text{heat}}$
$CuSO_4$

Cuprous ions (orange-red) + Oxidized Glucose
Cu_2O

FIGURE 10-4 *Interaction of copper sulfate with reducing substances such as glucose in the presence of an appropriate environment to induce a characteristic color change in the Clinitest®.*

necessary heat for reduction of cupric ions by sugar and other reducing substances in urine. The color of the final reaction is matched to a color scale ranging from blue through green and brown to orange, corresponding to 0, 250, 500, 750, 1000, and 2000 mg/dl of reducing substances.

The test can also be performed with 2 drops of urine and 10 drops of water. If the 2 drop technique is used, the color scale is different but the colors are similar. Colors ranging from green to orange correspond to concentrations of 1000, 2000, 3000, and 5000 mg/dl of reducing substance.

Close observation is required while the reaction boils since a phenomenon termed the "pass-through" may occur with large concentrations of glucose. A concentration of more than 2000 mg/dl causes a fleeting orange color, which fades back to brown. This phenomenon is caused by reoxidation of cuprous oxide to cupric oxide. Other cupric complexes may form that are green. Reoxidation may occur when there are large quantities of reducing substances or the reaction mixture is exposed to room air after the protective CO_2 blanket disperses. If this color change is not observed, the final reaction may be erroneously matched to the 1000 mg/dl color block. Addition of 2 rather than 5 drops of urine makes the test less sensitive and may be used to avoid the "pass-through" phenomenon, provided urine glucose concentration does not exceed 10 g/dl of urine. In addition, color changes after 15 seconds should be ignored.

Confirmatory Testing

When unexpected results or unusual test pad colors from highly pigmented urine occur, results can be confirmed by measurement of glucose in the urine and/or by testing urine for reducing substances (Clinitest®). Hexokinase- or glucose dehydrogenase–based techniques are recommended for quantitation of glucose in urine.[2] Sodium fluoride preservatives have been evaluated.[10]

Samples that give rise to false-positive test results by Clinitest® (modified Benedict's test) would be expected to be negative by hexokinase methodology.

Ascorbic acid would not be measured by hexokinase- or glucose dehydrogenase–based tests that measure NADH spectrophotometrically (if NADH is coupled with the indicator, then the result is ascorbic acid sensitive).

> When unexpected results or unusual test pad colors from highly pigmented urine occur, results can be confirmed by measurement of glucose in the urine and/or by testing urine for reducing substances.

Therefore glucose can be accurately quantitated.

Positive reagent strip test results may be confirmed with the Clinitest®. The 5 drop Clinitest® can be used to measure glucose and other reducing substances. False-positive reactions due to "color reversion" would be identified.

INTERPRETATION (see Table 10-5)
Specificity of Methods
Glucose Oxidase
Glucose-Specific Test

Tests based on glucose oxidase activity are specific for glucose and will not react with nonglucose-reducing substances.[1] Reagent strips are to be used according to the manufacturer instructions and by the expiration date. The strip should be removed from the bottle just before use. Undue exposure to room air, light, and humidity will cause erroneous results. Substances such as drugs containing azo dyes, nitrofurantoin, and riboflavin or other causes of pigmenturia (such as large quantities of bilirubin) may affect the readability of the reagent test pad and lead to misinterpretation.

False-Positive Reactions

Contamination of the sample or test system with small quantities of hydrogen peroxide (0.006%) will induce false-positive results, as will careless contamination with hydrochlorite, chlorine, or other strong oxidizing agents. An unidentified compound (termed "pseudoglucose") has been observed by one investigator in the urine of cats with urethral obstruction. In addition, exposure of glucose oxidase/peroxidase coupled with a potassium iodide chromogen to room air resulted in a false trace reaction after 7 days and a trace to 1+ reaction after 28 days (Multistix®).[3]

False-Negative Reactions

Numerous studies have indicated that ascorbic acid is capable of interfering with the test. The ascorbic acid interference on the reagent strips, however, occurs only for the lowest detectable levels of glucose (50 or 100 mg/dl). Outdated reagents or reagents exposed to sunlight may give erratic results.

Formaldehyde (generated from methenamine) will inhibit glucose oxidase and peroxidase. Moderately high ketone levels (40

TABLE 10-5

INTERPRETATION OF COMBINATION TEST RESULTS

Negative glucose oxidase test and negative copper reduction test = absence of significant quantities of glucose in urine

Positive glucose oxidase test and negative copper reduction test = less than 250 mg/dl of glucose in urine or a false-positive glucose oxidase reaction

Positive glucose oxidase test and positive copper reduction test = glucosuria in excess of 250 mg/dl

Negative glucose oxidase test and positive copper reduction test = nonglucose-reducing substances in urine

mg/dl) may cause false negatives for specimens containing small amounts of glucose (75–125 mg/dl). Acetoacetate in concentrations as low as 0.75 g/L interfered with the glucose reaction on the Hema-Combistix®.[13]

Large quantities of bilirubin have been reported to inhibit Clinistix®. Adding 300 mg of glucose to 10 ml of urine and retesting after 10 minutes may reveal some inhibitors. Reagent tapes have been observed to have a unique advantage over reagent pads when inhibitors are present. As urine ascends the tape by capillary action, inhibitor compounds adhere to the paper but glucose does not. The result is development of a line of color indicative of glucosuria at the solvent front.

The reactivity of the Multistix® glucose test area may decrease with increasing specific gravity.

Copper Reduction

Copper reduction methods are not specific for glucose. False-positive reactions may be caused by sufficient concentrations of reducing substances, including:

- *Glucose, fructose, lactose, galactose, maltose, and pentose.* If necessary, thin-layer chromatography may be used to specify the cause of mellituria.
- *Creatinine, homogentisic acid, and uric acid.* Although these are reducing substances, they do not affect Clinitest® reactions.
- *Ascorbic acid (endogenous and/or exogenous).* Although it is a reducing substance and may contribute to a positive reaction, it probably would not be found in a high enough concentration to cause a false-positive reaction in the absence of other reducing substances such as glucose. Unlike humans, dogs and cats normally synthesize and excrete varying quantities of ascorbic acid in their urine. The practical limit of sensitivity for scorbutic animals would be expected to be less than that in humans, primates, fruit-eating bats, and guinea pigs. Humans given massive doses of ascorbic acid (either 6 or 9 g twice a day) yielded only 2.7% trace test reactions

with the 2 drop Clinitest®.[14] Ascorbic acid is occasionally used as a urinary acidifier (although its efficacy is questionable).

- *Conjugated glucuronates.* Many compounds are conjugated with glucuronic acid in the liver prior to excretion. Conjugated bilirubin is commonly found in urine. Sufficient quantities of glucuronic acid will give a positive reaction with copper reduction tests.
- *Certain drugs and their metabolites.* Substances such as salicylates, penicillin (at large doses), sulfonamides, and chloral hydrate act as reducing agents and may contribute to the intensity of the color produced by copper reduction methods.
- *Cephalosporin and nalidixic acid.* These drugs can cause false-positive reactions to Clinitest® in humans.
- *Formaldehyde.* Formaldehyde may induce false-positive reactions with Clinitest® and therefore should not be used as a preservative for urine samples to be tested for glucose by this method.

Sensitivity of Methods (Table 10-4)

The sensitivity of all methods is influenced to varying degrees by urine specific gravity, adverse pH, interfering compounds, and suboptimum temperatures. Consult the manufacturers' product descriptions for further information.

Test methods are generally more sensitive to glucose in saline than glucose in urine. The term "practical sensitivity" has been defined as being the concentration of glucose that will be detected in 90% of a fairly large number of specimens under normal conditions. Lesser quantities of glucose may be detected in most urine samples; therefore the limits of detection given as "practical sensitivity" are intended as a general guideline only.

Chemstrip® 2GP, 4OB, 4, 6, 8, 9, and 10 with SG have been reported by the manufacturer to have a practical sensitivity of 40 mg/dl in urine samples free of ascorbic acid (i.e., human urine). Chemstrip® uG and uGK have a practical limit of sensitivity of 60 mg/dl.

Petstix™, Clinistix®, and Multistix® have a practical sensitivity of less than 100 mg/dl (i.e., 75 mg/dl, 90 mg/dl, and 85 mg/dl, respectively).

Clinitest® has a lower sensitivity equivalent to approximately 250 mg/dl for both the 2 drop and 5 drop techniques. Some investigators have observed a slightly lower limit of detection (150 mg/dl) for the 5 drop technique.

Ascorbic Acid versus Sensitivity

As previously discussed, ascorbic acid has the capacity to inhibit glucose oxidase test systems. However, since it is a strong reducing substance, it may cause or contribute to positive copper reduction tests.

The amount of ascorbic acid in urine influences the degree to which it alters tests for urine glucose. The greater the concentration of glucose in urine, the greater the quantity of ascorbic acid required to inhibit glucose oxidase tests. Likewise, the greater the concentration of ascorbic acid, the higher the reading of copper reduction test results. Ascorbic acid concentrations as low as 50 mg/dl can prevent detection of low concentrations of urine glucose by glucose oxidase tests. Ascorbic acid concentrations as high as 90 mg/dl have been detected in urine samples collected from dogs. We have observed an ascorbic acid concentration as high as 50 mg/dl in a cat with diabetes mellitus.

Ascorbic acid may be present in sufficient concentration to inhibit detection of low concentrations of urine glucose with glucose oxidase tests and result in underestimation of the quantity of urine glucose. Ascorbic acid concentrations sufficiently high to significantly alter copper reduction test results in dogs and cats have not been recognized in our hospitals. Ascorbic acid–induced variations in test results should be considered if urine glucose determined by glucose oxidase methods is used as an aid in titration of insulin dosage for patients with diabetes mellitus.

At one time, products differed in their sensitivity to glucose, partly because of various chemical modifications to avoid ascorbic acid interference. Manufacturers state that this problem has been corrected.

Automatic strip readers may appear to be less sensitive than visual readers. Using Multistix® 10SG with Clinitek® 200, urine spiked with 100 mg/dl resulted in a trace reading, while 90% of samples containing 50 mg/dl were negative. Visually, 50 mg/dl may read as positive, depending on the individual. This apparent discrepancy is due to the fact that the instrumental sensitivity is set by the manufacturer to meet product claims and contains no visual bias.

In a 1996 study of 138 and 55 cats, Multistix® 10SG (the same methodology is used in Petstix™ 8) glucose results obtained at the University of Minnesota and University of Guelph were compared to the hexokinase method on the Cobas analyzer (Roche Instruments). Agreement of the reagent strip with the reference method was 100% for glucose ≥70 mg/dl (incidence of positive glucose was 8% in dogs and 16% in cats).

Physiologic Glucosuria (Figure 10-1)

Because of its molecular characteristics (molecular weight = 180), glucose readily passes through glomerular capillary walls into glomerular filtrate. Almost all of the glucose in glomerular filtrate is actively reabsorbed by the proximal tubules. Only a small quantity (2 to 10 mg/dl or 100 to 200 mg/24 hours in humans) normally appears in urine.

Physiologic glucosuria may occur any time the quantity of glucose in glomerular filtrate exceeds the transport capacity (so-called "transport maximum" [T_m]) of the renal tubules for glucose. The T_m for urine glucose in dogs corresponds to a venous blood glucose concentration of approximately 170 to 180 mg/dl. The T_m for urine glucose in cats corresponds to a venous blood glucose of approximately 260 to 310

> **Ascorbic acid may be present in sufficient concentration to inhibit detection of low concentrations of urine glucose with glucose oxidase tests and result in underestimation of the quantity of urine glucose.**

> **Hyperglycemic glucosuria may occur following significant stress, especially in cats, even though the renal threshold for glucose in cats is relatively high.**

mg/dl. It is obvious that hyperglycemia of a lesser magnitude may exist without glucosuria.

Physiologic glucosuria is usually transient in duration. Hyperglycemic glucosuria may occur following significant stress, especially in cats, even though the renal threshold for glucose in cats is relatively high. This phenomenon is usually associated with the release of endogenous adrenaline and glucocorticoids and is thought to be dependent on mobilization of glycogen stored in the liver. Strong reactions for urine glucose due to diet, stress, or glucocorticoids (exogenous or endogenous) is unusual in most species. For example, if a strong glucosuria is encountered in a patient suspected of having hyperadrenocorticism, it is advisable to evaluate the patient for concurrent hyperglycemic disorders.

Hyperglycemic glucosuria has been reported in humans following consumption of unusually large quantities of glucose. We have not observed this phenomenon in dogs or cats. However, cats have been reported to have a limited capacity to metabolize dietary sugars.[8]

An increase in the amount of glucose lost per 24 hours has also been observed in pregnant humans.

Pharmacologic Glucosuria (Figure 10-1)

Consult the section on specificity of glucose interpretation tests for additional information about false-positive reactions associated with various glucose tests.

Hyperglycemic glucosuria may occur following parenteral administration of solutions containing sufficient quantities of glucose. Varying degrees of glucosuria may be induced by parenteral administration of glucocorticoids, but in our experience this is extremely uncommon in dogs and cats. Other pharmacologic agents that have been reported to have the potential to induce glucosuria include:

■ Adrenocorticotropic hormone
■ Glucagon
■ Adrenaline
■ Morphine
■ Phenothiazine
■ Progesterone

Pathologic Glucosuria (Figure 10-1)

Glucosuria is associated with hyperglycemic syndromes. Diagnosis of these syndromes is based on immunochemical determination of hormonal concentrations. Insulin and the insulin counterregulatory hormones interact in a number of disease situations to result in hyperglycemia. Glucagon, adrenaline, glucocorticoids, and growth hormone production are intimately involved in physiologic and disease processes. This concept is apparent in the following list of hyperglycemic physiologic situations and diseases.[5,9]

Hyperglycemic glucosuria may be induced by several disorders, including:

- Diabetes mellitus
- Acute pancreatitis (variable)
- Hyperadrenocorticism (variable)
- Central nervous system lesions (variable)
- Pheochromocytoma
- Glucagonoma[6]
- Acromegaly or progesterone administration
- Sepsis (some cases)
- Chronic liver disease (failure to clear glucagon)
- Extreme stress

Normoglycemic glucosuria may be induced by several disorders, including:

- Primary renal glucosuria
- Fanconi's syndrome
- Congenital renal disorders
- Acute renal failure associated with significant tubularlesions (variable)

Consequences of Glucosuria

Dehydration with azotemia can be a sequela to the osmotic-induced polyuria effect of glucosuria. In this situation, antidiuretic hormone will be functional, leading to an increased urine specific gravity. Dehydration characterized by a relatively high specific gravity for a polyuric state is expected.

Bacterial urinary tract infections are often associated with persistent glucosuria. Therefore examination of urine sediment is appropriate.

REFERENCES AND SUGGESTED READINGS

1. Adams EC, Burkhart E, Free AH: Specificity of a glucose test for urine glucose. Science 125:1082–1083, 1957.
2. Berg B, Hellsing K, Jagenburg R, Kallner A: IFCC Document: Guidelines for evaluation of reagent strips. Exemplified by analysis of urine albumin and glucose concentration using visually read reagent strips. Scand J Clin Lab Invest 49:689–699, 1989.
3. Cohen HT, Spiegel DM: Air-exposed urine dipsticks give false positive results for glucose and false negative results for blood. Am J Coll Physicians 96(3):398–400, 1991.
4. Daae LN, Juell A: Rapid diagnostic tests for glucosuria are still influenced by ascorbic acid. Scand J Clin Lab Invest 43(8):747–749, 1983.
5. Eigenmann JE: Diabetes mellitus in elderly female dogs: Recent findings on pathogenesis and clinical implications. JAAHA 17:805-812, 1981.
6. Gross TL, O'Brian TD, Davies AP, Long RE: Glucagon-producing pancreatic endocrine tumors in two dogs with superficial necrolytic dermatitis. JAVMA 15(12):1619–1990, 1990.
7. Juiell A: A new and more ascorbic acid resistant dipstick test for the detection of glucosuria has been introduced. Scand J Clin Lab Invest 45(3):289, 1985.
8. Kuienze E: Blood sugar levels and renal sugar excretion after the intake of high carbohydrate diets in cats. J Nutr 1245(12 Suppl):2563S–2567S, 1994.
9. Lager I: The insulin-antagonistic effect of the couterregulatory hormones. J Intern Med 735 (Suppl):41–47, 1991.
10. Lough S, et al: Efficacy of 1% sodium fluoride as a preservative in urine samples containing glucose and Candida albicans. J Forens Sci 38(2):266, 1993.
11. Miller E: Long term monitoring of the diabetic dog and cat: Clinic signs, serial blood glucose determinations, urine and glycated blood proteins. Vet Clin North Am Small Anim Pract 25(3):571–584, 1995.
12. Paquignon A, Tran G, Provost JP: Evaluation of the Cliniteck 200 urinary teststrip reader in the analysis of dog and rat urines in pre-clinical toxicology. Lab Anim 27(3):240–246, 1993.
13. Smally DL, Bradley ME: New test for urinary glucose (BM33071) evaluated. Clin Chem 31(1):90–92, 1985.
14. Smith D, Young WW: Effect of large dose ascorbic acid on the two-drop Clinitest® determination. Am J Hosp Pharm 34(2):134–139, 1977.
15. White-Stevens RH: Interference by ascorbic acid in test systems involving peroxidase. I. Reversible indicators and the effects of copper, iron and mercury. Clin Chem 28:578–588, 1982.
16. White-Stevens RH, Stover LR: Interference by ascorbic acid in test systems involving peroxidase. II. Redox-coupling indicator systems. Clin Chem 28:589–595, 1982.
17. Zweig MH, Jackson A: Ascorbic acid interference in reagent-strip reactions for assay of urinary glucose and hemoglobin. Clin Chem 32(4):674–677, 1986.

Section 3: Ketones

INDICATIONS

Ketone bodies include acetoacetic acid, acetone, and beta-hydroxybutyric acid. However, other chemical forms of ketones can be found in urine. Evaluation of urine for ketone bodies in patients with diabetes mellitus is especially important since diabetic ketonuria suggests development of diabetic ketoacidosis. Evaluation of urine for ketones may aid in differentiation of a diabetic coma from therapeutically induced insulin shock.

Detection of ketone body formation is indicated in diseases and conditions associated with increased gluconeogenesis and/or excessive catabolism of lipids. The physiology of ketonuria may be localized as: (1) impaired ability to utilize available carbohydrates (diabetes mellitus), (2) inadequate carbohydrate consumption (starvation, altered diets, strenuous exercise, exposure to a cold environment), and (3) loss of carbohydrates (renal tubular disorders and digestive disorders). Evaluation of urine for ketones in late gestation may aid in the detection of pregnancy toxemia and inadequate nutrition of gestational diabetes mellitus. It may also lead to detection of uncommonly recognized genetic diseases such as mitochondrial myopathy or Gierke's glycogen storage disease.

METHODOLOGY

Nitroprusside Tests

Available laboratory tests for ketonuria are designed to detect all three ketones. Most tests used as a part of routine complete urinalysis for detecting ketones are based on the reaction of acetoacetic acid and acetone with nitroprusside (also called sodium nitroferricyanide) in an alkaline environment to produce a deep purple-colored compound (Figure 10-5).

Petstix™, Multistix®, Ketostix®, Keto-Diastix®, Labstix®, and Chemstrip® contain test pads impregnated with sodium nitroprusside, glycine (aminoacetic acid), and an alkaline phosphate buffer (disodium hydrogen phosphate). The buffer provides an optimum pH for the reaction. The interaction of these reagents with ketones is depicted in Figure 10-5. The reaction will not detect beta-hydroxybutyric acid, and it is much more sensitive to acetic acid than to acetone. The results of one study illustrate the variable sensitivity of the sodium nitroprusside reaction for different ketones in urine (Table 10-6).

Reaction of Strip and Tablet Tests (Acetest®) for Ketonuria

$$\text{Acetoacetic Acid + Sodium Nitroprusside + Glycine and Acetone} \xrightarrow[\text{(NaOH)}]{\text{alkaline pH}} \text{Purple-colored complex}$$

FIGURE 10-5 *Reagents and biochemical events associated with positive strip and tablet tests for ketonuria.*

After the immersion of the reagent strip in urine the color of the reagent pad should be examined at the appropriate time (40 seconds for Petstix™ and Multistix® and 60 seconds for Chemstrip®). The color of the test strips should be compared to the color scale on the label. Color changes from beige (buff) to purple are indicative of ketonuria. The intensity of the color is proportional to the quantity of ketones present. Some reports claim a trace sensitivity at 5 mg/dl rather than a 1+ reaction and a 1+ reaction at 10 mg/dl or greater.

Acetest® is a tablet test based on the same reactions as those described for reagent strips. In addition, lactose is added to enhance the quality of color changes.

The test is performed by placing a reagent tablet on a white, square piece of filter paper and placing one drop of urine (or serum, plasma, or whole blood) on the tablet (not the paper). Thirty seconds later the color of the tablet should be compared to the color scale supplied by the manufacturer. A positive reaction, indicated by a lavender to deep purple color, is dependent on the quantity of the ketones present.

Acetest® is more sensitive than dipsticks. It will detect 5 mg/dl of ketones in urine versus about 10 mg/dl for the Ketostix® dipstick. It will detect about 10 mg/dl of ketones in blood, serum, or plasma.

Confirmatory Testing

Trace quantities found by dipstick are "confirmed" by retesting the sample with the more sensitive Acetest®. The results are reported as trace regardless of the degree of reaction of the Acetest®.

False-positive reactions may occur with highly pigmented urines or urines containing phthaleins or compounds with sulfhydryl groups. Often the color is not typical and can be recognized as not being attributable to ketone bodies. The color of the test strip is removed by the addition of one drop of glacial acetic acid to the reaction pad. Unusually high concentrations of the free sulfhydryl compounds may require dilution of the urine to read as moderate to small on the reading area of the pad before addition of acid. A definite color develops instantly but fades and usually disappears by the recommended time of 30 seconds. The ketone bodies induce and inten-

sify color for about 60 seconds. Read the test at 60 seconds. These times deviate from the manufacturer's recommended reading times.

Addition of 4 N NaOH dropwise to alkalinize a small subsample of the urine will turn it reddish orange if phthalein dyes are present.

INTERPRETATION
Specificity

The nitroprusside reaction can detect acetoacetic acid and, to a lesser degree, acetone but will not react with beta-hydroxybutyric acid. Approximately 96% of the total color is due to acetoacetic acid.

If toluene is the urine preservative, it should be used sparingly because acetone is more soluble in toluene than urine. However, toluene is not generally recommended as a preservative.

Because of volatilization of acetone at room temperature, specimens should be immediately tested or refrigerated. The concentration of ketones has been reported to decrease in vivo as a result of urinary tract infection and in vitro as a result of bacterial contamination. Bacteria may reduce the quantity of acetoacetic acid but not acetone.

The ketone portion of a dipstick is sensitive to the effects of moisture, heat, or light. Therefore the dipstick container lid must be replaced immediately after a test strip is removed to minimize false-negative results due to improper management of reagents.

Substances with a keto, aldehyde, or sulfhydryl group have the potential for reacting with nitroprusside to produce a color reaction. Pyruvate, a ketone, has the potential to cause an unusual blue color change. It may be present in urine in sufficient concentration to interfere with detection of ketones.

TABLE 10-6

SENSITIVITY OF SODIUM NITROPRUSSIDE REACTION FOR DIFFERENT KETONES IN HUMAN URINE

Color	β-Hydroxybutyric Acid	Acetoacetic Acid	Acetone
Neg	Negative	<5 mg/dl	<70 mg/dl
Weak	Negative	10–25 mg/dl	100–400 mg/dl
Moderate	Negative	25–50 mg/dl	400–500 mg/dl
Strong	Negative	50–150 mg/dl	800–2000 mg/dl
Very strong	Negative	>150 mg/dl	>2000 mg/dl

Although excretion of phenylketones in urine in concentrations equal to or greater than 100 mg/dl will cause false-positive color reactions (orange-red), phenylketonuria of this magnitude is uncommon in humans and has not been reported in animals. Red-orange to red color shades produced by phenylketone compounds are usually readily distinguishable.

Agents that contain free sulfhydryl groups may cause false-positive results. These include captopril, d-penicillamine, 2-mercaptopropionyl glycine (tiopronin), and cystine (an amino acid).

Administration of sulfobromophthalein dye to evaluate liver function may result in production of a color (reddish) that mimics a positive reaction for ketonuria in alkaline urine. Similar reactions with phenolsulfonphthalein would be expected. Colors produced by phthalein compounds are usually readily distinguishable.

Levodopa has been reported to cause false-positive results in humans (brownish-violet color). When unusual or positive test results occur in animals receiving known interfering compounds, confirmatory testing should be attempted.

Sensitivity

The manufacturers indicate that the lower limit of sensitivity of these tests is approximately 5 to 10 mg/dl for acetoacetic acid and approximately 70 mg/dl for acetone. Beta-hydroxybutyric acid will not contribute to color development (Table 10-6).

It is possible to estimate crudely the quantity of ketones present by using the limit of detection (sensitivity) and diluting the test sample until only a trace reaction can be identified. For example, a urine sample is diluted by mixing one drop of urine with nine drops of water (1:10) dilution and the test indicates a trace of ketones. The actual quantity of ketones present may be calculated by multiplying the dilution factor (10) by the lowest limit of sensitivity (5 mg/dl):

$$5 \text{ mg/dl} \times 10 = 50 \text{ mg/dl of ketones}$$

Applied Physiology

During normal metabolism, fatty acids are almost completely converted via the Krebs cycle to carbon dioxide, water, and energy in the liver. In the process, however, small quantities of ketone bodies are formed. These intermediary metabolites are metabolized by peripheral tissues of the body at a limited rate. Acetone is irreversibly formed from acetoacetic acid by decarboxylation, whereas beta-hydroxybutyric acid is reversibly formed from acetoacetic acid.

Inadequate consumption of dietary carbohydrates, impaired endogenous utilization of carbohydrates, and/or excessive loss of carbohydrates results in a shift to increased oxidation of fatty acids as the primary metabolic substrate. When the proportion of fatty acids metabolized for energy becomes large, utilization by the Krebs cycle becomes incomplete and excessive quantities of ketone bodies are formed. As a result, mitochondria, especially those in the liver, begin active ketogenesis. Catabolism of the

> **The concentration of ketones has been reported to decrease in vivo as a result of urinary tract infection and in vitro as a result of bacterial contamination.**

amino acids leucine, tyrosine, and phenylalanine may also result in increased production of acetoacetic acid. When production of these metabolites exceeds the capacity of tissues to oxidize them, they accumulate in plasma (ketonemia), in milk (ketolactia), and in urine (ketonuria). Acetone expired by the lungs may cause a characteristic odor to the breath.

Ketone bodies are cleared from blood by glomerular filtration. There is a low renal threshold for ketone bodies because the tubular transport mechanism is easily saturated. Even at low plasma concentrations, ketone bodies will appear in the urine. The primary reabsorption mechanism is by diffusion back into the renal interstitium. There is no maximum (i.e., the more there is in urine, the more it will be reabsorbed). Although ketones are excreted in urine in different relative proportions (78% beta-hydroxybutyric acid, 20% acetoacetic acid, and 2% acetone), detection of one indicates the presence of the others.

Ketones are said to be mildly toxic. However, the toxicity seems to be more related to the production of acidosis and not directly due to the ketones. Uric acid excretion is reported to be hindered by ketone bodies.

Significance of Ketonuria

Ketonuria is not common in dogs (1.9%) and cats (2.6%) but is quite common in dairy cattle and somewhat common in swine.[1]

Ketonemia, ketolactia, and ketonuria may be caused by any disorder associated with a significant shift of energy production from carbohydrates to fats. Gluconeogenesis depletes oxaloacetate, which forces acetyl coenzyme A into ketone body production. Increases in reduced nicotine amide adenine dinucleotide/nicotine amide adenine dinucleotide ratios (reductive environment) is also associated with oxaloacetate depletion. By either or both mechanisms, depletion of oxaloacetate is associated with increased gluconeogenesis. The rate-limiting factor appears to be carnitine acyltransferase. This enzyme system is responsible for mitochondrial uptake of free fatty acid, which is increased in diabetes mellitus, for example, and contributes to ketogenesis.

Production of ketone bodies leads to metabolic acidosis. The high proton concentration displaces potassium out of cells and into plasma. This leads to depletion of potassium from the body.

Uncontrolled diabetes mellitus is the most commonly encountered form of ketonuria in dogs and cats. Urinary excretion of ketones induces systemic electrolyte losses including hypokalemia and hyponatremia. The loss of potassium, sodium, and ketones in urine contributes to the increased osmolality of the urine due to glucose and therefore increases the magnitude of polyuria associated with diabetes mellitus. Severe dehydration leading to poor tissue perfusion and hypoxia may result in an increase quantity of beta-hydroxybutyric acid. In this situation, severe ketosis could occur with minimal ketonuria detected by nitroprusside test methods.

TABLE 10-7

CONDITIONS/SUBSTANCES ASSOCIATED WITH KETONURIA AND/OR FALSE-POSITIVE RESULTS

Diseases/Physiologic States
Carbohydrate restriction
Diabetes mellitus
Fever
Frequent vomiting
Growth hormone administration
Gierke's glycogen storage disease
High fat diets
High protein diets
Hyperthyroidism
Lactation
Methylmalonic acidemia
Persistent vomiting
Postpancreatectomy
Pregnancy (terminal trimester)
Renal glucosuria
Starvation
Thyrotoxicosis

Drugs/Toxins
Butyric acid
Captopril
Cysteine
Cysteamine
Dimercaprol
3-Hydroxybutyrate
Ifosfamide
2-Mercaptoethane sulfonate sodium
Mercaptopropionyl glycine
Levodopa
Methyldopa
Paracetamol
Paraldehyde
d-Penicillamine
Phenylketone
Pyruvate

Dyes (color interference)
Sulfobromophthalein
Phenolsulfonphthalein

ciated with pyruvate excretion, and pituitary adenomas, adrenal tumors, insulinomas, and glucagonomas may be associated with ketone body production. In humans, methylmalonic acidemia has been associated with ketonuria.

Examples of physiologic states, diseases, drugs, toxins, and dyes associated with ketonuria and/or false-positive results are shown in Table 10-7.

REFERENCES AND SUGGESTED READINGS

1. Almond GW, Stevens JB: Urinalysis techniques for swine practitioners. *Compend Contin Educ Pract Vet* 17(1):121–129, 1995.
2. Free AH, Free HM: Nature of nitroprusside reactive material in urine ketosis. *Am J Clin Pathol* 30(1):7–10, 1958.
3. Eigenmann JE: Diabetes mellitus in elderly female dogs: Recent findings on pathogenesis and clinical implications. *JAAHA* 17:805–812, 1981.
4. Gross TL, O'Brian TD, Davies AP, Long RE: Glucagon-producing pancreatic endocrine tumors in two dogs with superficial necrolytic dermatitis. *JAVMA* 15(12):1619–1990, 1990.
5. Lager I: The insulin-antagonistic effect of the counterregulatory hormones. *J Intern Med* 735(Suppl):41–47, 1991.

Section 4: Bilirubin

INDICATIONS

Because detection of bilirubinuria by routine urinalysis may precede clinical recognition of jaundice in most species, bilirubinuria may be an early indicator of naturally occurring disorders with the potential to induce jaundice. Lack of bilirubinuria does not exclude disorders associated with bilirubin metabolism, however.

In addition to simple glomerular filtration, the canine kidney produces bilirubin and causes it to appear in urine. This phenomenon disassociates serum bilirubin as the only cause of bilirubinuria in dogs. Therefore the high rate of positive tests for bilirubinuria in the absence of disorders that have the potential to produce icterus renders the test nonspecific as a screening test in dogs.

Detection of abnormal quantities of bilirubin in urine may be used as a crude index of hepatotoxicity caused by potentially toxic therapeutic agents.

METHODOLOGY

Tests designed to detect bilirubin are based on an azo-coupling reaction with a diazonium salt in an acid medium to form an azodye. Color changes vary from light tan to beige or light pink. Tests differ from one another by the diazonium salt used. Do not use reagent strips or tablets after the expiration date printed on the label. See Table 10-8 for instructions on how to perform three of the most common tests.

Ictotest®

Ictotest is a tablet test based on a diazotization reaction and color change that are proportional to the quantity of bilirubin present in urine. The tablets contain the following ingredients: 2,4-dichlorobenzene diazonium tetrachlorozincate and sulfosalicylic acid. Sulfosalicylic acid provides an acid environment that promotes the reaction. A bluish-violet color develops as a result of the reaction.

Starvation and low carbohydrate–high fat diets (ketogenic diets) may also induce ketonuria.

Counterregulatory hormones (cortisol, epinephrine, somatostatin, and glucagon) contribute to several syndromes by increasing gluconeogenesis and lipase activity. Hormone-sensitive lipase (different from lipoprotein lipase) increases with decreased insulin activity. These hormones have an antagonistic effect on insulin. The role these hormones play in ketogenesis has not been fully worked out. However, in such conditions as pyometra, acromegaly, and old dog diabetes, they may play a role.[3–5]

Immature animals are more likely than adults to develop ketonuria as a result of starvation. Exercise may be followed by a positive test for ketonuria. Mitochondrial myopathy may be asso-

TABLE 10-8

SAMPLE PROCEDURES TO SCREEN FOR BILIRUBIN

Ictotest®
- Place 10 drops of urine on a square of the special test mat. Wait for each drop to be absorbed before proceeding with the next.
- Place a reagent tablet on the center of the moistened area of the mat.
- Allow one drop of water to flow over the tablet. Wait 5 minutes and then place a second drop of water on the tablet so that water runs off the tablet onto the mat.
- Evaluate the test mat for a color change that develops within 60 seconds.
- Lack of color change and pink or red colors indicate a lack of bilirubin. A positive result is indicated by a blue or purple color on the mat around the tablet. The speed and intensity of color development are proportional to the degree of bilirubinuria.
- Color changes affecting the tablet or those following a lapse of 60 seconds should not be interpreted as positive or negative results.
- CAUTION: Avoid use of discolored tablets or tablets exposed to moisture.

Petstix™ and Multistix®
- Immerse the reagent pad of the strip into the urine sample and remove it immediately.
- Draw the edge of the strip along the rim of the container to remove excess urine.
- After 30 seconds compare the color of the reagent pad to the color scale provided by the manufacturer.
- A negative reaction is indicated by a pale lemon color (the pad is beige-colored when dry). Under favorable conditions positive reactions are indicated by light tan (+ = small; ++ = moderate) and light brown (+++ = large). Careful color comparisons are recommended by the manufacturer since color changes may be subtle.
- CAUTION: Urine samples that are concentrated or discolored may be unsuitable for evaluation by this method. Questionable results should be verified by a different test method.

Chemstrip®
- Immerse the reagent pad of the strip into a fresh urine sample and remove it immediately.
- Draw the edge of the strip along the side of the container to remove excess urine.
- After 30 to 60 seconds compare the color of the reagent pad to the color scale provided by the manufacturer.
- A negative reaction is indicated by no color change. A change in color of the test zone from white to beige-pink indicates bilirubinuria. Varying shades of beige-pink to pale red-violet indicate slight (+ or 0.5 mg/dl), moderate (++ or 1.0 mg/dl), and heavy (+++ or 2.0 mg/dl) bilirubinuria.

A special cellulose mat is included with the tablet; its adsorbent qualities allow bilirubin to be concentrated at its surface.

Petstix™ and Multistix®

Reagent strips contain stabilized diazotized 2,4-dichloroaniline. When bilirubin is present in sufficient quantities, it reacts with this reagent to form azobilirubin and is associated with a change in color from buff to light tan or light brown. The degree of color change is dependent on the degree of bilirubinuria.

Conjugated bilirubin is much more reactive with these reagents than free bilirubin. Biliverdin cannot be detected by this method. Since bilirubin glucuronide spontaneously hydrolyzes to free bilirubin in urine samples allowed to remain at room temperature for long periods following collection, it is important to examine fresh or properly preserved specimens.

Chemstrip®

Chemstrip® 6, 7, 8, and 10 with SG contain 2,6-dichlorobenzene-diazonium-tetrafluoroborate, a buffer, and nonreactive ingredients. The test is based on the coupling reaction of the diazonium salt with bilirubin in an acid medium, which yields a pink to red-violet reaction, proportional to the total bilirubin concentration.

Confirmatory Testing

Trace positive reactions by dipsticks should be confirmed with the more sensitive Ictotest®. However, the dipstick results and not those obtained with Ictotest® are the ones that should be reported.

INTERPRETATION
General

The diazotization reaction is more reactive with conjugated bilirubin (which is more soluble) than free bilirubin (which is less soluble). Conjugated bilirubin may spontaneously hydrolyze to free bilirubin at room temperature.

Bilirubin is an unstable compound that may spontaneously oxidize to biliverdin, especially if allowed to stand at room temperature (Figure 10-6). Biliverdin cannot be detected by the diazotization reaction. For this reason urine should not be shaken. Unpreserved urine should be evaluated within 30 minutes from the time of collection.

Light degrades bilirubin. Exposure to light results in formation of products such as dipyrroles that color the urine but are not detected by the diazotization reaction.

Selective glomerular capillary permeability to plasma proteins does not significantly alter tests for bilirubinuria. The common tests are designed to detect conjugated bilirubin primarily. In addition, the amount of free bilirubin carried on albumin would be insignificant unless the concentration of bilirubin was extremely high and the amount of albumin was at an extreme (see section on interpretation for additional information).

Specificity

Indoxyl sulfate (indican) can alter the dipstick reading strip color sufficiently to mask a weak bilirubin-positive reaction. Indoxyl sulfate was found in about 50% of human bilirubin-positive urine.[9]

Urine should not be filtered or centrifuged prior to exami-

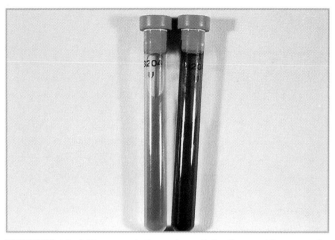

FIGURE 10-6 *Urine sample from a dog with dirofilariasis. The green color is characteristic of biliverdin. (Courtesy of Dr. Ralph Richardson, Purdue University, West Lafayette, Indiana).*

nation for bilirubin since precipitates of calcium carbonate and calcium phosphate may absorb varying quantities of bilirubin.

Drugs that color urine red in an acid medium (e.g., phenazopyridine) may cause false-positive reactions. Large quantities of chlorpromazine metabolites may directly react with the diazonium salt and cause a false-positive reaction.

Ictotest®

Large quantities of ascorbic acid decrease the sensitivity of the test. Because ascorbic acid is a strong reducing agent, it readily reacts with diazonium salts and removes them from sequences of reactions essential to the test. A colorless dehydroascorbate forms, explaining why the test pad does not change color. Drugs that have the capacity to change urine color may also interfere with recognition of test results (e.g., phenazopyridine may cause an orange to red color change). However, drugs containing phenothiazine do not affect this test unless present in very large quantities.

A common strategy used to avoid false-positive results due to interfering compounds is to test a urine sample for bilirubin with a dipstick technique. If the test is positive, it can be confirmed with Ictotest® but the level of positivity found with the dipstick should be reported.

Multistix®

Phenazopyridine may cause an orange to red color change, and very large doses of phenothiazine drugs (e.g., chlorpromazine) have been reported to give false-positive results in humans. The manufacturer also reports that ascorbic acid at concentrations of 25 mg/dl or greater may cause false-negative results. Bilirubin in concentrations of 6.4 mg/dl has been reported to result in a positive test for hemoglobin. Experience with Petstix™ is not yet sufficient to make generalizations.

Chemstrip®

Large quantities of ascorbic acid in the urine may decrease the sensitivity of the test. In humans, sensitivity of the test was also reduced by elevated concentrations of

nitrite induced by urinary tract infections. Drugs such as phenazopyridine that can color the urine red or that have an intrinsic red color in acid urine may give false-positive readings.

Sensitivity

As with all semiquantitative tests for urine analytes, always interpret the significance of test results in light of urine specific gravity. The tests are manufactured for use in humans, in whom urine can be concentrated to only 1.035 in contrast to 1.080 in cats. (Consult the section on glucose interpretation for definitions of "practical" and "absolute" sensitivity.)

Ictotest®

The practical limit of sensitivity is 0.1 mg/dl. Under ideal conditions the test may detect as little as 0.05 mg/dl of bilirubin in urine.

Petstix™ and Multistix®

According to the manufacturer, the lower limit of sensitivity is 0.4 to 0.8 mg/dl. When canine urine was spiked with bilirubin at 0.4 and 0.8 mg/dl bilirubin, 5 of 10 samples and 1 of 10 samples, respectively, gave negative values with an automated urine test strip reading device.[7] The manufacturer cautions that Ictotest reagent tablets should be the method of choice when very small amounts of bilirubin in urine are sought.

Applied Physiology

Bilirubin, an intensely orange-yellow metabolite, is derived primarily from the catabolism of the heme component of hemoglobin in reticuloendothelial cells of the body. Smaller quantities are derived from nonerythroid sources in the liver, preerythroid bone marrow sources, bone marrow metabolism, and other heme-containing proteins such as myoblobin. Once heme has been liberated, it is normally catabolized to bilirubin in approximately 3 hours. The iron is bound to transferrin and returned to the body's iron stores. The protein is returned to the amino acid pool for reutilization.

Bilirubin formed as a result of degeneration of hemoglobin by reticuloendothelial cells is water insoluble and becomes reversibly bound to albumin and transported via the circulation. Albumin-bound bilirubin is more soluble. Albumin-bound bilirubin cannot enter cells, where it would be toxic. One form of protein-bound bilirubin is commonly referred to by a variety of names, including unconjugated bilirubin, free bilirubin, indirect bilirubin, slow-reaction bilirubin, and hemobilirubin. Because it is bound to protein, it cannot pass through normal glomerular capillary walls.

Another form is tightly bound and is referred to as delta-bilirubin. This form is generally found in low concentrations and is not easily removed from the blood by the liver.

The liver removes loosely protein-bound bilirubin from the circulation and conjugates it with glucuronic and sulfuric acids. Conjugated bilirubin (also called walter-soluble bilirubin, direct bilirubin, bilirubin glucuronide, and cholebilirubin) is water soluble and readily passes through glomerular capillary walls.

> Healthy dogs tend to have bilirubinuria even when serum bilirubin concentrations are normal.

A great majority of conjugated bilirubin is transported to the intestinal tract in bile via the biliary system; however, a small amount escapes from the liver directly into the blood vascular system. Bilirubin excreted into the small intestine is converted to urobilinogen (a colorless tetrapyrrole pigment) by intestinal bacteria. Most of the urobilinogen is ultimately oxidized to urobilin, which imparts the characteristic dark color to feces. Urobilin cannot be resorbed. Some of the urobilinogen, however, is reabsorbed and excreted in urine (consult the section on urobilinogen for additional details).

Conjugated bilirubin that escapes through glomeruli may appear in urine. The renal threshold for clearance of conjugated bilirubin apparently varies from species to species. The quantity of bilirubin excreted in normal feline urine is insufficient to give a positive result.

Studies performed in dogs have revealed that bilirubin may also be formed in the renal tubules. The capacity to reform tubular-derived bilirubin from hemoglobin was found to be greater in males than females. Since tubular epithelial cells of dogs have been shown to contain glucuronyl transferase, the capacity of these cells to conjugate bilirubin appears probable. In addition, the enzyme heme oxidase has been shown to be inducible in rats. Heme oxidase degrades heme to bile pigment.[8]

Normal dogs excrete bilirubin in excess of creatinine, which suggests that the normal dog kidney functions in some respects like the normal liver in the processing of effete hemoglobin (the urine is somewhat like bile in this respect). Therefore healthy dogs, especially intact males but also females, tend to have bilirubinuria even when serum bilirubin concentrations are normal.

A variety of disorders may result in abnormal production of unconjugated and/or conjugated bilirubin, hyperbilirubinemia, and bilirubinuria. Abnormal quantities of conjugated bilirubin in urine may be associated with:

- Increased production of conjugated bilirubin as a result of abnormal red blood cell destruction, hepatocellular disease, and/or bile duct obstruction.
- The rat kidney has been shown to adapt to chronic hemolysis through enzyme induction to increase hemoglobin catabolism with time.[8]
- The combined occurrence of these disorders and renal dysfunction may lead to difficulties in quantitative interpretation of bilirubinuria because of alteration in the renal threshold for excretion of bile pigments.[3,4] Abnormal quantities of unconjugated bilirubin would be expected to occur in conditions associated with hyperbilirubinemia (i.e., hemolytic disease). This hypothesis has not been substantiated in animals with experimentally induced or spontaneously occurring diseases, however.

Significance

Because of the high false-positive and false-negative rates, the commonly available tests for bilirubinuria are not reliable as

> **Bilirubinuria in healthy cats is uncommon. When discovered as a part of routine urinalysis, it should not be ignored.**

screening tests in the dog. These tests have utility in cats, however.

In Dogs

Small quantities of bilirubin are commonly observed in urine samples obtained from normal dogs. This observation had been attributed to a low renal threshold for bilirubin. Currently, the presence of bilirubin in urine in the face of a normal serum bilirubin is attributed to catabolism of hemoglobin by the kidney with subsequent excretion of conjugated bilirubin in the urine.

Unpublished data obtained at North Carolina State University College of Veterinary Medicine indicate that over 60% of male dogs had 1+ or greater Ictotest® reactions, even when serum bilirubin was within the normal range. Reactions for bilirubin were relatively common even when the urine specific gravity was low. When male dogs with normal serum bilirubin values were evaluated, almost 50% had 1+ or greater Ictotest® results and about 25% were positive on the Chemstrip® test.

A high percentage of dogs with negative tests for bilirubinuria were found to actually have elevated serum bilirubin concentrations. Unpublished data indicate that the false-negative rate is 48% for Ictotest® (n = 854) and 31% for Chemstrip® (n = 343). This suggests that there is some unidentified inhibitor to the test reaction. Ascorbic acid does inhibit the detection of bilirubin.

N-Multistix® produced an atypical visual response to indoxyl sulfate that may mask bilirubin. This emphasizes the importance of using a more specific confirmatory test (e.g., Ictotest®) whenever dip and read tests for bilirubin are inconclusive.

In Cats

Bilirubinuria in healthy cats is uncommon. Retrospective evaluation of clinical cases admitted to the University of Minnesota Veterinary Hospital revealed that bilirubinuria was not a finding in normal cats, even in highly concentrated urine samples. When discovered as a part of routine urinalysis, it should not be ignored.

In the University of Minnesota series, feline bilirubinuria was associated with a variety of diseases, including primary hepatic diseases, diabetes mellitus, feline infectious peritonitis, and feline leukemia–related disorders.

Detection of bilirubin in less concentrated urine samples, or persistent bilirubinuria, should prompt consideration of disorders characterized by prehepatic, hepatic, or posthepatic disorders of bile metabolism. Bilirubinuria may precede hyperbilirubinemia. A variable degree of bilirubinuria may be associated with intravascular hemolysis of sufficient magnitude to exceed the hemoglobin-binding capacity of haptoglobin. In this situation in the cat, bilirubinuria is associated with increased production of conjugated bilirubin from hemoglobin. The liver increases the release of conjugated bilirubin into the blood and hence into the urine. Although damage to glomeruli may be associated with subsequent loss of unconjugated bilirubin, this mechanism is unlikely to be of clinical significance because of the magnitude of proteinuria that would be required to deliver a detectable quality of bilirubin in urine.

Bilirubinuria of the greatest magnitude is usually associated with peripheral lobular hepatocellular diseases (intrahepatic) or disorders that obstruct bile ducts (extrahepatic). A significant degree of liver disease can exist, however, in the absence of bilirubinuria.

Sixty percent of sick cats with bilirubinuria were males. The true significance of this is not known, but this finding implies a sex predilection in cats similar to that in dogs.

REFERENCES AND SUGGESTED READINGS

1. DeSchepper J: Degradation of hemoglobin to bilirubin in the kidney of the dog. *Tigdschr Diergeneesk* 99:699–707, 1974.
2. DeSchepper J, VanDerStock J: Influence of sex on the urinary bilirubin excretion at increased free plasma hemoglobin levels in whole dogs and in isolated normothermic perfused dog kidneys. *Experentia* 27:1264–1265, 1971.
3. Fulop M, Brazeau P: The renal excretion of bilirubin in dogs with obstructive jaundice. *J Clin Invest* 43:1192–1202, 1964.
4. Fulop M, Brazeau P: Impaired renal function exaggerates hyperbilirubinemia in bile-duct ligated dog. *Dig Dis* 15:1067–1072, 1970.
5. McDonald A, Spencer WW: Falsely positive results for bilirubin with Ames' "Clini-Tek." *Clin Chem* 25:813–814, 1979 (letter).
5a. Lees GE, Hardy RM, Stevens JB, Osborne CA: Clinical implications of feline bilirubinuria. *JAAHA* 20:765–771, 1984.
6. Osborne CA, Stevens JB, Lees GE, et al: Clinical significance of bilirubinuria. *Compend Contin Educ Pract Vet* 2:897–902, 1980.
7. Paquignon A, Tran G, Provost JP: Evaluation of the Clinitek 200 urinary test-strip reader in the analysis of dog and rat urines in pre-clinical toxicology studies. *Lab Anim* 27:240–246, 1993.
8. Primestone NR: Renal degradation of hemoglobin. *Semin Hematol* 9(1):31–42, 1972.
9. Skjold AC, Frwitag JF, Stover LR, Berry HK: Indoxyl sulfate interference with dip-and-read urinary bilirubin estimate. *Clin Chem* 26:1368–1369, 1980.

Section 5: Occult Blood, Hemoglobin, and Myoglobin

INDICATIONS

Common urine tests for blood are designed to detect concentrations of red blood cells, hemoglobin, or myoglobin that are not visible to the human eye. These tests may aid in identifying the cause of abnormal urine color. The presence or absence of red blood cells, hemoglobin, or myoglobin may be of value in localizing the source of proteinuria.

Detection of hemoglobin by chemical means may aid in the interpretation of the significance of urine sediment. Since microscopic examination of urine sediment will not detect free hemoglobin released from lysed red blood cells, total reliance on sediment examination for semiquantitation of hematuria may result in gross underestimation of the degree of hematuria.

The tests may aid in differentiation of microhematuria from hemoglobinuria and myoglobinuria through chemical means. They may also assist in the evaluation of muscle damage associated with release of myoglobin.

METHODOLOGY
Overview

The common tests depend on detection of pseudoperoxidase activity of the heme moiety of hemoglobin and myoglobin in urine and, in some cases, feces (Figure 10-7). The iron-containing porphyrin compounds, commonly referred to as heme (ferriheme or ferroheme), act as a peroxidase in a buffered environment with a variety of peroxide substrates to catalyze oxidation of a test substance. The test substance (benzidine, tetramethylbenzidine, o-toluidine, o-dianisidine, or guaiac) develops various intensities and shades of color depending on the reagent, concentration of heme or other peroxidase and other coloring matter, and the presence or absence of inhibitors. Newer generations of test substances prevent or are more resistant to interference by reducing metabolites such as ascorbic acid, homogentisic acid, and 5-hydroxyindole acetic acid.

The maximum test sensitivity is reagent dependent, with benzidine being the most sensitive and guaiac being the least sensitive. However, benzidine cannot currently be used because of its known carcinogenic properties. Nontheless, manufacturers have fine-tuned current reagents to deliver the required sensitivity.

Myoglobin, like hemoglobin, will cause a positive reaction. Porphyrin without iron will not react with these tests. Intestinal bacterial enzymes may remove the iron from the heme moiety, leaving porphyrin.

For screening tests, evaluations should be performed on well-mixed noncentrifuged samples. See Table 10-9 for instructions on how to perform the most common tests.

Hematest®

Hematest® tablets were developed for feces, in contrast to more sensitive reagent strips, which were developed for urine. The substrate is strontium peroxide; the chromogen is tetra-

Basic Reaction for Detection of Red Blood Cells, Hemoglobin, or Myoglobin

$$\text{Organic } H_2O_2 + \text{Chromogen} \xrightarrow[\text{activity}]{\text{pseudoperoxidase}} \text{Oxidized Chromogen} + H_2O$$
$$\text{(orange through green to blue)}$$

FIGURE 10-7 *Basic biochemical reaction associated with strip and tablet tests for red blood cells, hemoglobin, and myoglobin.*

methylbenzidine. A red dye is present to mask discoloration of the tablet. A mixture of tartaric acid and calcium acetate is also present to buffer the reaction. Sodium bicarbonate is added so that when the tablet is moistened, it will react with tartaric acid to cause effervescence, which aids in solubilizing the reagents and rupturing red blood cells. Small square filter papers are supplied to provide a white background color.

In the presence of hemoglobin (released from lysed red blood cells, free hemoglobin, or myoglobin), monomolecular oxygen is liberated from strontium peroxide and oxidizes the chromogen to produce a blue color change on the white paper background.

Petstix™, Hemastix®, and Multistix®

Like the Hematest® reagent tablets, these reagent strip tests are based on the pseudoperoxidase activity of hemoglobin or myoglobin. Cumen hydroperoxide is the source of peroxide; tetramethylbenzidine is the chromogen. Positive test results may be caused by free hemoglobin, myoglobin, or lysis of numerous red blood cells.

The color of certain test strips (Multistix® and N-Multistix®) can be read by a reflectance meter (Clinitek®) rather than visually. The instrument sensitivity to intact red blood cells is less than that achievable by direct visual observation.

Chemstrip® 4OB, 6, 7, 8, 9, and 10 with SG

This reagent strip test is also based on the pseudoperoxidase activity of red blood cells, hemoglobin, and myoglobin. Each strip contains tetramethylbenzidine (chromogen), 2,5-dimethyl-2,5-dihydroperoxyhexane (peroxide substrate), and a buffer. Release of monomolecular (nascent) oxygen by the action of the pseudoperoxidase on the substrate oxidizes chromogen into a green-blue dye, which, in turn, causes the yellow test zone to turn green.

Chemstrip® may permit differentiation of intact red blood cells from hemoglobinuria through the use of separate color comparison blocks, but there is only one test pad on the strip (as with Multistix®). Hemolysis of a small number of previously intact red blood cells on the test pad initiates production of green spots of varying numbers at that site. If large numbers of intact red blood cells are present, the test zone will become homogeneously green. In this situation the manufacturer suggests that the sample be diluted with physiologic saline solution

TABLE 10-9

SAMPLE PROCEDURES TO SCREEN FOR OCCULT BLOOD, MYOGLOBIN, AND HEMOGLOBIN

Hematest®
- For the screening test, place a drop of well-mixed urine on a piece of square filter paper (or smear a small amount of feces across the test pad).
- Place a reagent tablet in the middle of the moistened area or the area discolored by the feces and then add two drops of water at 5 second intervals in such a fashion as to cause the water to run over the tablet onto the filter paper.
- A positive reaction is indicated by development of a distinct blue ring of color on the paper around the tablet within 2 minutes. The speed and intensity of color development are related to the quantity of red blood cells, hemoglobin, and/or myoglobin in the sample. In our laboratory the time it takes to develop the blue color is recorded according to the following schedule:
  — Negative = no color
  — Trace = slight blue color at 120 seconds
  — 1+ = blue color at <120 seconds
  — 2+ = blue color at <90 seconds
  — 3+ = blue color at <60 seconds
  — 4+ = blue color at <30 seconds
- Color changes that develop after 2 minutes should be ignored. Likewise, the color of the tablet should be ignored, even if it turns slightly blue.

Hemastix®, Multistix®
- Dip the test strip into a well-mixed urine sample and remove it immediately.
- Draw the edge of the strip along the edge of the container top to remove excess urine.
- After 60 seconds, compare the color of the test strip to the color scale on the label.
- A positive reaction is indicated by a color change from colorless to green. With very high concentrations color development may go to blue. Based on the intensity of color change, test results may be recorded as small, moderate, or large.
- Hemolyzed blood or myoglobin appears as a more homogenous green to blue color. Nonhemolyzed red blood cells appear as green dots. High numbers of red blood cells result in a confluent color indistinguishable from free hemoglobin or myoglobin.

to aid in differentiation of intact red blood cells from hemoglobinuria.

A uniformly green coloration of the test pad may be caused by free hemoglobin, myoglobin, or lysis of numerous red blood cells. Partial hemolysis of red blood cells may result in a diffuse green coloration of the test pad in addition to green spots produced by individual cells. In such circumstances the test result may be verified by repeating the procedure using a fresh urine sample.

INTERPRETATION
Specificity
False-Positive Reactions

Peroxidase enzymes in bacteria, white blood cells, epithelial cells, and spermatozoa are potential but very unlikely causes of false-positive reactions. Studies performed using human urine have indicated a high degree of improbability that these sources of peroxidase would cause false-positive reactions.

Feces contain meat and blood products originating from the diet. Heating the sample to 90°F will destroy plant peroxidases but will decrease the amount of positivity of heme by only a small amount. Test the diet before testing feces. If the diet is positive for blood, interpretation of the test result in feces is compromised. Some dog and cat foods are negative, but others are positive.

Contamination of urine with large quantities of iodide or bromide is also a potential, but extremely unlikely, cause of false-positive results. Likewise, contamination with residues of oxidizing agents in disinfectants used to clean tabletops or collection containers may also be associated with false-positive reactions.

Commercially available bilirubin added to dog and rat urine caused false-positive reactions for blood. Bilirubin concentration that are ≥ 64 mg/L and ≥8 mg/L in dog and rat urine, respectively, resulted in a false-positive blood test result.[17] It is possible to get false-positive blood results with commercial bilirubin if it is contaminated with blood. A blood-free bilirubin can be obtained from Kodak.

False-Negative Reactions

Failure to resuspend red blood cells that have settled to the bottom of the collection container may reduce or inhibit positive results. Because of the rapid sedimentation of red blood cells in urine, this is perhaps the most common reason for disparity between sediment examination and chemical test strip results.

Although unlikely to occur, large quantities of nitrite produced by bacteria causing urinary tract infections may delay the reaction. Likewise, large quantities of endogenous or exogenous ascorbic acid (urinary acidifiers, vitamin therapy, drug preservatives, etc.) may interfere with the intensity of the color reaction. Ascorbic acid is a strong reducing agent that reacts directly with H_2O_2 in the reagent pad with the result that H_2O_2 is eliminated from the desired reaction. Use of formalin as a preservative may also cause false-negative results.

Multistix® may permit differentiation of hemoglobin from intact red blood cells. Trace concentrations of hemoglobin (0.015 to 0.062 mg/dl) are equivalent to about 5 to 20 red blood cells. Proportionally more spots will be observed with increasing numbers of red blood cells.

Chemstrip® may permit differentiation of low (10 RBC/μl), moderate (50 RBC/μl), and high (250 RBC/μl) numbers of red blood cells from hemoglobinuria. According to the manufacturer, differentiation at higher numbers may be aided by serial dilution of the sample with physiologic saline solution.

Sensitivity

Visual detection of blood in urine requires about 0.5 ml blood per liter of urine. This corresponds to approximately 2500 red blood cells per microliter.

Hematest® is reported by the manufacturer to have a practical sensitivity of approximately 6 mg of hemoglobin per gram of feces. Other investigators have found the test to be far less sensitive.

For Hemastix® and Multistix® the absolute sensitivity for intact red blood cells is 1 red blood cell per microliter, while the practical sensitivity is 5 to 20 red blood cells per microliter. The sensitivity for free hemoglobin is 0.015 to 0.062 mg/dl, which is also equivalent to 5 to 20 intact red blood cells per microliter. Because of the optical system used in automated reading devices, sensitivity is less for intact red blood cells than it is for hemolyzed blood.

TABLE 10-10

HAPTOGLOBIN BINDING CAPACITIES FOR CATS, DOGS, AND HUMANS

| Species | Capacity | |
	Mean	Range
Cat	111	31–216
Dog	104	14–252
Human	89	30–161

For Chemstrip® the practical sensitivity for red blood cells is 5 red blood cells per microliter and that for free hemoglobin is equivalent to 10 red blood cells per microliter. The concentration of red blood cells on the surface of the test pad from the urine absorbed on the test pad increases the sensitivity for red blood cells over free hemoglobin. The practical sensitivity for myoglobin is not well established.

Correlation of sensitivities between various test methods, including hemocytometer counts and sedimentation examinations, are not good at the very lowest levels.[1]

Applied Physiology
Red Blood Cells

A few red blood cells are often present in the urine of normal dogs and cats. In humans up to 5 red blood cells per microliter (so-called physiologic microhematuria) is normal. Similar quantitative determinations have apparently not been established for normal dogs or cats. Refer to the discussion of red blood cells in Chapter 11 for additional details.

Hemoglobin

Intravascular hemolysis from any cause results in release of free hemoglobin into plasma. Hemoglobin forms a complex with haptoglobin. Haptoglobin binding capacity is variable (see Table 10-10). Once haptoglobin is saturated, free tetrameric hemoglobin (MW = 69,000) appears in the blood, divides into dimeric subunits (MW = 32,000), and is cleared from the blood by the kidneys. Unbound feline hemoglobin is cleared more rapidly then canine hemoglobin. Some unbound plasma hemoglobin releases ferriheme, which reversibly binds to either albumin (methemalbumin) or hemopexin, a plasma protein. Free hemoglobin, hemoglobin-haptoglobin complex, hemoglobin subunits, methemalbumin, ferriheme-hemopexin complex, and bilirubin all contribute to the color of plasma. Hemoglobin complexes in concentrations above about 50 mg/dl of plasma are detectable as pink plasma. Hemopexin and methemalbumin are cleared more slowly from plasma than hemoglobin-haptoglobin.

Hemoglobin is recovered and metabolized by proximal renal tubule cells. This mechanism contributes to bilirubinuria and diminishes urine hemoglobin concentration. Only after the renal tubular uptake mechanism is saturated will hemoglobin protein appear in urine, resulting in hemoglobinuria.

Large quantities of free hemoglobin may also escape into urine if significant numbers of red blood cells undergo lysis within the excretory pathway. Hemolysis results when the urine specific gravity is approximately 1.008 or lower. Alkaline urine contributes to red blood cell lysis in vivo or in vitro.

Myoglobin

Myoglobin is the oxygen-carrying pigment of muscle. Although it is similar to hemoglobin, it has some different physical, chemical, and immunologic properties.

Myoglobinemia of sufficient magnitude to permit detectable myoglobinuria is abnormal. Myoglobinemia and myoglobinuria may occur as a result of traumatic, toxic, or ischemic injury and necrosis (rhabdomyolysis) of muscle cells.

Because of its molecular characteristics, myoglobin readily passes through glomerular capillary walls (MW = 17,000). In contrast to hemoglobin, myoglobin released from damaged muscle does not bind to serum proteins. It is rapidly cleared by the liver and kidney. Therefore detectable myoglobinuria may occur when the plasma concentration of myoglobin reaches 15 to 20 mg/dl. However, this concentration will not cause a color change in plasma.

SIGNIFICANCE
Interpretations and Misinterpretations

Always interpret test results in association with urine specific gravity as well as with microscopic evaluation of urine sediment. A positive chemical test for blood associated with lack of identification of red blood cells in urine sediment might indicate:

- Hemoglobinuria or myoglobinuria
- Generalized hemolysis following hematuria caused by dilute and/or alkaline urine
- A false-positive chemical reaction
- Misidentification of red blood cells in urine sediment as bubbles or fat droplets, for example

A negative chemical test for blood associated with the detection of red blood cells in urine sediment might indicate:

- Use of outdated reagents
- Chemical evaluation of a poorly mixed or centrifuged urine sample
- Conceptually, failure of small numbers of red blood cells to hemolyze
- Misidentification of red blood cells in urine sediment
- A false-negative chemical reaction

Addition of 5% sulfosalicylic acid to red, brown, or black urine with a negative blood test may help differentiate false-negative blood tests from non–heme-containing chromogens. A negative

> **Alkaline urine contributes to red blood cell lysis in vivo or in vitro.**

test for blood in red, brown, or black urine suggests a chromogen other than blood or myoglobin. If addition of 5% sulfosalicylic acid yields a white sediment after centrifugation, nonhemoglobin or myoglobin chromogens are suggested. Precipitate with a red/brown/black color suggests a false-negative test for blood or myoglobin.

Differentiation of hematuria from hemoglobinuria and myoglobinuria is of obvious importance. Centrifugation of an aliquot of a visibly discolored sample and comparison of the supernatant to an uncentrifuged aliquot of the sample may be of value. The supernatant of samples with significant hemoglobinuria or myoglobinuria will remain equally discolored. The supernatant of samples with significant hematuria will be normal in color or far less discolored.

The solubility test for myoglobinuria may aid in its differentiation from hemoglobinuria but is not definitive. To perform the test, adjust the urine pH to 7.5 to 8.0 with NaOH. To 5 ml of urine, add 2.8 g of ammonium sulfate and dissolve by mixing. This will create an 80% solution. Centrifuge or filter the mixture. If the centrifugate or filtrate has an abnormal color, myoglobin is present. If only a normal color is present, the precipitated pigment is hemoglobin. If the centrifugate and precipitated pigment are abnormally colored, both are probably present.

Observation of plasma may aid in differentiation of myoglobinuria from hemoglobinuria. Clear plasma suggests myoglobinuria or hematuria. Hemoglobinuria without icterus suggests acute hemolytic anemia, while both signs suggest chronic hemolytic anemia.

Pink plasma with a positive test for blood in urine suggests intravascular hemolysis. Chocolate-colored whole blood with a positive test for blood in urine suggests specific hemolyzing methemoglobin-producing toxins (oxidants).

A likely chemical cause of a false-positive result is urine contamination with an oxidant. False-positive urine test results for heme may be suggested by clear plasma, normal serum creatine kinase enzyme activity, and lack of protein in urine (see below).

Haptoglobin is an acute phase protein and tends to be elevated in inflammatory disease. However, chronic hemolysis may result in lowering of plasma haptoglobin concentration. Visualization of pink plasma is dependent on sufficient haptoglobin concentrations to bind free hemoglobin. Concentrations of free hemoglobin plus hemoglobin bound to haptoglobin in plasma must exceed 50 mg/dl before they can be seen. Free hemoglobin is rapidly cleared. Therefore it is not as likely to significantly contribute to plasma color.

Other methods that have been used to identify myoglobinuria include:

- Electrophoresis and immunoelectrophoresis
- Spectroscopic analysis
- Ultracentrifugation
- Millipore filtration

Hematuria

Hematuria is a nonspecific indicator of disease of the urinary

TABLE 10-11
CAUSES OF NONURINARY HEMOGLOBINURIA

Genetic and Congenital Causes
Pyruvate kinase deficiency
Phosphofructokinase deficiency[7,8,19]
Old English sheepdog exertional lactic acidosis
Copper-associated liver disease[13]
Methemoglobinemia[6a]

Toxins/Drugs
Chlorates
Benzocaine[11]
Copper
Dimethyl sulfoxide
Ioxosceliem (brown recluse spider)
Menadione (vitamin K_3)
Methionine[16]
Methylene blue[20]
Mercury
Milbemycin (caval syndrome)
Nitrates/Nitrites
Phenazopyridine
Paracetamol (acetaminophen)[6,12]
Phenylhydrazine
Propylene glycol
Propylthiouracil
Snake venom (Elapidae)
Zinc[15]

Poisonous Plants
Onions (dogs)

Physical Agents
Burns (severe)
Crush injury
Electric shock
Extreme exercise/azoturia[9]
Heatstroke
Microangiopathy (caval syndrome, disseminated intravascular coagulation)

Infectious Agents
Babesiosis
Hemobartonellosis (rarely causes intravascular hemolysis)[2]
Leptospirosis (*Leptospira icterohaemorrhagiae*)

Immune-Mediated Causes
Idiopathic immune-mediated hemolytic anemia[14]
Incompatible blood transfusion[4]
Isoerythrolysis (cats)
Systemic lupus erythematosus

Deficiencies
Hypophosphatemia (induced by hyperalimentation or diabetes mellitus)[18]

---

tract. Once its presence has been verified, the next priority of clinical investigation is to localize its source. Possibilities include:

■ Coagulation defects (acquired and genetic)
■ Disseminated intravascular coagulation (shock, pancreatitis, septicemia, etc.)
■ Trauma
■ Neoplasia
■ Infectious diseases
■ Iatrogenic causes

Refer to the discussion about hematuria in Chapter 11 for additional details.

Hemoglobinuria

Hemoglobinuria may have a nonurinary or urinary origin. Nonurinary hemoglobinuria is associated with hemoglobinemia (see examples in Table 10-11). Urinary hemoglobinuria may be caused by extravascular hemolysis induced by dilute and/or alkaline urine.

Myoglobinuria

Myoglobinuria has been an uncommonly encountered disorder in dogs and cats. This may be related, at least in part, to the fact that commonly used screening tests do not permit differentiation between myoglobinuria and hemoglobinuria.

Myoglobinuria may be caused by traumatic, toxic, or ischemic disorders of muscles.

REFERENCES AND SUGGESTED READINGS

1. Bee DE, James GP, Paul KL: Hemoglobinuria and hematuria: Accuracy and precision of laboratory diagnosis. *Clin Chem* 25(10):1696–1699, 1979.
2. Bellamy JC, MacWilliams PS, Searcy GP: Cold agglutinin hemolytic anemia and *Haemobartonella canis* infection in a dog. *JAVMA* 173(4):397–410, 1978.
3. Breitschwerdt EB, Kornegay JN, Wheeler SJ, et al: Episodic weakness associated with exertional lactic-acidosis and myopathy in Old English Sheepdog littermates. *JAVMA* 201:731–736, 1992.
4. Callan MB, Jones LT, Giger U: Hemolytic transfusion reactions in a dog with an alloantibody to a common antigen. *J Vet Intern Med* 9(4):277–279, 1995.
5. Fernandez et al: Dog: Menadione Vit K3: *JAAHA* 20:711–720, 1984.
6. Finco DR, Duncan JR, Schall WD, Prasse KW: Acetaminophen toxicosis in the cat. *JAVMA* 166:469–472, 1975.
6a. Fine DM, Eyster GE, Anderson LK, et al: Cyanosis and congenital methemoglobinemia in a puppy. *JAAHA* 35:33–37, 1999.
7. Giger U, Harvey JW: Hemolysis caused by phosphofructokinase deficiency in English Springer Spaniels: Seven cases (1983–1986). *JAVMA* 191:453–459, 1987.
8. Giger U, Harvey JW, Yamaguchi RA, et al: Inherited phosphofructokinase deficiency in dogs with hyperventilation-induced hemolysis. Increase in vitro and in vivo alkaline fragility of erythrocytes. *Blood* 65(2):345-351, 1985.
9. Glauser SC, Wagner H, Glaucer EM: *Am J Med Sci* 264:135. Blood and myoglobin same color. Hemopexin, 80,000 Heme transport. Greyhound Medicine and Surgery: The T. G. Hungerford Refresher Course for Veterinarians Proc. 12225–12229, Sept 1989, 1972.

10. Greene CE, Cook JR Jr, Mahaffey EA: Clindamycin for treatment of toxoplasma polymyositis in a dog. JAVMA 187(6):631–634, 1985.
11. Harvey JW, Sameck JH, Burgard FJ: Benzocaine-induced methemoglobinemia in dogs. JAVMA 175:1171–1175, 1979.
12. Harvey JW, French TW, Senior DF: Hematologic abnormalities associated with chronic acetaminophen administration in a dog. JAVMA 189:1334–1335, 1986.
13. Hultgren BD, Stevens JB, Hardy RM: Bedlington Terr. Am J Vet Res 47:365, 1986.
14. Klag AR, Giger U, Shofer FS: Idiopathic immune mediated hemolytic anemia in dogs: 42 cases. JAVMA 202(2):783–788, 1993.
15. Luttengen PJ, Whitney MS, Wolf AM, Scruggs DW: Heinz body anemia associated with a high plasm zinc. JAVMA 197(10):1347–1350, 1990.
16. Maede Y, Zhoshino T, Inaba M, Namioka S: Cat: Methionine. Am J Vet Res 48:289–292, 1987.
17. Paquignon A, Tran G, Provost JP: Evaluation of the Clinitek 200 urinary test strip reader in the analysis of dog and rat urine in preclinical toxicology studies. Lab Anim 27:240–246, 1993.
18. Perman V, Shall WD: in Ettinger SJ (ed): Textbook of Veterinary Internal Medicine: Disease of the Dog and Cat, ed 2. Philadelphia, WB Saunders, 1983, pp 1938–2000.
19. Rand JS, O'Brien PJ: Exercise-induced malignant hyperthermia in an English Springer Spaniel. JAVMA 190(8):1013–1014, 1987.
20. Schalm OW: Dog. Methylene blue. Canine Pract 5(2):20–25, 1978.

Section 6: Proteinuria

INDICATIONS

Overview

The quantity and composition of urine proteins vary in normal and abnormal states. Evaluation of urine for protein is included as a part of complete routine urinalysis, because when interpreted in conjunction with other clinical and laboratory findings, test results often aid in detection, localization, and occasionally specific identification of underlying disorders.

Definitions[25,33]

Proteinuria is defined as the detection of protein in urine. Urine proteins are composed of variable quantities of plasma proteins, proteins derived from the urinary tract, and, depending on the method of collection, proteins derived from the genital tract. Proteinuria is normally used to imply the presence of an abnormal quantity (greater than 20 mg/kg/day) of protein in urine.[25] It is a laboratory finding associated with a variety of causes. The term "proteinuria" is preferable to "albuminuria" since more than 40 proteins have been found in normal urine and they may also be present in disease states associated with albuminuria.[1,2,34]

Bence Jones proteinuria is the presence of Bence Jones proteins in urine. These small (MW = 22,000 to 44,000) proteins are named after the English physician Henry Bence Jones, who described their ability to precipitate when urine is gradually warmed (45° to 70°C) and subsequently to redissolve as urine is heated near boiling. Bence Jones proteins are identical to immunoglobulin light chains (compare with paraproteinuria) and may be observed in the urine of patients with neoplastic disorders of plasma cells (multiple myeloma).[35]

Clinically significant proteinuria warrants further investigation of its cause and biologic behavior. It is persistent and exceeds that associated with normal excretion.

Functional proteinuria may occur in association with stress, exercise, fever, seizures, exposure to extremes of temperature, and venous congestion in the kidneys. Although glomerular function is temporarily altered, the process is rapidly reversible. The exact mechanisms are not clear but may be related to changes in glomerular blood flow or in the permeability of capillary walls of glomeruli. Although it must be differentiated from other forms of proteinuria, functional proteinuria has no apparent clinical significance.

Glomerular proteinuria results from pathologic damage to various components of glomerular capillary walls. Glomerular proteinuria is typically persistent and usually involves albumin (66,000 Daltons) and other proteins of high molecular weight (see Table 1-3). Glomerular proteinuria may result in hypoalbuminemia.

Glomerular overload proteinuria (also called protein overload proteinuria) has been experimentally induced in dogs by parenteral administration of large quantities of plasma proteins. As serum protein concentrations rise, large quantities of albumin and other proteins of high molecular weight are excreted in urine. Glomerular morphology is reversibly altered during abnormal protein excretion. Glomerular overload proteinuria should be considered as a cause of proteinuria in dogs with severe hyperproteinemia (greater than 9 g/dl).[25]

Paraproteinuria is a form of overload proteinuria that may occur when complete immunoglobulins, immunoglobulin fragments, macroglobulins, or cryoglobulins produced by neoplastic plasma cells reach abnormally high concentrations in plasma. If readily filtered through glomerular capillary walls, these proteins attain abnormally high concentrations in the urine.

Postglomerular proteinuria results from protein loss arising within the urogenital tract but below the level of the glomerulus. Protein exudation is commonly the result of inflammatory, neoplastic, ischemic, or traumatic diseases. Examples include pyelonephritis, urocystitis, prostatitis, urolithiasis, acute tubular necrosis, and transitional cell carcinomas. Tubular proteinuria may be considered as a form of renal proteinuria (e.g., renal proteinuria may be divided into glomerular and tubular forms), or it may be considered as a form of postglomerular proteinuria.

Preglomular proteinuria refers to proteinuria resulting from abnormalities in systems other than the urogenital tract. Examples include functional proteinuria and overload proteinuria.

Selective proteinuria may occur in association with mild to moderate glomerular pathology. Minimally damaged glomerular capillary walls allow passage of plasma proteins within a narrow range of molecular weights (approximately 60,000 to 80,000 Daltons; Table 1-3). If glomerular lesions worsen, however, plasma proteins of all sizes and weights easily pass through the capillary walls (i.e., nonselective proteinuria).

Tubular proteinuria is characterized by excretion of plasma proteins of low molecular weight (1,500 to 45,000 Daltons) as a result of defective resorption by proximal tubules. Protein electrophoresis may reveal prominent alpha and beta bands, which are characteristic of tubular proteinuria. In humans, excreted proteins typically include beta-2-microglobulin, lysozyme, alpha-microglobulin, and alpha-acid glycoprotein in addition to many amino acids (Table 1-3).[35] Tubular diseases do not cause hypoalbuminemia.

Tubular overload proteinuria may be associated with excessive production of serum proteins of low molecular weight (less than 45,000 Daltons). Such proteins easily pass through

TABLE 10-12
SAMPLE PROCEDURES TO SCREEN FOR PROTEINURIA

Sulfosalicylic Acid Turbidimetric Test
- Prepare a 3% to 5% solution from reagent grade powder. A 5% solution is preferred for veterinary application.
- Place 10 drops of clear urine into a clean, dry test tube and add an equal amount of sulfosalicylic acid solution. If the urine is very alkaline, add 20 drops of sulfosalicylic acid. To clear a cloudy urine sample, first centrifuge or filter it. Alternatively, heat it to 38° to 40°C to clear it.
- Thoroughly mix the solution and determine the degree of turbidity according to the following list (applicable only when an equal volume of urine is mixed with an equal volume of test reagent):
  — No turbidity = Negative (less than 10 mg/dl)
  — Trace = Faint precipitate visible against a black background (10 mg/dl)
  — 1+ = Small degree of turbidity (10 to 50 mg/dl)
  — 2+ = Moderate turbidity (50 to 200 mg/dl)
  — 3+ = Heavy turbidity (200 to 500 mg/dl)
  — 4+ = Heavy flocculation (greater than 500 mg/dl)
- If turbidity in the original sample cannot be eliminated, compare a tube containing 10 drops of the original urine plus 10 drops of water to the tube containing the 10 drops of urine plus 10 drops of test solution.

Dipstick Colorimetric Tests
- Immerse the dipstick into the urine sample and remove it immediately.
- Compare the color of the test strip to the color chart:
  — Trace = 5 to 20 mg/dl
  — 1+ = 30 mg/dl
  — 2+ = 100 mg/dl
  — 3+ = 300 to 500 mg/dl
  — 4+ = 600 to 2000 mg/dl

Bence Jones Protein Heat Test
- Place 4 ml of urine into a test tube.
- Add 1 ml of acetate buffer and mix. The final pH should be 4.9 ± 0.1. To make acetate buffer (pH 4.9 2M), place 17.5 g of sodium acetate trihydrate into a volumetric flask, add 4.1 ml of glacial acetic acid, and add water to 100 ml.
- Heat for 15 minutes in a 56°C water bath. Formation of a precipitate is indicative of Bence Jones proteinuria.
- If there is turbidity or a precipitate at 56°C, heat the same tube in a boiling water bath for 3 minutes and check for a decrease in the amount of precipitate or turbidity. Bence Jones proteins will redissolve at 100°C.
- An increase in turbidity or precipitate at boiling temperatures indicates the presence of globulins or albumin and will mask the presence of dissolving Bence Jones protein. If this occurs, filter the contents of the tube taken directly from the boiling water bath and observe the filtrate as it cools. If it is initially clear, becomes cloudy as it cools, and then becomes clear at room temperature, the test is positive for Bence Jones protein.
- A heavy precipitate of Bence Jones protein may not redissolve on boiling. In this instance the test should be repeated with dilute urine.
- The urine specimen should be fresh or refrigerated since heat-coagulable protein will denature or decompose when allowed to remain at room temperature. The altered proteins may give a false-positive result.

---

glomerular capillary walls and overload tubular resorptive mechanisms. The result is protein loss through the kidneys. Examples of this condition include hemoglobinuria, myoglobinuria, and paraproteinuria.

METHODOLOGY[32,33]
Generalities

There are a number of reasons why it is more difficult to measure and identify urine proteins than serum proteins:

- Urine proteins are often present in very small quantities.
- There is a large sample-to-sample variation in the amount and composition of urine protein.
- Protein in urine is derived from plasma, the urinary tract, and sometimes the genital tract.
- Protein degradation products are concentrated by the kidney and may be measured along with intact proteins.

Qualitative, semiquantitative, and quantitative methods are available for analysis of protein. Most tests employed in conjunction with routine urinalyses provide qualitative and semiquantitative results. Methods to identify and quantify urine proteins, including protein electrophoresis, gel filtration, and immunochemical techniques, have been described.[35]

Sample Collection

As with all diagnostic tests of routine urinalyses, analyses should be performed only on samples collected prior to administration of diagnostic or therapeutic agents. Although screening tests for protein are commonly performed on uncentrifuged samples, turbidimetric tests should be performed using the supernatant of centrifuged samples to eliminate positive results caused by proteinaceous material commonly found in urine sediment (red blood cells, white cells, epithelial cells, casts, etc.).

Either fresh or refrigerated samples may be used. In one study no significant change in protein concentration was detected in urine samples preserved by refrigeration at 4° to 10°C for 4 weeks. However, this observation is not a recommendation for use of samples refrigerated for more than 24 to 48 hours.

Procedures for commonly used tests are shown in Table 10-12.

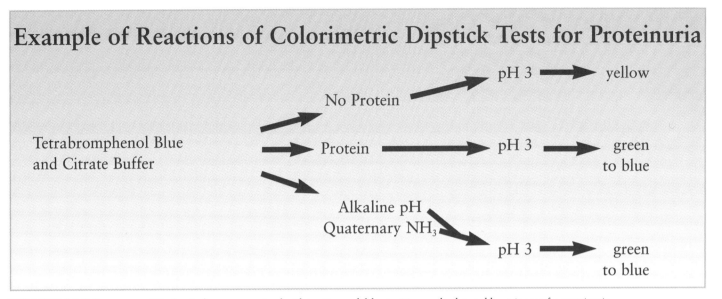

FIGURE 10-8 *Reagents and biochemical events associated with positive and false-positive results detected by strip tests for proteinuria.*

Sulfosalicylic Acid Turbidimetric Test

This test is based on the fact that sulfosalicylic acid will precipitate urine protein with resultant turbidity that is approximately equal to the quantity of protein present. It is less convenient than dipstick tests for urine protein. The results are semiquantitative since not all proteins form the same type of precipitate in terms of the quantity of precipitate per milligram of protein. Test results may also be altered if urine turbidity is caused by nonprotein substances. This problem may be minimized by use of aliquots of supernatant following centrifugation of urine. A 3% to 7% solution of sulfosalicylic acid from reagent grade powder[a] mixed with an equal volume of urine is commonly used. The magnitude of turbidity should be compared to the magnitude of turbidity in a "control" sample containing an aliquot of urine supernatant to which water has been added rather than sulfosalicylic acid.

Dipstick Colorimetric Test

This test is based on the phenomenon called the "protein error of pH indicator dyes" (Figure 10-8). In simple terms the test is based on the ability of amino groups of proteins to bind with and alter the color of some acid-base indicators even though the sample pH remains constant by way of a buffer in the test pad. When some indicator dyes react with proteins (anions), they release hydrogen ions and cause a change in color. Binding of the dye is dependent on the number of free amino groups of each protein. Albumin has more free amino groups than globulins, hemoglobin, Bence Jones proteins, and mucoproteins. In one study it was found that the development of the same color change as that caused by a certain albumin concentration required a globulin concentration two times as high and a mucoprotein concentration three times as high.[16] Because of reduced capacity to detect globulins, Bence Jones proteins, hemoglobin, and mucoprotein, test results are semiquantitative.

Tetrabromphenol blue or tetrachlorophenol-tetrabromosulfonphthalein are yellow at a pH of 3. At a pH of 4 they are blue or green. Commercially prepared strips are impregnated with the indicator dye and citrate buffer, which maintains a pH of 3. Addition of protein in varying concentrations will result in an increasing color change from yellow to greenish-blue to blue or yellow to light green to green even though the pH remains at 3.

Commercial strips include Albustix®, Bili-Labstix®, Combistix®, Hema-Combistix®, Labstix®, Multistix®, Petstix™, Uristix®, and Chemstrip®.

Although the protein reagent is the least sensitive to environmental factors, it is wise to protect strips from prolonged exposure to excessive heat, humidity, and light. Because the test is based on a buffer system, the strips should be protected in their original container. The cap of the storage bottle should be replaced immediately following use.

Bence Jones Proteinuria

The Bence Jones heat test is based on the unusual thermosolubility properties of Bence Jones proteins. Electrophoretic and immunoelectrophoretic methods provide the best results.

Albumin and globulins do not coagulate and precipitate out of solution until they are heated to a temperature of 56° to 70°C. The degree of turbidity may increase as the temperature rises. Bence-Jones proteins precipitate at 40° to 60°C and redissolve as the temperature rises to 85° to 100°C. As the temperature cools, Bence-Jones proteins may reprecipitate at 40° to 60°C and redissolve at lower temperatures. Because of this unique heat solubility, Bence Jones proteins are sometimes called "pyroglobulins."

Twenty-Four Hour Urine Protein Determination

The protein concentration in urine may vary widely from specimen to specimen. Because of the unpredictable variability of protein excretion throughout the day, quantitative determinations should be based on 24 hour aliquots. Samples should be collected with the aid of a metabolism cage. Preservatives such as toluene are satisfactory, but the aliquot for analysis should be taken from below the toluene-layered surface of the 24 hour sam-

TABLE 10-13
EQUATIONS[a] FOR CALCULATION OF DAILY URINE PROTEIN EXCRETION[25]

Method of Analysis	Regression Equation (protein mg/kg/day)
Coomassie brilliant blue (Dog)	3.1 + (19.2 × UP/UC)
Trichloroacetic acid–Ponceau-S (Dog)	2.8 + (28.72 × UP/UC)
Coomassie brilliant blue (Cat)	29.39 (UP/UC)+ 0.18

UP/UC = protein-creatinine ratio of urine.
[a]Equations used to determine urine protein loss were constructed from previously reported values by designating the urine protein-creatinine ratio as the dependent variable in a linear regression analysis.

ple. The Coomassie brilliant blue and trichloroacetic acid–Ponceau-S of protein in biologic fluids are recommended to measure urine protein concentration. They are precise and sensitive methods requiring spectrophotometric analysis.

Urine Protein-Creatinine Ratios

Twenty-four hour urinary protein excretion may also be reliably estimated by determining urine protein-creatinine ratios.[25] Urine samples submitted for analysis should be collected by cystocentesis or during midstream voiding. The sample should then be centrifuged to separate particulate matter (cells) from dissolved substances (protein). The supernatant is saved for determination of protein and creatinine concentrations. The sediment and remaining supernatant should be used for routine urinalysis. The urine protein-creatinine ratio is obtained by dividing the protein concentration (mg/dl) by the creatinine concentration (mg/dl). The result is a unitless ratio:

■ Less than 0.5 = normal
■ 0.5 and 1.0 = questionable
■ Greater than 1.0 = abnormal

Unlike the qualitative dipstick tests, the ratio is not affected by urine concentration and volume. Petstix™ 8, a new urinalysis reagent strip from Bayer, has a test zone for creatinine that can be used to obtain semiquantitative protein-creatinine ratios. Unpublished data from a University of Minnesota study have shown a 92% agreement between strip and reference ratio in the negative population (ratio <0.5).

Urine protein-creatinine ratios of single, randomly collected urine samples have excellent correlation with the protein content of 24 hour urine samples obtained from normal dogs and from dogs with glomerular dysfunction. These observations indicate that when renal function is stable, glomerular filtration and tubular concentration mechanisms affect protein and creatinine

similarly. Consequently, urine protein-creatinine ratios offer the accuracy of 24 hour urine protein measurements.

Equations used to determine daily protein loss (mg/kg) in urine were constructed from previously reported values by designating the urine protein-creatinine ratio as the dependent variable in a linear regression analysis (Table 10-13). Daily protein loss in urine can be calculated by solving the equation once the urine protein-creatinine ratio has been determined. Knowledge of the laboratory method used to determine urine protein concentration is essential for selection of the correct equation. The daily urine protein loss may also be interpolated from published charts.[19,40]

Urine protein-creatinine ratios may be used to help confirm significant proteinuria. Urine protein concentrations that persistently exceed normal limits are clinically significant.

Screening tests (dipstick dye or sulfosalicylic acid) used to detect urine protein are sensitive to protein concentrations between 5 and 30 mg/dl. In dilute urine, significant concentrations of protein may remain undetectable by these procedures or may appear to be so low that they are misinterpreted as insignificant. Because urine protein-creatinine ratios are unaffected by urine concentration and volume, they aid in the accurate assessment of urine protein loss in patients with urine of low specific gravity.

Urine protein-creatinine ratios may be used to help differentiate preglomerular, glomerular, and postglomerular proteinuria.[25] In general, urine protein-creatinine ratios are relatively low in urine of patients with preglomerular and postglomerular proteinuria and some patients with primary glomerular disease. If hyperproteinemia is not present and there are no abnormal cells in urine sediment, an elevated urine protein-creatinine ratio is strong evidence of glomerular dysfunction. Most of the patients with urine protein-creatinine ratios greater than 5.0 have primary glomerular disease.[25]

Urine protein-creatinine ratios may be markedly elevated in patients with significant hemorrhage or inflammation affecting urine that passes through the excretory pathway. We have observed protein/creatinine ratios greater than 10 in urine of dogs with staphylococcal infection of the lower urinary tract. Therefore urine protein-creatinine ratios should always be interpreted with knowledge of results of complete urinalysis.

INTERPRETATION
Overview

Interpretation of proteinuria is dependent on:

■ Knowledge of types and quantities of proteins normally present in urine

> Urine protein-creatinine ratios offer the accuracy of 24 hour urine protein measurements.

- Conceptual understanding of methods used to detect urine proteins
- The etiology and pathophysiology of disorders associated with proteinuria

Collect urine samples for detection of urine protein prior to the administration of diagnostic and therapeutic agents. Because mild proteinuria may be transient and of little clinical significance, verify its existence and persistence before pursuing potentially costly and time-consuming diagnostic plans to determine its cause and before initiating therapy to control or correct it.

Always interpret qualitative and semiquantitative tests in light of urine specific gravity. Most screening tests for proteinuria are performed on a small volume of urine without regard to the rate of formation of urine or total volume. For example, mild proteinuria (1+) in the presence of a low specific gravity (i.e., 1.005) implies a greater loss of protein than mild proteinuria (1+) in a more concentrated sample (i.e., specific gravity of 1.040).

Before considering the underlying cause of significant proteinuria, try to localize its source. Localization is aided by knowledge of the method of urine collection and the composition of urine sediment (Table 2-3).

Because of significant discrepancies among various laboratory tests for proteinuria, its clinical significance should always be interpreted in association with other clinical and laboratory findings. The absence of proteinuria does not eliminate the presence of renal disease or renal failure. Likewise, the severity of proteinuria is not a reliable index of the severity or reversibility of the underlying disorder.

Specificity of Tests[32,33]
Sulfosalicylic Acid Turbidimetric Test

Sulfosalicylic acid will precipitate urine protein with resultant turbidity that is approximately equal to the quantity of protein present. False-positive results or overestimated positive results may be obtained if an aliquot of centrifuged urine is not used.

Radiopaque contrast agents that are excreted in urine will give a false-positive reaction; radiopaque contrast agents will also increase urine specific gravity. Massive doses of penicillin, cephalothin, cephaloridine, and sulfisoxazole have been reported to give a false-positive reaction for protein with sulfosalicylic acid in humans. Highly buffered alkaline urine may give false-negative reactions (especially if a 3% rather than a 5% solution is used).

Because measurement of the degree of turbidity (i.e., 1+ to 4+) is not standardized, variability in test results between individuals and different laboratories may occur.

The preservatives thymol and para-amino salicylic acid may give a false-positive protein reaction with this test. Unlike colorimetric tests, however, sulfosalicylic acid will detect Bence Jones proteins in urine.

Dipstick Colorimetric Test

Results are not affected by urine turbidi-

ty. The urine pH of all domestic animals is 4.5 to 5.0 or higher. Changes of pH within physiologic ranges of dilute urine usually do not affect test results. Highly alkaline dilute urine or moderately alkaline concentrated urine may induce false-positive results. The buffer capacity of concentrated urine, as is often found in dogs and cats in contrast to humans, can exceed the buffer capacity of the reagent strip, even when the pH is not extremely alkaline. The increase in pH will result in a false-positive reaction. Acidification of urine for the purpose of preventing false-positive results should be avoided, since it will require a considerable amount of acid that will either dilute the urine (if added in a dilute form) or precipitate the protein and damage other analytes (if added in a concentrated form). When a false-positive result is suspected, it should be confirmed with another method. The Petstix™ 8 strip is likely to minimize misinterpretation of false-positive protein results by providing a creatinine ratio. As with all tests, false-positive results could also occur if the strip were allowed to remain in the urine sample for a sufficient period for the test reagents to be leached out.

As described above, colorimetric reagents are more sensitive to albumin than globulins, including hemoglobin and myoglobin. They may not detect Bence-Jones proteins unless they are present in large quantities.

Negative results are usually significant, with the notable exception of pure Bence-Jones proteinuria. False-negative results may occur if a sample is acidified following collection as the protein may precipitate out of solution.

Benzalkonium (Zephiran®), a cationic quaternary ammonium surface-acting antimicrobial agent, and chlorhexidine may give false-positive results if sufficient residues remain in collection containers.[19] Phenazopyridine may cause false-positive reactions with Chemstrip®, and infusion of polyvinyl pyrrolidone as a plasma expander has been reported to cause false-positive reactions with this product in humans.

Sensitivity of Tests

For the sulfosalicylic acid turbidimetric procedure the test range is between trace (5 mg/dl) and 5000 mg/dl or greater. For the dipstick colorimetric procedure the test range is between trace (approximately 5 to 30 mg/dl) and 1000 mg/dl+. Trace positive results are commonly encountered in concentrated urine samples obtained from normal dogs and cats. Consult Table 10-14 for additional information.

Reactions of 4+ detected by colorimetric dipstick and turbidimetric tests occur with as little as 0.5 to 1.0 g/100 ml but cannot be used by themselves to estimate the exact quantity of protein, however. We have evaluated dogs with generalized glomerular disease characterized by 4+ dipstick and sulfosalicylic test reactions that have excreted as little as 1 g and as much as 35 g of protein in their urine over 24 hours. Quantitation of 4+ screening test reactions for urine protein requires use of urine protein-creatinine ratios or determination of the quantity of protein excreted in urine over 24 hours.

> **Albumin constitutes approximately 40% to 60% of the total protein normally excreted in urine because it is not completely resorbed by renal tubule cells.**

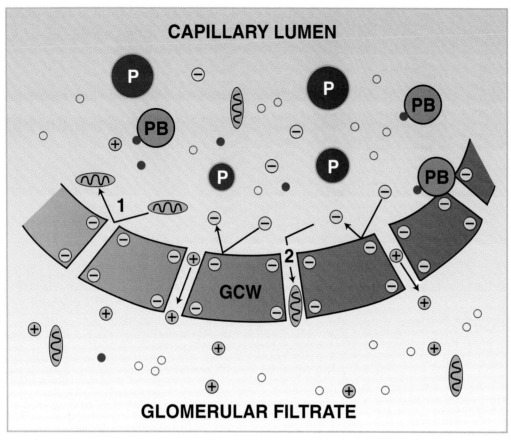

CAPILLARY LUMEN

GCW

GLOMERULAR FILTRATE

FIGURE 10-9 *Schematic illustration of some factors influencing the selective permeability of glomerular capillary walls to filtration of protein molecules. 1 = viscous drag associated with friction caused by passage of protein molecule through glomerular pores; 2 = steric hindrance caused by malalignment of elongated protein molecules with glomerular pores; P = large protein molecule. PB = increased size associated with binding of small and large molecular weight proteins. The small, negatively charged protein molecules in the glomerular capillary lumen are repelled by the negatively charged capillary wall. In contrast, small, positively charged protein molecules in the glomerular capillary lumen are attracted by the negatively charged capillary wall and pass into glomerular filtrate.*

Applied Physiology
Renal Handling of Protein

Although the precise mechanism by which proteins are handled by the kidneys are still not completely understood, the major variables involved are:

■ Glomerular selective permeability
■ Tubular reabsorption and disposal of absorbed proteins

Glomerular Permeability (Figure 10-9)

The capillary walls of glomeruli are semipermeable filters that retain most of the plasma proteins in the vascular compartment. Glomerular capillary walls are composed of the following three layers: capillary endothelial cells, noncellular basement membranes, and cytoplasmic processes (extensions) of renal epithelial cells (podocytes). The processes wrap around portions of capillary loops. Collectively, these three layers form the functional units (the so-called filtration barrier) of glomeruli.

As blood flows through glomeruli, a large quantity of an acellular, low protein ultrafiltrate is formed. The degree to which individual proteins are normally filtered through glomerular capillary walls is a function of their plasma concentration and their molecular size, shape, and charge.[10] In other words, the primary factors that influence the movement of proteins across glomerular capillaries are the size-selective properties of glomeruli, the charge-selective properties of glomeruli, and hemodynamic forces operating across glomerular capillary walls.

In general, transport of protein molecules through glomerular capillary walls progressively diminishes as protein size (as estimated from molecular weight) increases (Table 1-3). Normally, proteins of high molecular weight (e.g., immunoglobulin M, which has a molecular weight of 900,000 Daltons) do not appear in glomerular ultrafiltrate in detectable amounts.

Even though plasma contains high concentrations of albumin, small quantities of albumin are normally present in glomerular ultrafiltrate, partly because albumin has a molecular weight of approximately 66,000 to 68,000 Daltons. In addition, fixed negative charges on glomerular capillary walls impede the passage of negatively charged plasma molecules, such as albumin. Plasma proteins with molecular weights of 1,500 to 45,000 Daltons pass through more readily but appear in urine in lower concentrations because of their relatively low concentrations in plasma and tubular recovery from glomerular filtrate.

Although hemoglobin has a small molecular size, it normally does not enter glomerular ultrafiltrate because it is usually bound to haptoglobin, which is a larger plasma protein (Table 1-3). This phenomenon is called protein binding.

Peptides (including several hormones) appear in glomerular ultrafiltrate, but are reabsorbed by the renal tubules.

Tubular Reabsorption and Disposal of Absorbed Protein

Normally, only a small quantity of protein is present in glomerular filtrate. In one study in dogs the quantity of protein in proximal tubular fluid was 10 to 15 mg/dl or less.[13]

The proportion of filtered plasma proteins ultimately excreted in urine depends on the extent of resorption by renal tubules. Albumin constitutes approximately 40% to 60% of the total protein normally excreted in urine because it is not completely resorbed by renal tubule cells.[21,37] In contrast, plasma proteins of low molecular weight are actively resorbed from tubular filtrate, catabolized by proximal tubular cells, and returned to the blood as amino acids. The renal tubules also degrade a variety of peptide hormones, including parathormone, insulin, growth hormone, and thyrotropic hormone. Distal renal tubule cells secrete small amounts of protein (Tamm-Horsfall mucoprotein and possibly secretory immunoglobulin A), which add to the final urine protein concentration.[35,38]

Proteins Originating from the Urinary Tract

It has been estimated that 40% to 60% of the proteins normally present in urine originate from the distal tubules and collecting ducts (Tamm-Horsfall mucoprotein), the epithelial lining of the lower urinary tract, and the genital tract (prostatic, semen-related, and vaginal secretions).[35] Tamm-Horsfall protein has been reported at a concentration of 0.5 to 1.0 mg/dl in canine urine.[37] The urothelium may also secrete immunoglobulins, especially IgA, as a part of local host defenses against ascending urinary tract infections.[35]

Normal Urine Protein Concentration

Few investigators have performed controlled studies of large numbers of dogs and cats to assess normal daily excretion of protein in urine. Additional confusion concerning normal protein excretion exists because various methods used for protein determination give significantly different results. In one study, for example, the Coomassie brilliant blue method consistently yielded higher protein concentrations than were obtained by use of the trichloroacetic acid–Ponceau-S method on identical samples.[21] Differences were greater with higher protein concentrations. Likewise, two groups of investigators using the same method to determine urine protein concentration (Coomassie brilliant blue method) reported different values for normal dogs. Grauer et al. reported that young adult beagles excreted 0.6 to 5.1 mg/kg/day of protein.[19] This value is lower than that reported by McCaw et al., who determined that normal canine outpatients ranging in age from 0.5 to 10 years excreted protein at a rate of 1.8 to 22.4 mg/kg/day.[26] Using the trichloroacetic acid–Ponceau-S method for urine protein determination, Center et al. and White et al. found similar results (maximum protein excretion was 11.7 mg/kg/day).[8,44]

Biewenga et al. evaluated 29 clinically normal dogs of various breeds, sexes, and ages and reported a range of 2.7 to 23.3 mg/kg for daily protein excretion.[2] Although the subjects were clinically and biochemically normal, immunofluorescent staining methodology revealed immune deposits of glomeruli in about half of the dogs. The significance of these deposits was not determined.

Seventeen dogs (6 males and 11 females) evaluated by DiBartola et al. had urine protein excretion of 4.55 to 28.3 mg/kg/day.[12] Dogs with active urine sediment (more than five white cells per high power field and/or more than five red blood cells per high power field) were included in this group, which may account for the higher protein excretion values than those reported by other investigators. The 24 hour urine protein excretion by male dogs (16.5 ± 10 mg/kg/day) was not significantly different from that of female dogs (12.4 ± 6.1 mg/kg/day) in the small sample of dogs evaluated.

On the basis of these observations, we concluded that a urine protein concentration in adult dogs in excess of 20 mg/kg/day evaluated by either the Coomassie brilliant blue method or trichloroacetic acid–Ponceau-S is abnormal.[25] This value corresponds to a urine protein-creatinine ratio between 0.67 and 0.96 according to the linear regression equations established for dogs.[19,44]

Physiologic proteinuria occurs in the neonate of many species including puppies and kittens but not in human infants. Proteinuria peaks within 20 hours and persists for 10 days for puppies.[4,24] The proteinuria coincides with the absorption of protein from the gut.

Hoskins et al. found that mean 24 hour urine protein excretion values for 4 to 30 week old kittens (range of 2.54 ± 1.81 mg/kg at 4 weeks to 11.39 ± 7.61 mg/kg at 14 weeks) varied from week to week of age.[22] Urine protein was determined by the Coomassie brilliant blue dye–binding method.

The sensitivity of commonly used tests for proteinuria is below the protein content of most normal urine samples. Therefore persistent proteinuria of sufficient quantity to be detected by the usual laboratory tests should be investigated. Trace and 1+ results are commonly observed with colorimetric dipstick tests on concentrated urine samples obtained from normal dogs and cats. If reagent strip tests are used as screening tests for proteinuria, positive findings may be confirmed with a test based on different biochemical reactions, such as the sulfosalicylic acid test.

Abnormal Urine Protein Concentration (Tables 10-14 and 10-15 and Figure 10-10)

Proteinuria may be classified (localized) as preglomerular, glomerular, or postglomerular.[25]

Preglomerular Proteinuria

Preglomerular proteinuria results from abnormalities of systems other than the urogenital tract. Preglomerular proteinuria can be further subdivided into functional proteinuria and overload proteinuria.

Functional proteinuria is sometimes associated with strenuous exercise, extremes of heat and cold, stress, fever, seizures, or venous congestion.[9] In humans functional proteinuria apparently results from alterations in glomerular blood flow or in permeability of glomerular capillary walls.[11] Decreased tubular resorption of filtered proteins can also occur.[36] Although glomerular function is temporarily altered, the process is rapidly reversible. Functional proteinuria typically consists of mild, transient albuminuria.

Tubular overload proteinuria is associated with excessive production of plasma proteins of low molecular weight (e.g., immunoglobulin fragments, myoglobin, or hemoglobin) or the reduction in available binding sites on carrier molecules (e.g., haptoglobin for hemoglobin).[17,31,41] When

> Albumin constitutes approximately 40% to 60% of the total protein normally excreted in urine because it is not completely resorbed by renal tubule cells.

TABLE 10-14

EXAMPLES OF DIFFERENT CAUSES OF PROTEINURIA

Factors	Cause					
	Normal Concentrated Sample	Contaminated With Hypaque[a]	Glomerular Disease	Urinary Tract Infection	Hemoglobinuria	Hemorrhage
Color	Yellow	Yellow	Yellow	Yellow	Red	Reddish
Turbidity	Clear	Slightly cloudy	Clear	Cloudy	Clear	Cloudy
Specific gravity	1.060	1.065	1.026	1.018	1.035	1.035
pH	6.5	6.0	6.5	8.0	6.5	6.0
Glucose	Negative	Negative	Negative	Negative	Negative	Negative
Acetone	Negative	Negative	Negative	Negative	Negative	Negative
Bilirubin	Trace	Negative	Negative	Negative	Negative	Negative
Protein	1+	3+	4+	3+	2+	2+
Occult blood	Negative	Negative	Negative	3+	3+	4+
Red blood cells/hpf	1–2	Negative	Negative	100+	None	Too numerous to count
White cells/hpf	0–1	None	0–1	Too numerous to count	None	1–3
Casts/lpf	None	None	1–3 hyaline	None	1–3 granular	None
Epithelial cells	Occasional	Occasional	Occasional	Many	Occasional	Moderate
Bacteria	None	None	None	Many rods	None	None
Crystals	None	None	None	Struvite	None	Occasional amorphous urate

[a]Sulfosalicylic acid.

plasma concentrations of proteins that weigh less than 45,000 Daltons (and that therefore easily pass through glomerular capillary walls) are increased, the resorptive mechanisms of the tubules become overloaded. Detectable quantities of protein then appear in urine.

Glomerular overload proteinuria (also called protein overload proteinuria) has been experimentally induced in dogs and rats by parenteral administration of large quantities of plasma proteins.[23,40,42] When plasma protein concentrations were above 9 g/dl, large quantities of albumin and other proteins of high molecular weight were excreted in urine. Alterations in glomerular morphology were detected in rats during episodes of hyperproteinemia and proteinuria.[30,43] Glomerular abnormalities consisted of numerous protein resorption droplets as well as swelling and obliteration of the foot processes of epithelial cells. These changes completely reversed after resolution of hyperproteinemia and proteinuria. Glomerular overload proteinuria should be considered to be a cause of proteinuria in animals with severe hyperproteinemia (e.g., in patients with multiple myeloma or ehrlichiosis or after overzealous administration of plasma).[5,7,27–29,39]

Glomerular Proteinuria

Glomerular proteinuria is the most commonly recognized and potentially most severe form of renal proteinuria. It results from disease-induced alterations of glomerular capillary barriers, which normally prevent loss of larger plasma proteins into glomerular infiltrate. Damage can be characterized by loss of the fixed negative charges of glomerular capillaries. In addition, structural changes in filtration barrier may result from primary disorders (e.g., antiglomerular basement membrane disease, inflammation, or neoplasia) or secondary disorders (e.g., immune complex deposition, amyloidosis, hyperfiltration, or hyperadrenocorticism). Protein in the urine of patients with these forms of glomerular dysfunction primarily consists

TABLE 10-15

MAGNITUDE OF PROTEINURIA COMMONLY ASSOCIATED WITH SELECTED URINARY AND NONURINARY DISORDERS

Disorder	Reaction of Urine to Strip Tests or Sulfosalicylic Acid			
	Trace to 100 mg	100–500 mg	500–1000 mg	>1000 mg
Nonurinary				
Strenuous exercise	±			
Fever	±			
Hyperproteinemia (>10 g/dl)	±	±	Uncommon	
Congestive heart failure	±			
Inflammatory or hemorrhagic diseases of the genital system	+	+	±	±
Urinary: Renal				
Glomerular	+	+	+	+
Tubular	+	±		
Inflammatory	+	+	+	±
Hemorrhagic	+	+	+	±
Urinary: Ureter, Bladder, Urethra				
Inflammatory	+	+	+	±
Hemorrhagic	+	+	+	±

of albumin and varying quantities of proteins of high molecular weight (e.g., immunoglobulins and coagulation proteins).

Although the origin of protein cannot be consistently predicted on the basis of the quantity of protein detected by urinalysis, persistent proteinuria in moderate to large quantities that occurs in the absence of hematuria or pyuria indicates generalized glomerular disease.

Postglomerular Proteinuria

In postglomerular proteinuria, plasma or tissue proteins gain access to urine after it has passed through the glomeruli. Postglomerular proteinuria can result from normal genital secretions or from disruption of the epithelial linings of the urogenital tract by inflammation, neoplasia, ischemia, or trauma. Occasionally, the disorder results from defects in proximal tubular resorption of proteins of between 1,500 and 45,000 Daltons; this condition is called tubular proteinuria.[20] In humans almost 50 proteins have been identified in patients with tubular proteinuria (including enzymes, polypeptide hormones, immunoglobulin fragments, and microglobulins).[35] This form of proteinuria is typically mild and may not be detected by qualitative screening tests for proteinuria. Familial (e.g., Fanconi's syndrome) and acquired (e.g., gentamicin toxicity) causes of tubular proteinuria have occurred in dogs.[3,6,15]

Postglomerular proteinuria can usually be differentiated from glomerular proteinuria by evaluating clinical signs and urine sediment. The disorder is often associated with leukocyturia and/or erythrocyturia or both; leukocytes and erythrocytes are typically absent in the urine of patients with glomerular proteinuria.

It may be difficult to recognize a combination of glomerular proteinuria and postglomerular proteinuria. The combination may have been present if cell-free proteinuria persists after successful treatment of postglomerular inflammation or hemorrhage. If successful treatment of postglomerular proteinuria is not possible, detection of high concentrations of albumin in urine should prompt consideration of concurrent glomerular dysfunction, especially if hypoalbuminemia is also detected.

Since dipstick tests for protein are performed with uncentrifuged urines, they are also a highly sensitive indicator of casts, although they cannot differentiate between proteinuria and casts.

Pseudoproteinuria (False-Positive Proteinuria)

False-positive reactions for protein detected by colorimetric dipsticks include:

- Highly alkaline-buffered urine as might result after administration of alkalinizing drugs or following degradation of urea to ammonia by urease-producing bacteria
- Loss of reagents from the dipstick as a result of prolonged immersion in the urine sample
- Contamination of the sample with quaternary ammonium compounds (e.g. disinfectants)

False-positive reactions for protein detected by sulfosalicylic acid include:

- Turbid urine prior to initiation of the test
- Radiopaque contrast agents excreted in urine[16]
- Excretion of large quantities of penicillin, cephaloridine, or sulfisoxazole
- Contamination of the test sample with thymol, a urine preservative

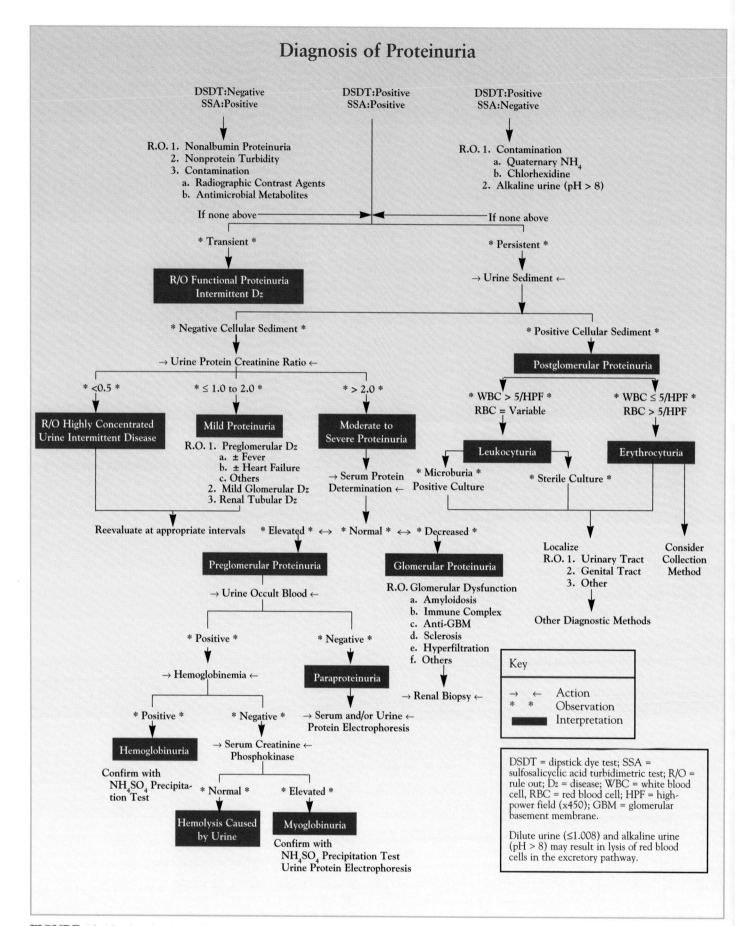

FIGURE 10-10 *Algorithm for the diagnosis of proteinuria. (From Lulich JP, Osborne CA: Interpretation of urine protein-creatinine ratios in dogs with glomerular and nonglomerular disorders. Compend Contin Educ Pract Vet 12:59, 1990.)*

■ Coprecipitation of crystals caused by sulfosalicylic acid–induced change in urine pH
■ Any substance precipitated by acid

False-Negative Proteinuria

False-negative reactions for protein detected by colorimetric dipsticks include:

■ Low to moderate amounts of Bence Jones proteins
■ Examination of a urine sample that has been acidified following collection (protein precipitates as a result of acidity)

False-negative reactions for proteins detected by sulfosalicylic acid include:

■ Evaluation of highly buffered alkaline urine
■ Inability to read the results because of evaluation of turbid uncentrifuged urine.

aSigma Chemical Co., St. Louis, MO.
bWinthrop, New York, NY.

REFERENCES AND SUGGESTED READINGS

1. Berggard I: Plasma proteins in normal human urine, in Manuel Y, Revillard JP, Betuel H (eds): *Proteins in Normal and Pathological Urine*. Basel, Karger, 1970, pp 7–19.
2. Biewenga WJ, Gruys E, Hendricks HJ: Urinary protein loss in the dog. Nephrological study of 29 dogs without signs of renal disease. *Res Vet Sci* 33:366–374, 1982.
3. Bovee KC, Joyce T, Blazer-Yost B, et al: Characterization of renal defects in dogs with a syndrome similar to the Fanconi syndrome in man. JAVMA 174:1094–1099, 1979.
4. Brambell FWR: The passive immunity of the young mammal. *Biol Rev* 33:488–531, 1958.
5. Breitschwerdt EB, Woody BJ, Zerbe CA, et al: Monoclonal gammopathy associated with naturally occurring canine ehrlichiosis. *J Vet Intern Med* 1:2–9, 1987.
6. Brown SA, Rakich PM, Barsanti JA, et al: Fanconi syndrome and acute renal failure associated with gentamicin therapy in a dog. JAAHA 22:635, 1986.
7. Center SA, Smith JF: Ocular lesions in a dog with serum hyperviscosity secondary to an IgA myeloma. JAVMA 181:811–813, 1982.
8. Center SA, Wilkinson E, Smith CA, et al: 24-hour urine protein-creatinine ratio in dogs with protein-losing nephropathies. JAVMA 187:820–823, 1985.
9. Coye RD, Niehoff R, Rammer M, et al: Proteinuria associated with experimentally produced abscesses and fever in dogs. *AMA Arch Path* 68:126–133, 1959.
10. Deen WM, Satvat B: Determinants of the glomerular filtration of proteins. *Am J Physiol* 241:F162–F170, 1981.
11. Dennis VW, Robinson RR: Proteinuria, in Seldin DW, Giebisch G (eds): *The Kidney: Physiology and Pathophysiology*. New York, Raven Press, 1985, pp 1805–1816.
12. DiBartola SP, Chew DJ, Jacobs G: Quantitative urinalysis including 24-hour protein excretion in the dog. JAAHA 16:537–546, 1980.
13. Dirks JH, Clapp JR, Berliner RW: The protein concentrations in the proximal tubule of the dog. *J Clin Invest* 43:916–921, 1964.
14. Easley JR, Breitschwerdt EB: Glucosuria associated with renal tubular dysfunction in three basenji dogs. JAVMA 168:938–943, 1976.
15. Feeney DA, Walter PA, Johnston GR: The effect of radiopaque contrast media on the urinalysis, in Kirk RW (ed): *Current Veterinary Therapy IX*. Philadelphia, WB Saunders, 1986, pp 1115–1117.
16. Free EL, Rupe CO, Metzler I: Studies with a new colorimetric method for proteinuria. *Clin Chem* 3:716, 1957.
17. Giger U, Harvey JW: Hemolysis caused by phosphofructokinase deficiency in English springer spaniels. JAVMA 191:453–459, 1987.
18. Glover JF, Wallach J: Positive dipstick test for albumin when other renal function tests are normal. JAMA 223:928, 1973.
19. Grauer GF, Thomas CB, Eicker SW, et al: Estimation of quantitative proteinuria in the dog using the urine protein-to-creatinine ratio from a ran-

dom voided sample. *Am J Vet Res* 46:2216–2119, 1985.
20. Hall CW, Chung-Park M, Vacca CV, et al: The renal handling of beta 2-microglobulin in the dog. *Kidney Int* 22:156–161, 1982.
21. Harvey DG, Hou CM: The use of paper eletrophoresis for routine identification of urinary proteins in the dog. *J Small Anim Pract* 7:431–440, 1966.
22. Hoskins JD, Turnwald GH, Kearney MT, et al: Quantitative urinalysis in kittens from four to thirty weeks after birth. *Am J Vet Res* 52:1295–1299, 1991.
23. Lambert PP, Gassee JP, Askenasi R: Physiologic basis of protein excretion, in Manuel Y, Revillard JP, Betuel H (eds): *Proteins in Normal and Pathological Urine*. Basel, Karger, 1970, pp 67–82.
24. Loh SW, Bourne FJ, Curtis J: Urine protein levels in the pig. *Anim Prod* 15:273–283, 1972.
25. Lulich JP, Osborne CA: Interpretation of urine protein ratios in dogs with glomerular and nonglomerular disorders. *Compend Contin Educ Pract Vet* 12:59–72, 1990.
26. McCaw DL, Knapp DW, Hewett JE: Effect of collection time and exercise restriction on the prediction of urine protein excretion using urine protein-creatinine ratio in dogs. *Am J Vet Res* 46:1665–1669, 1985.
27. Matus FE, Leifer CE, Gordon BR, et al: Plasmapheresis and chemotherapy of hyperviscosity syndrome associated with monoclonal gammopathy in the dog. JAVMA 183:215–218, 1983.
28. Matus FE, Leifer CE, MacEwen EG, et al: Prognostic factors for multiple myeloma in the dog. JAVMA 188:1288–1292, 1986.
29. Miller C, Fish MB, Danelski TF: IgA multiple myeloma with multisystem manifestations in the dog: A case report. JAAHA 18:53–56, 1982.
30. Mori H, Yamasshita H, Nakanishi C, et al: Proteinuria induced by transplantable rat pituitary tumor MLT SAS. *Lab Invest* 54:636–644, 1986.
31. Nelson DA, Davey FR: Erythrocyte disorders, in Henry JB (ed): *Clinical Diagnosis and Management by Laboratory Methods*. Philadelphia, WB Saunders, 1984, pp 652–703.
32. Osborne CA, Stevens JB: Clinical significance of proteinuria. Proceedings of the 45th Annual Meeting of the American Animal Hospital Association, Salt Lake City, 1978, pp 527–543.
33. Osborne CA, Stevens JB: *Handbook of Canine and Feline Urinalysis*. St. Louis, Ralston Purina, 1981.
34. Pesce AJ: Methods used for analysis of proteins in urine. *Nephron* 13:93–104, 1974.
35. Pesce AJ, First MR: *Proteinuria: An Integrated Review*. Marcel Dekker, New York, 1979.
36. Poortman JR: Post exercise proteinuria in humans. JAMA 253:236–240, 1985.
37. Porter P: Comparative study of the macromolecular components excreted in urine of dog and man. *J Comp Path* 74:108–118, 1964.
38. Schenk EA, Schwartz RH, Lewis PA: Tamm-Horsfall mucoprotein. I-Localization in the kidney. *Lab Invest* 25:92–95, 1971.
39. Shull RM, Hayden DW, Johnston GR: Urogenital blastomycosis in a dog. JAVMA 171:730–735, 1977.
40. Terry R, Hawkins DR, Church EN, et al: Proteinuria related to hyperproteinemia in dogs following plasma given parenterally. *J Exp Med* 87:561–573, 1948.
41. Torrance AG, Fulton RB: Zinc-induced hemolytic anemia in a dog. JAVMA 191:443–444, 1987.
42. Vernier RL, Papermaster BW, Olness K, et al: Morphologic studies of the mechanism of proteinuria. *Am J Dis Child* 100:476–478, 1960.
43. Weening JJ, VanGuildener C, Daha MR, et al: The pathophysiology of protein-overload proteinuria. *Am J Pathol* 129:64–73, 1987.
44. White N, Oliver NB, Reimana K, et al: Use of protein-to-creatinine ratio in a single urine specimen for quantitative estimation of canine proteinuria. JAVMA 185:882–883, 1984.

Section 7: Urobilinogen

INDICATIONS

Urobilinogen is a colorless tetrapyrrole metabolite of bilirubin, produced by the action of anaerobic bacteria.

Evaluation of urine for urobilinogen is typically used as a screening test of human patients for:

■ Hepatic disorders
■ Hemolytic disorders
■ Patency of the bile ducts

Unlike the situation in humans, we have not found routine examination of urine for urobilinogen to be particularly useful. Because this test is commonly included with multiple test reagent strips designed for testing human urine (Multistix®, Chemstrip®, etc.), we have included a discussion of this procedure. Tests for urine urobilinogen are not included in the Petstix™ reagent strip system. We do not routinely test for urobilinogen as a part of routine complete urinalyses in our clinical laboratories.

A computer search of 10,787 canine urinalysis records yielded only 0.015% positive urobilinogen tests. Of these only 0.006% were equal to or greater than 1+. Of 2070 feline urine samples only 0.015% were positive and only 14 were equal to or greater than 1+.

METHODOLOGY[1,2]

Because urobilinogen is very unstable, meaningful results can only be obtained by analysis of fresh urine samples. Urobilinogen may be oxidized to urobilin (a dark greenish compound) in the bladder if urine is acid or if it is exposed to light following collection.

Urobilin will not result in a positive reaction with commonly used screening tests for urobilinogen (see Table 10-16).

Multistix® SG, 9, 10SG, N-Multistix®, N-Multistix® SG

These reagent strip tests are based on a modification of the standard Ehrlich's aldehyde reaction. The test pad contains strongly acid-buffered paradimethylaminobenzaldehyde and a color enhancer (Figure 10-11). Urobilinogen reacts with this reagent to form a pink-red condensation product.

Chemstrip® 8, 9, 10 SG

The reagent test pad on these strips is impregnated with a diazonium salt (p-methoxybense-benzene diazofluoroborate) and a strong acid buffer. Urobilinogen reacts with the diazonium salt to form a red azo dye.

Confirmatory Testing

The Watson-Schwartz test is used to confirm the color developed on the reagent strip and to extract colors caused by urobilinogen into a chloroform layer. Colors caused by porphobilinogen and other Ehrlich's reactive compounds will not be extracted. This procedure is recommended for use only by chemists.

One part urine is mixed with an equal volume of Ehrlich's reagent (0.7 g p-dimethylamineobenzaldehyde, 150 ml concentrated HCl, and 100 ml distilled water). Add two parts of saturated sodium acetate and mix well. A light pink to red color is positive.

TABLE 10-16

SAMPLE PROCEDURES TO SCREEN FOR UROBILINOGEN

Multistix® SG, 9, 10SG, N-Multistix®, N-Multistix® SG
- Immerse the reagent pad into a fresh urine sample and rapidly remove it.
- Compare the color of the test strip to the color scale after 1 minute. The scale comprises five color blocks (from light yellow to dark brown) corresponding to 0.2, 1, 2, 4, and 8 Ehrlich units. One Ehrlich unit is equivalent to 1 mg/dl. The test cannot be relied on to detect the complete absence of urobilinogen.

Chemstrip® 8, 9, 10 SG
- Immerse the test pad in a fresh urine sample and rapidly remove it.
- After 30 to 60 seconds compare the test pad to the color scale composed of five colors (from white to pink to red) corresponding to normal urobilinogen concentration in urine and to pathologic values of 1, 4, 8, and 12 mg/dl. Intermediate values may be estimated by interpolation. No color change or colors paler than the color for 1 mg/dl indicate a normal human urobilinogen concentration. The color for the normal value corresponds to a urine urobilinogen concentration of approximately 0.4 mg/dl.

Add a small volume of chloroform and mix. Color caused by urobilinogen will be extracted into the chloroform.

INTERPRETATION
Specificity
Multistix®

Metabolites of para-amino salicylic acid, sulfonamides (specifically sulfisoxazole), and other compounds with aromatic amines may cause false-positive reactions. They usually form brown to red condensation products. Phenazopyridine may result in production of a red color because of marked acidity of the buffer in the reagent pad.

Metabolites normally found in varying quantities in urine (including indole, skatole, and indican) may cause a false-positive reaction. On the other hand, oxidation of urobilinogen in stale urine samples may inhibit or reduce a positive reaction.

Formaldehyde at concentrations of 200 mg/dl or higher inhibit the reaction in human beings. Sources include urine preservatives and methenamine (a urinary antiseptic).

Reaction of Multistix® for Urobilinogen

p-Diethylaminobenzaldehyde + Color Enhancer + Urobilinogen $\xrightarrow{\text{strong acid pH}}$ Pink Compound

FIGURE 10-11 *Reagents and biochemical events associated with positive Multistix® test for urobilinogen.*

A sufficient concentration of nitrite will depress or inhibit the reaction as a result of oxidation of urobilinogen to urobilin. Urobilin will not react with these reagents to produce a characteristic color change.

Chemstrip®

This test is reported to have greater specificity than tests based on Ehrlich's aldehyde reaction. It is not affected by indole, skatole, or indican in physiologic or pathologic concentrations.

As for Multistix®, phenazopyridine may result in production of a red color because of the marked acidity of the buffer in the reagent pad and oxidation of bilirubin in stale urine samples may inhibit or reduce a positive reaction.

High concentrations of formaldehyde will inhibit or depress positive reactions. Nitrites have less tendency to interfere with this test than those based on Ehrlich's aldehyde reaction, although they still have the potential to do so at concentrations greater than 5 mg/dl.

Bilirubin occasionally produces a pale grayish-green color after 1 minute (possibly due to biliverdin).

Sensitivity

Renal excretion of urobilinogen is pH dependent, being augmented in alkaline and suppressed in acid urine. Urine urobilinogen excretion may be enhanced by administration of alkalinizing agents such as sodium bicarbonate. Urine urobilinogen excretion may be reduced by administration of urinary acidifiers.

Oral administration of antimicrobial agents may reduce the population of enteric bacteria and therefore interfere with conversion of bilirubin to urobilinogen.

Multistix®

These tests are not capable of detecting reduced quantities or absence of urine urobilinogen. The color block equivalent to 0.1 Ehrlich unit may be caused by urea.

In the absence of nitrite a negative reaction eliminates pathologic urobilinogenuria. A positive reaction requires further investigation because of its nonspecificity.

Chemstrip®

This test is not capable of detecting reduced quantities or absence of urine urobilinogen. The practical limit of sensitivity is 1.0 mg dl; the absolute limit of sensitivity is 0.4 mg/dl.

Applied Physiology

Following excretion into the small intestine, conjugated bilirubin is reduced to several colorless chromogens called urobilinoids by anaerobic bacteria. One of these metabolites is urobilinogen.

Most of the urobilinogen is excreted in the feces; however, some (an estimated 10% to 20%) is absorbed into the portal venous system. Most of the absorbed urobilinogen is reexcreted into the intestinal tract by the liver (an estimated 80%). This phenomenon is sometimes referred to as the enterohepatic circulation. A small quantity gains access to the systemic circulation; if it is not bound to carrier proteins, it is filtered by glomeruli.

In addition to glomerular filtration, urobilinogen may gain access to the urinary tract by proximal tubular secretion. Urobilinogen present in tubular lumens may be reabsorbed by pH-dependent nonionic diffusion in the distal tubules.

The concentration of urobilinogen in urine is dependent on:

- Quantity of conjugated bilirubin transported to the intestine in bile
- Efficiency of bacterial conversion of bilirubin to urobilinogen
- Quantity of urobilinogen absorbed from the intestine
- Efficiency of the liver in removing urobilinogen following absorption

REFERENCES AND SUGGESTED READINGS

1. Kutter D et al.: Usefulness of a new test strip for detecting urobilinogen in urine. *Deutsch Med Wochenschr* 98:112, 1973.
2. Levy M, Lester R, Levinsky NG: Renal excretion of urobilinogen in the dog. *J Clin Invest* 47:2117-2124, 1968.

Section 8: Nitrituria

Nitrate is a normal constituent of urine and is of dietary origin. Normally, nitrite, the reduced form of nitrate, is not found in urine. However, nitrite is produced by some bacteria.

Significant bacteriuria is usually defined in terms of quantitative cultures. However, the nitrite detection method was suggested as a screening method for detection of bacteriuria. A positive result suggests significant bacteriuria.

Clinical evaluation of this test in dogs and cats revealed that it will not consistently detect significant bacteriuria; therefore it is unsuitable for use in these species.

Section 9: Leukocytes

INDICATIONS

Significant numbers of white cells (leukocyturia) indicate active inflammatory lesions somewhere along the urinary or genital tract that has come in contact with urine. Active inflammation is associated with an underlying cause(s) of disease which may or may not be associated with microbial infections.

METHODOLOGY

The leukocyte reagent strips detect leukocyte esterases found in cytoplasmic azurophilic granules of granulocytes (neutrophils, eosinophils, and basophils), monocytes, and macrophages. Lymphocytes are not detected by this reagent strip method.

The reagent pad contains an ester (derived pyrrole amino acid ester in Multistix®, and indoxylcarbonic acid ester in Chemstrip®), a diazonium salt, and a buffer. Esterases in leukocytes hydrolyze the ester to an aromatic compound (3-hydroxy-5-phenyl pyrrole in Multistix®). An azo-coupling reaction immediately occurs between the liberated pyrrole and the diazonium salt to produce a purple color. Using a standard color chart supplied by the manufacturer, color changes are interpreted visually as negative (beige) to varying shades of violet recorded as trace, 1+, 2+, or 3+.

Tests for detection of esterase activity in leukocytes are insensitive in dogs. A leukocyte esterase test strip was found to be specific (93.2%) but insensitive (46%) when used to evaluate canine urine specimens for pyuria.[1] In studies performed at the University of Minnesota, the sensitivity of this test for leukocytes was 75 cells/µl (very poor), but the specificity was 100%. Although the leukocyte esterase test pad has a low sensitivity in dogs (25 to 75 leukocytes/microliter), it has a high specificity for bacteriuria. Unpublished data from the University of Minnesota and University of Guelph Veterinary Teaching Hospitals using the Multistix® 10SG leukocyte reagent revealed 62% sensitivity with 100% specificity for bacteria in 111 urine samples obtained from dogs. In other words, when the leukocyte reagent pad was positive for white cells, quantitative bacterial cultures of urine samples were also positive.

Leukocyte esterase tests for urine white cells are positive in most feline urine samples that do not contain leukocytes; therefore the leukocyte esterase reagent strip test is of no diagnostic value in this species. When used to evaluate feline urine specimens for pyuria, a leukocyte esterase test was observed to be moderately sensitive (77%) but highly nonspecific (34%) compared with microscopic sediment evaluation.[2]

The mechanism(s) associated with false-positive reactions to this test in cats is unknown. However, freezing cat urine samples eliminates the false-positive reactions. It is possible that feline esterases of non-leukocyte origin hydrolyze the leukocyte esterase test strip reagent. Perhaps these esterases contribute to the innate resistance that cats have to bacterial UTI.

INTERPRETATION

The test for leukocytes is limited to detection of cells containing esterase enzyme activity (granulocytes and macrophages, but not lymphocytes). Detection of granulocytes (neutrophils, eosinophils, and basophils) is typically an indication of inflammatory disease. White cells associated with bacteria, fungi, or parasite ova in sufficient number to be seen by light microscopic examination of urine sediment indicate that the inflammatory lesion has been caused or complicated by urinary tract infection.

More than five white cells per high power field is generally considered to be abnormal, and is called pyuria. However, the total number of white cells found in urine is affected by many factors including method of collection, method of preservation, sample volume and concentration (i.e., specific gravity), magnitude of white cell destruction following collection, and technique of detection.

White cells rapidly lyze in alkaline or hypotonic urine. This phenomenon could produce a positive leukocyte esterase test result in the absence of significant microscopic pyuria. Consult the section entitled White Cells in Chapter 11 for further details about factors that influence white cell numbers in urine.

Urine white cell numbers may be reduced if patients with inflammatory disorders of the urinary tract are given glucocorticoids or nonsteroidal antiinflammatory drugs.

Substances that color urine red in an acid medium, such as

phenazopyridine or nitrofurantoin, may alter the color of the reagent pad so that its color resembles a positive reaction.

Detection of significant numbers of white cells in samples collected by cystocentesis localizes the site of inflammation to at least the urinary tract. However, it does not exclude the urethra or genital tract. White cells may reflux from the urethra into the urinary bladder of dogs with inflammatory prostatic disease.

REFERENCES AND SUGGESTED READINGS

1. Vail DM, Allen TA, Weiser G: Applicability of leukocyte esterase test strip in detection of canine pyuria. JAVMA 189:1451–1453, 1986.
2. Holan KM, Kruger JM, Gibbons SN, Swenson CL: Clinical evaluation of a leukocyte esterase test-strip for detection of feline pyuria. *Vet Clin Path* 26:126–131, 1997.

Section 10: Urine Specific Gravity

INDICATIONS

Unlike the situation in humans, we have not found urine specific gravity reagent pads included on some urine diagnostic test strips to be reliable. We do not recommend currently available products for use in dogs or cats.

METHODOLOGY

Indirectly measuring urine specific gravity with test strips is based on the change in pK (the pH at which acid is 50% ionized) of a polyelectrolyte in the test pad in relation to the concentration of ionic solutes in urine.[1] This method is not influenced by nonionic urine analyses, such as urea, glucose, or protein.

The test pad is impregnated with a polyelectrolyte (polymethylvinyl ether/maleic acid in Multistix®, and ethyleneglycol-bis tetra-acetic acid and in Chemstrip®), and a pH indicator (bromthymol blue) and is maintained at an alkaline pH. When the test pad is immersed in urine, the pKa of the polyelectrolyte reagent decreases, thus releasing protons in proportion to the concentration of urine ionic analytes. The protons released from the polyelectrolyte decrease the pH of the test pad causing a color change in the indicator dye from dark blue-green (SG = 1.000) to yellow-green (SG = 1.030). Consult the section on methodology of urine specific gravity in Chapter 9 for additional details.

INTERPRETATION

Because the highest value that these reagent strips can detect is approximately 1.025 to 1.030, they are unsatisfactory for detection of adequate renal concentrating capacity in dogs or cats. We have also found them to be unreliable in less concentrated urine samples because urine from these species have greater buffering capacity than human urine.

REFERENCES AND SUGGESTED READINGS

1. Cialla AP, Newsome B, Kaster J: Reagent strip method for specific gravity. *Lab Med* 16:38–40, 1985.

Chapter 11

Ultimately, compassion can be measured only by the action it prompts.

C.A.O.

Urine Sediment: Under the Microscope

INDICATIONS

The value of microscopic examination of urine sediment in the interpretation of urinalysis is comparable to microscopic examination of blood smears in the interpretation of hemograms. Interpretation of urine color, specific gravity, turbidity, protein, occult blood, and pH test results of routine analyses is enhanced by knowledge of the composition of urine sediment. For example, a moderate degree of proteinuria in the absence of significant numbers of red and white cells usually indicates proteinuria of glomerular origin; in contrast, a moderate degree of proteinuria associated with hematuria and pyuria indicates an inflammatory response somewhere along the urinary and/or genital tract. If proteinuria is detected without knowledge of hematuria and/or pyuria, it may be erroneously assumed that protein originated from lesions in glomeruli or tubules.

Examination of urine sediment is especially important in the detection and evaluation of crystals, white cells, various types of epithelial cells, casts, bacteria, yeast cells or hyphae, and parasites. These elements cannot reliably be detected by "dipstick" analysis.

Examination of urine sediment may be considered to be a form of biopsy (exfoliative cytology). Like other techniques of exfoliative cytology, the morphologic characteristics of cells, casts, crystals, bacteria, and the like provide useful information, but frequently they do not permit establishment of a specific

Most figures in this chapter appear in the color plate section following p. 150.

diagnosis (Table 11-1). Although disease states may be established on the basis of positive findings, they cannot always be eliminated by exclusion on the basis of negative findings. Therefore the results of examination of urine sediment must be interpreted in combination with other clinical data, including the physical and chemical characteristics of urine.

A frequently asked question is whether or not microscopic examination of urine sediment should be performed on all urine specimens submitted for diagnostic analysis. The question is primarily one related to economics as microscopic evaluation of sediment is the most time consuming part of urinalysis. Therefore, the answer is not "always" or "never." The answer is related to the goal of evaluating the urine sample. If all components of multiple test reagent strips are normal for nonturbid urine obtained from a patient without any evidence of current or previous urinary tract disease, the microscopic evaluation of sediment will also, in all probability, be normal. In this instance, in our opinion it would be acceptable not to evaluate urine sediment by microscopy.

METHODOLOGY

To minimize variations in sediment examination from sample to sample, it is recommended that all personnel be trained to follow a standard sequence of steps. Even with standardization of technique, reproducible semiquantitative results are often difficult to obtain. The procedure to be followed for preparation of urine sediment for microscopic examination with a bright field microscope is outlined in Table 11-2.

TABLE 11-1

CORRELATION OF SOME COMMON URINARY TRACT DISEASES WITH EXPECTED MICROSCOPIC FINDINGS IN URINE SEDIMENT

Diseases[a]	RBCs	WBCs	Hyaline Casts	Granular Casts	WBC Casts	Epithelial Cells	Bacteria	Struvite Crystals	Urate Crystals	Ca-Ox Crystals
Glomerular amyloidosis	0	0	1+ to 2+	0 to 1+	0	0 to 1+	0	0	0	0
Chronic renal failure	0 to 1+	0 to 1+	0 to 1+	0 to 1+	0	0 to 1+	0	0	0	0
Chronic E. coli pyelonephritis[b]	0 to 3+	0 to 3+	0	0 to 2+	0	0 to 2+	0 to 2+	0	0	0
Acute Proteus spp. pyelonephritis	2+ to 4+	2+ to 4+	0	1+ to 4+	0 to 2+	1+ to 4+	1+ to 4+	2+ to 4+	0	0
Lower urinary tract E. coli infection[b]	3+ to 4+	3+ to 4+	0	0	0	3+ to 4+	3+ to 4+	0	0	0
Portovascular shunt and urate urocystoliths[c]	0 to 4+	0 to 4+	0	0	0	0 to 3+	0	0	0 to 4+	0
Calcium oxalate urocystoliths[c]	0 to 4+	0 to 4+	0	0	0	0 to 3+	0	0	0	0 to 4+
Struvite urocystoliths with staphylococcal urinary tract infection	3+ to 4+	3+ to 4+	0	0	0	3+ to 4+	3+ to 4+	3+ to 4+	0	0
Idiopathic feline lower urinary tract disease[b]	3+ to 4+	0 to 1+	0	0	0	0 to 1+	0	1+	0	0

[a]Based on the assumption that other concomitant diseases are not present.
[b]Assuming concomitant uroliths are not present.
[c]Assuming secondary bacterial urinary tract infection is not present.
0 = negative; 1+ = occasional; 2+ = few; 3+ = moderate; 4+ = many.

Microscopes

The availability of a quality microscope greatly enhances evaluation of urine sediment. In addition to standard light microscopy, other microscopic techniques may be of value. Phase contrast microscopy, based on conversion of differences in refractive index to differences in contrast, facilitates more detail of structures with a refractive index similar to that of urine. Polarizing light microscopy is useful in evaluation of urine crystals and identification of cholesterol.

Sample Collection

Strive to collect uncontaminated urine samples in an appropriate container. Good test results cannot be obtained from poor samples. Be sure to accurately label the body of the container (not the lid).

Because the nature of urine sediment may be altered to a variable and unpredictable degree following elimination from the body, analysis of a freshly voided sample provides the most reliable results. One of the most detrimental alterations that occurs when urine is allowed to remain at room temperature following collection is a variable change in pH secondary to proliferation of bacterial contaminants and escape of CO_2 from urine into the atmosphere

Urease-producing bacteria alkalinize urine; alkaline urine promotes disruption, fragmentation, or lysis of red blood cells, casts, and especially white cells within a few hours and may alter crystal composition as well. Some bacteria produce acidifying metabolites and lower urine pH. These changes may be minimized by the addition of preservatives such as toluene or formaldehyde, but preservatives interfere with one or more chemical test results.

Preservation of Sample

Delay in examination may also result in loss of cellular detail due to degenerative mechanisms. If urinalysis cannot be performed within 30 minutes following collection, the sample should be immediately refrigerated to minimize changes caused by bacterial contaminants and autolysis. Refrigerated but not frozen samples are suitable for sediment examination several hours after collection.

Mixing Sample

Before transferring an aliquot of urine into a test tube for centrifugation, properly mix the entire sample. Failure to adequately mix a urine specimen before removing an aliquot for centrifugation may result in loss of formed elements, which rapidly settle to the bottom of the collection container.

TABLE 11-2
PROCEDURE FOR PREPARATION OF URINE SEDIMENT

- Collect urine specimen in appropriate container.
- Mark the body of the container with appropriate identification.
- If analysis cannot be performed within 30 minutes of time of collection, refrigerate sample.
- Thoroughly mix specimen, and transfer a standard volume (we prefer 5 ml) to a conical tip centrifuge tube.
- Centrifuge the sample for 3 to 5 minutes at 450g (1500 to 2000 rpm).
- Remove the supernatant with a transfer pipette or by decanting, and save for chemical analysis. Allow a standard volume (approximately ½ ml) of supernatant to remain in the test tube.
- Thoroughly resuspend the urine sediment in the remaining supernatant by agitation of the tube or "finger-flipping" of the tube.
- Transfer a drop of reconstituted sediment to a microscope slide with a transfer pipette, and place a coverslip over it.
- Subdue the intensity of the microscope light by lowering the condenser and closing the iris diaphragm.
- Systematically examine the entire specimen under the coverslip with the low power objective, assessing the quantity and type (casts, cells, crystals, etc.) of sediment.
- Examine the sediment with the high power objective to identify the morphology of elements, and to detect bacteria.
- Record the results.

If the specimen is very turbid, centrifugation may yield too much sediment for proper evaluation. In this circumstance examination of a noncentrifuged aliquot should be considered. Alternatively, a portion of the sediment may be diluted with physiologic saline solution.

Standardized Volume to Be Centrifuged

Although some authors recommend the transfer of 10 to 15 ml of urine to a conical tip centrifuge tube, the actual volume is not critical. More important is the use of a consistent volume of urine each time so that the diagnostician can develop some perspective of normal and abnormal findings at that volume. Charts of normal or expected results should indicate the volume of urine used to prepare the sediment from which the data were generated. We routinely use 5 ml of urine because of difficulties associated with consistently obtaining larger volumes from companion animals. The volume of urine should be recorded on the urinalysis results form. Normal reference values in this manual are based on 5 ml samples.

Centrifuge Tubes

Although round tip centrifuge tubes may be used, conical tip tubes are recommended because they facilitate removal of

the supernatant by decanting. Different types of centrifuge tubes should not be intermixed because different tubes may affect the quantity of sediment formed and thus results of sediment evaluation.

Centrifugation

The sample should be placed in a capped centrifuge tube that is centrifuged at a relatively low rate of speed (or relative centrifugal force) for approximately 5 minutes. Centrifugation at high gravitational force or for prolonged periods may induce artifacts in cells, casts, and other structures.

In context of standardizing technique, the concept of relative centrifuge force rather than revolutions per minute should be adopted because it eliminates variables associated with different models of centrifuges such as varying length of centrifuge arms. Centrifugation of urine at a relative centrifuge force of 450 is recommended. However, the speed in rpm required to obtain a "g" force of 450 varies with different centrifuges.

The revolutions per minute on the centrifuge tachometer can be converted to relative centrifuge force by using the following formula:

$$\text{Relative centrifuge force} = 1.118 \times 10^{-5} \times \text{Radius of the centrifuge arm (cm)} \times \text{Revolutions per minute}$$

The radius of the centrifuge arm is equal to the length of the rotor from its center to the outermost portion of the test tube cup when it is in the horizontal position.

The duration of centrifugation is less important than the speed of centrifugation, although it is recommended that both be standardized. We recommend a duration of 5 minutes.

Caution: When the power to the centrifuge stops after 5 minutes, rapidly slowing the rotor arm to a stop with a brake is not recommended because it may result in resuspension of a portion of the sediment. This would result in an erroneous decrease in the number of structures in the sediment preparation.

If the urine is centrifuged at high speeds, the sediment may become distorted as a result of packing in the bottom of the tube. When the packed sediment is forcefully resuspended in the supernatant, fragile formed elements may fragment.

It is noteworthy that there may be a wide variation in recovery of cells following centrifugation. In one human study only 50% of erythrocytes and 40% of leukocytes present in urine before centrifugation could be recovered afterward.[10]

Removing Supernatant

The supernatant should be carefully removed from the test tube by decanting (inverting the tube and pouring off the supernatant) or transferring it with a disposable pipette. It should be saved for chemical determinations. Care should be used not to disturb the sediment.

Since the concentration of formed elements detected by microscopy is significantly influenced by the volume of supernatant allowed to remain in the test tube, this portion of the procedure should be standardized. We recommend that ½ ml of urine be allowed to remain in the tube.

Resuspending Sediment

The next step is to manually resuspend (or "reconstitute") the sediment. Sediment may not be grossly visible. Whether or not a button of sediment in the bottom of the centrifuge is observed, the tube should be thoroughly mixed with the remaining supernatant by flipping the tube with a finger or by gentle aspiration and discharge from a disposable pipette. If the sediment is not thoroughly reconstituted, heavy elements, such as casts, may remain in the bottom of the tube and escape detection. If special water-soluble stains (e.g., Kova stain[a] or Sedistain[b]) are to be used, they should be added before the sediment is resuspended (refer to the following section describing sediment stains). One drop of stain is usually mixed with one drop of sediment.

If a sufficient quantity of sediment is available, it is recommended that a portion be saved for unstained examination and another for staining. Use of stains dilute the sediment and alter semiquantitative evaluation of results.

Standardizing Sediment Aliquot

Next, the quantity of resuspended sediment to be examined should be standardized. A drop of reconstituted sediment should be transferred to a clean microscope slide with a disposable pipette. An automatic pipette with polypropylene tip is superior to a manual pipette. The drop to be examined should be standardized and sufficiently large to include the entire area under the coverslip but not so large that it would cause the coverslip to float. If disposable pipettes are used to transfer sediment to the microscope slide, different sizes and brands should not be used interchangeably.

The coverslip is then placed over the preparation. The use of a glass coverslip is recommended because it:

- Promotes the formation of a uniformly thin layer of sediment
- Prevents contact of the microscope objectives with the sediment
- Permits examination of the sediment under oil immersion when necessary
- Reduces the rate of evaporation of water
- Minimizes movement of sediment

A short time should be allowed for heavier elements to gravitate to the surface of the microscope slide and for fat droplets to float to the undersurface of the coverslip.

The refractive index of many formed elements (for example, hyaline casts) in unstained urine sediment is similar to the surrounding medium. Therefore for the examination of unstained specimens it is recommended that the intensity of the microscope be subdued to improve contrast. If necessary, the intensity of the light may be increased. If excessive light is used, however, many objects may be obscured. Reduced illumination may be accomplished by lowering the microscope condenser and/or closing the substage iris diaphragm.

> A drop of reconstituted sediment should be transferred to a clean microscope slide with a disposable pipette. An automatic pipette with polypropylene tip is superior to a manual pipette.

Standardizing Sediment Preparation With Specialized Sediment Systems

Variations in supplies and technique from person to person affect the reproducibility of results of urine sediment evaluation. To promote consistency several systems for preparation of urine sediment have been developed. They are superior to the uncontrolled method of using a drop of urine on a glass slide and covering it with a coverslip. These systems are designed with the goal of (1) standardizing the volume of urine used to obtain the sediment and (2) standardizing the volume of sediment used for microscopic examination. They also facilitate using the same types of centrifuge tubes, transfer pipettes, and microscope slides.

Each manufactured system contains a disposable plastic centrifuge tube marked with gradations to facilitate measurement of urine volume. The tubes are transparent to allow evaluation of the macroscopic appearance of the specimen. The conical tip of the tubes facilitates preparation of a pellet of sediment by centrifugation.

The Kova system utilizes a pipette designed to fit the centrifuge tube, and to allow 1 ml of urine to remain in the tube after the supernatant is removed. The pellet of sediment can thus be resuspended in a constant volume of urine.

All components of these systems need not be purchased to standardize the method of urine sediment preparation. For example, the Petstix™ 8[c] urinalysis system contains Kova Glasstic Slide

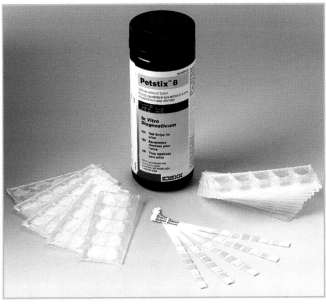

FIGURE 11-1 *The Petstix™ 8 urinalysis system contains reagents strips as well as a microscopy slide system (Kova Glasstic Slides) for in-clinic urinalysis on dogs and cats.*

10 With Grids in addition to diagnostic reagent strips. This combination microscope slide and coverslip system contains 10 separate sample chambers, each of which holds exactly 6.6 microliters (a microliter is 0.000001 liter) of urine sediment. Thus each slide could be used to examine 10 sediment samples. A total of 6.6 microliters of urine sediment will be drawn into the specimen chamber by capillary action, resulting in a homogeneous suspension of sediment.

The conventional method of counting structures in sediment and reporting them per high power magnification or low power magnification does not provide reproducible results. As a result, it is difficult to generate reliable data about the number of red blood cells, white cells, casts, etc. that are normal or abnormal. If the numbers of various structures were expressed in a standardized volume of urine (e.g., cells, crystals, or casts per microliter) rather than per high or low power field, comparisons of normal and abnormal data generated by different laboratories would be enhanced. The 0.33 square millimeter grids incorporated into the Kova Glasstic slides facilitate counting various structures under low or high power magnification. Directions to determine the number of cells, crystals, casts, etc. per microliter of urine are contained in the Petstix™-8 product insert.

Examination of Sediment

Visualization of formed and unformed elements in the sediment will be aided by continuously varying the fine focus adjustment of the microscope while the sediment is being examined. In addition, phase contrast microscopy and polarized light microscopy may be considered.

Initially, the entire sample should be systematically scanned with the aid of the low power objective (10×) to assess the quantity of sediment present and the suitability of the preparation. The fine adjustment should be continuously moved clockwise and then counterclockwise to visualize the three dimensional size of objects and to detect structures located at different planes. Good preparations are characterized by a relatively even distribution of elements without excessive overlapping.

If the amount of material in the sediment appears to be excessive, it may be diluted with supernatant or physiologic saline solution. However, this will alter semiquantitative interpretation of results. If excessive numbers of red blood cells continue to interfere with evaluation of the sediment, addition of a 2% to 5% acetic acid solution will cause hemolysis of the cells without destroying most other elements. However, it may alter urine crystals.

Semiquantitation of the contents of the sediment may be obtained by counting structures in at least 10 to 15 fields and averaging the number of individual elements seen per low power field (the same concept applies to counting per high power field). We emphasize that this method, although convenient, is not precise.

Examination under low power magnification aids in detection of elements (i.e., casts, crystals, bile pigment) that may be present in only a few microscopic fields. Heavier elements, especially casts, often accumulate near the edges of coverslips, especially if excess fluid is placed on the slide. Therefore, to identify larger structures, first examine the edge of the coverslip using low power magnification. Then move to the center

TABLE 11-3
SOURCES OF TECHNICAL ERROR

To obtain meaningful results, the following should be avoided:

- Examination of a contaminated sample
- Examination of unrefrigerated, stale urine
- Failure to thoroughly mix the sample prior to its transfer to the centrifuge tube or failure to properly resuspend the centrifuged sediment prior to examination
- Failure to use a constant volume of centrifuged urine for each sample examined
- Failure to standardize test tubes and transfer pipettes
- Failure to centrifuge urine at a standardized relative centrifugal force.
- Allowing the sediment to dry on the microscope slide
- Use of too much microscope light
- Careless reconstitution of sediment following centrifugation
- Use of dirty or scratched microscope slides and coverslips
- Use of low power or high power magnification only
- Failure to standardize number of microscope fields examined to determine number of red blood cells, white cells, casts, etc.
- Failure to consider the effect of dilution as a result of addition of vital stains to sediment on the numbers of structures detected

of the coverslip and continue the examination.

Following examination of the specimen under low power magnification, it should be examined under high power magnification (40×). With the aid of increased magnification the morphologic characteristics of cells (red blood cells, white cells, and epithelial cells), casts, and crystals can often be seen. The presence of bacteria, yeasts, and lipid droplets may also be detected. Continuous focusing with the fine adjustment will aid in detection of these elements.

If uncentrifuged urine specimens are visibly bloody or very turbid, the dipstick chemical analysis on the supernatant should be repeated. If excessive sediment interferes with microscopic evaluation, the following steps can be considered:

- Dilute the sediment further with urine supernatant.
- Dilute the sediment with physiologic saline solution.
- Add 2% to 10% acetic acid to lyse red blood cells and improve nuclear detail of white blood cells.

Technical errors to be avoided are listed in Table 11-3.

With experience and proper preparation and illumination it is usually possible to evaluate most details of formed elements in urine sediment in an unstained sample. However, some elements may be more easily recognized following staining. Nev-

TABLE 11-4
RECOMMENDED STAINS

For General Use (wet preparations)
- Sternheimer-Malbin stain
  - —Crystal violet and safranin stains
  - —Precipitates in highly alkaline urine
- Sedistain (a stabilized modification of the Sternheimer-Malbin stain)
- Kova stain (a specifically modified form of Sternheimer-Malbin stain)
- Toluidine blue (0.5%)
  - —Metachromatic stain
  - —Facilitates differentiation of nucleus from cytoplasm

For Cellular Elements (air-dried preparations; facilitate evaluation by oil immersion light microscopy)
- New methylene blue
- Wright's stain
- Diff-Quik®a

For Special Needs
- Gram's stain (for confirmation and classification of bacteria. Since a dry preparation is used, it can be evaluated with the aid of oil immersion.)
- Sudan III or IV or Oil Red O (triglycerides and neutral fats stain orange to red)
- Papanicolaou's stain
- Acetic acid (2% to 10%)—accentuates nucleus of leukocytes

*American Scientific Products.

TABLE 11-5
QUALITATIVE RESULTS: NORMAL AND ABNORMAL

Qualitative Results
Normal Urine
- A few red blood cells (less than 5/hpf?)
- A few white cells (less than 5/hpf?)
- A few transitional, squamous, and/or tubular epithelial cells
- A few hyaline casts and/or a few granular casts
- A variety of crystals
- Spermatozoa
- Fat droplets
- Artifacts and contaminants

Findings Warranting Further Investigation
- More than a few red blood cells
- More than a few white cells; clumps of white cells
- Hyperplastic and/or neoplastic epithelial cells
- More than a few hyaline or granular casts
- Cellular (red blood cell, white cell, epithelial cell) casts, fatty casts, waxy casts, hemoglobin casts, and the like
- Any number of cystine, tyrosine, and leucine crystals (consult the section on crystalluria)
- Large numbers of any type of crystal, in properly prepared samples, especially if aggregated together
- Parasite ova and microfilaria
- Bacteria in properly collected, transported, and prepared specimens
- Large numbers of yeast or hyphae

ertheless, even with stains it is not possible to identify all elements in urine sediment.

Sediment Stains

Several stains have been recommended as shown in Table 11-4. Consult clinical pathology textbooks for specific recommendations concerning preparation of stains, fixation of specimens, and staining technique.

It is important to ensure that the bottle of stain is not contaminated with bacteria. As mentioned, if a sufficient quantity of sediment is available, it is recommended that a portion be saved for unstained examination and another for staining.

Use of stains such as Sedistain or Kova stain will dilute the sediment and alter semiquantitative evaluation of results. Some stains applied to air-dried films of sediment (e.g., Gram's or Wright's stain) may require special preparation such as heat fixation or protein coating of slides; others (e.g., Papanicolaou's stain) require wet fixation. These procedures require several staining and washing steps and may result in loss of variable quantities of sediment from the slide.

For supravital staining (wet mounts), one strategy is to place a drop of unstained sediment and a drop of stained sediment adjacent to each other on the same microscope slide. The stained preparation may be used to identify various structures. Once they have been identified, the undiluted unstained preparation may be used to determine the numbers of various structures.

INTERPRETATION
Overview
Expectations

Meaningful evaluation of urine sediment is dependent on recognition of cellular elements, casts, crystals, and other objects. Identification of various structures in urine sediment preparations is often more difficult than evaluation of blood smears or cytologic preparations from other organs of the body, partly due to the fact that cells in varying stages of development may originate from the vascular system, interstitial tissue, or epithelial surfaces located in different areas of the urinary and/or genital tract. In addition, urine is an "unphysiologic" medium for most cells. Cells present in urine are subjected for varying periods to osmotic and pH changes that may be markedly different from their normal environment. They may also be exposed to enzymes or toxic concentrations of other metabolites excreted in urine or produced by pathogenic organisms. As a result they undergo changes in size, structure, and transparency.

TABLE 11-6

FACTORS INFLUENCING SEDIMENT COMPOSITION

- Volume of urine formed
- Method of urine collection
- Method of urine preservation
- Lysis of cells, crystals, and casts by changes in pH and/or the degree of dilution of the sample
- Volume of urine centrifuged
- Sedimentation force (dependent on speed of centrifugation, radius of the centrifuge arm, and duration of centrifugation)
- Volume of urine in which the sediment is resuspended and the thoroughness of reconstitution of the sediment
- Size of drop of sediment transferred to microscope slide
- Quantity of sediment transferred to the microscope slide and subsequently examined (i.e., thickness of the film of the slide preparation); the volume of urine covered by a standard 22 mm coverslip and scanned under one high dry objective field (570×) is about 1/30,000 ml
- Dilution of the reconstituted sediment by addition of stains (Sedistain, Kova stain, etc.) or preservatives
- Staining procedures that may result in loss of variable quantities of sediment during counterstaining and washing
- Ability to recognize various structures and to differentiate among various types of cells, casts, crystals, and the like

Perspectives

To minimize degenerative changes caused by exposure of elements in sediment to urine, urine may be centrifuged as soon as possible after voiding, following which the sediment is immediately examined. Alternatively, it may be maintained with an appropriate preservative. Mucolexx®d is an effective preservative of casts and cells but not all crystals (refer to the section on urine preservatives).

Because knowledge of urine specific gravity provides useful information regarding the relative concentrations of water and elements in urine sediment, urine sediment results should always be interpreted in conjunction with urine specific gravity. In addition, dilute urine (specific gravity less than 1.008) may cause cell lysis.

The significance of cells, bacteria, and amorphous debris should always be interpreted with knowledge of the method of sample collection. Cells and bacteria in noncatheterized samples may originate from the urethra and/or genital tract as well as the bladder, ureters, or kidneys. Red blood cells may occur in catheterized samples, samples obtained by digital compression of the bladder, or samples obtained by cystocentesis as a result of trauma induced by the collection technique. Knowledge of the collection method is also an important aid in localization of abnormalities.

Qualitative and Quantitative Results (see Table 1-1)

There is no precise reproducible information as to the upper limit of normal of many structures found in urine sediment. Typical qualitative (based on centrifugation of 5 ml of urine) results are listed in Table 11-5. Likewise, large numbers of variables alter the quantitative composition of urine sediment (Table 11-6), making stringent quantitative interpretations meaningless.

Conventionally, the number of red blood cells and the number of white cells are counted in each of at least 10 to 15 microscopic fields and are reported as the average number per high power microscope field (40×). Casts are conventionally reported as the average number per low power field (10×), although their identity may be determined at higher magnifications. Bacteria, parasites, crystals, sperm, and other elements are usually reported as few, occasional, frequent, or many. Because of the variables just described, the numbers of cells, casts, and other elements observed represent a crude semi-quantitative value at best.

As with all components of routine complete urinalysis, results of examination of urine sediment should be interpreted in combination with clinical observations and other laboratory, radiographic, or biopsy data.

Red Blood Cells

Appearance (Plates 1 through 4, 11, and 14)

Because of their small size, red blood cells are best evaluated at high magnification. The appearance of red blood cells is variable depending on specific gravity (osmolality), pH, and sometimes the presence of bacteria. In fresh urine with a specific gravity of approximately 1.010 to 1.020, red blood cells typically appear as moderately refractile, pale yellow, smooth homogeneous anuclear disks that are 6 to 7 microns in diameter and of uniform round shape.

Red blood cells that have been in urine for a time may appear colorless as a result of loss of hemoglobin in the surrounding medium (so-called ghost cells). They are smaller than leukocytes, contain no internal structures, and may be biconcave. In concentrated urine they may become smaller, crenated, and distorted due to dehydration. As they lose water, their biconcave shape disappears and spicules and crenations appear (crenations are abnormal notches in red blood cells caused by shrinkage in hypertonic solutions such as urine).

In dilute urine they may appear larger, swollen, and globular. In very dilute or alkaline urine, red blood cells appear as faint colorless circles (ghost cells) or undergo lysis and become invisible. The probability of hemolysis cannot be precisely predicted from knowledge of specific gravity or osmolality because these measurements are influenced by the concentration of urea and other nonelectrolytes that have a negligible effect on osmotic equilibrium between red cells and the surrounding medium. In vitro and in vivo studies indicate that significant osmotic-induced hemolysis usually occurs in urine samples with a specific gravity of 1.008 or less.

Because red cells have no internal structure, they sometimes resemble fat droplets, yeast cells, air bubbles, and amorphous urates. In this situation, the reagent strip test for occult blood would be negative, provided RBCs are not also present. In contrast to red blood cells, however, fat droplets are variable in size

TABLE 11-7

PROBABLE LOCALIZATION OF GROSS HEMATURIA

Hematuria Throughout Micturition

Rule Out	Diagnostic Tests
Renal disorder	Abdominal palpation; survey and contrast radiography; ultrasonography; biopsy; exploratory surgery
Diffuse bladder lesions	Abdominal palpation; examination of urine sediment; survey and contrast radiography; ultrasonography; catheter biopsy; cystoscopy and biopsy; exploratory surgery
Focal ventral or ventrolateral bladder lesions in active patients	Abdominal palpation; examination of urine sediment; survey and contrast radiography; ultrasonography; catheter biopsy; cystoscopy and biopsy; exploratory surgery
Severe prostatic or urethral lesions	Rectal and abdominal palpation; survey and contrast radiography; ultrasonography; catheter biopsy; aspiration biopsy; exploratory surgery
Hemoglobinuria	Examination of urine sediment for red blood cells; hemogram
Systemic clotting effect	Clotting profile, platelet count; evaluation of other body systems for hemorrhage

Hematuria Independent of or at the Beginning of Micturition

Rule Out	Diagnostic Tests
Urethral lesions	Rectal and abdominal palpation; comparison of analysis of urine samples collected by voiding and cystocentesis; survey and contrast radiography; catheter biopsy; exploratory surgery
Genital disease	Abdominal, rectal, and vaginal palpation; vaginal cytology; comparison of analysis of urine samples collected by voiding and cystocentesis; survey and contrast radiography; ultrasonography; endoscopy; exploratory surgery

Hematuria at End of Micturition

Rule Out	Diagnostic Tests
Focal ventral or ventrolateral lesions in inactive patients	Abdominal palpation; examination of urine sediment; survey and contrast radiography; ultrasonography; catheter biopsy; cystoscopy and biopsy; exploratory surgery
Renal disorder with intermittent hematuria in inactive patients	Abdominal palpation; survey and contrast radiography; ultrasonography; biopsy; exploratory surgery

Modified from Osborne CA, Klausner JS: A problem specific data base for urinary tract infections. Vet Clin North Am 9:783, 1979.

and highly refractile. Fat droplets are often out of the plane of focus of other elements in the sediment because they tend to float rather than sink and often have a dark appearance when examined by subdued illumination. Yeast cells frequently contain buds, vary in size, are colorless, and are usually ovoid rather than round in shape. Amorphous urates may be tan or brown in color but are typically darker than red blood cells. In addition, amorphous urates are variable in size and often are present in very large quantities. Addition of acetic acid will lyse red blood cells but leave oil droplets, yeast cells, and amorphous urates intact.

White cells can be difficult to differentiate from RBCs in very concentrated samples. In this situation, acetic acid may be used to accentuate the nuclei of white cells and to lyse RBCs.

Significance of Hematuria
Gross Hematuria (Table 11-7)

If gross hematuria has been observed, determining when

during the process of micturition its intensity was most severe may be helpful in localizing the source of hemorrhage.

Hematuria Throughout Micturition—Patients with persistent gross hematuria caused by renal disease often void urine containing blood throughout the entire period of micturition. This occurs because the ureters enter the caudodorsal portion of the bladder and because boluses of urine are periodically discharged from the ureters into the bladder lumen. Hematuria that occurs throughout micturition may also be observed in association with diffuse bladder lesions or when blood originating from severe prostatic or proximal urethral lesions refluxes from the prostatic urethra into the bladder (e.g., in patients with systemic clotting defects). Caution must be used to distinguish hematuria from hemoglobinuria.

Hematuria at the End of Micturition—Blood observed predominantly at the end of micturition suggests a focal lesion in the ventral or ventrolateral aspect of the urinary bladder. This pattern of hematuria is frequently associated with large uroliths and may be related to the fact that uroliths in the dependent portion of the bladder continually traumatize this area. It may also be associated with polyps.

This type of hematuria occurs in dogs that are sufficiently inactive, allowing most of the red blood cells in the urine to remain in the dependent portion of the bladder lumen; since urine contained in the uppermost portion of the bladder is forced into the urethra first, the bloody urine that has accumulated at the bottom of the bladder is voided last. This pattern of micturition could also be observed in dogs with *intermittent* gross hematuria of renal origin.

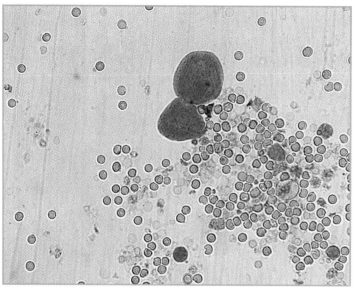

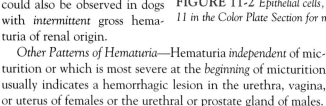

FIGURE 11-2 *Epithelial cells, red blood cells, and white cells. (See Plate 11 in the Color Plate Section for more details.)*

Other Patterns of Hematuria—Hematuria *independent* of micturition or which is most severe at the *beginning* of micturition usually indicates a hemorrhagic lesion in the urethra, vagina, or uterus of females or the urethral or prostate gland of males.

Microscopic Hematuria

Unlike white cells, all red cells originate from the blood vascular system, thus the name red blood cells. Since not all white cells in urine originate from the blood vascular system, it is technically a misnomer to call them all white blood cells.

Results of examination of sediment for red blood cells should be correlated with results of chemical evaluation of urine for blood. Refer to the section on occult blood for further information. Depending on the magnitude of hematuria, the hemoglobin released from RBCs may not contribute substantially to reagent strip tests for protein. The sensitivity of most reagent strip protein tests is 5 to 20 mg/dl. If the reagent strip test for occult blood is less than 3+, it is unlikely that hemoglobin would substantially affect the strip test for protein. The positive protein test associated with hematuria is more likely to be caused by loss of plasma proteins along with RBC into urine.

It has been reported that during centrifugation, only 50% of the red blood cells are recovered.[8]

Hemolyzed red blood cells often cannot be detected by sediment evaluation. It has been reported that red cells in urine with a specific gravity below 1.010 are difficult to see; at a specific gravity below 1.005, the cells disintegrate and cannot be detected.[10]

Low numbers of red blood cells (less than 5 per high power field?) are often observed in the urine sediment of normal patients. Larger numbers of red blood cells in a high power microscopic field indicate hemorrhage, inflammation, necrosis, trauma, or neoplasia somewhere along the urinary tract (or urogenital tract in voided samples).

In humans some investigators have reported that erythrocytes of glomerular origin are often small, fragmented, and variable in size and shape (so-called dysmorphism), while red

blood cells of nonglomerular origin are normal in size and shape. The explanation for this difference is that red blood cells apparently become deformed if they pass through the glomerular capillary wall.[30]

Disorders associated with hematuria are listed in Table 11-8.

White Cells
Appearance (Plates 5 through 8, 14, and 20)

Urine sediment may contain neutrophils, eosinophils, lymphocytes, and monocytes/macrophages. Not all white cells in urine originate from the blood vascular system, and therefore are not referred to as WBCs. The appearance of white cells is variable, being dependent on the type of cells and the influence of specific gravity (osmolality), pH, and toxin-producing bacteria on their morphology.

In fresh urine samples white cells that are primarily neutrophils typically appear as spherical cells with characteristic cytoplasmic granules and lobed or segmented nuclei. They are about 1½ to 2 (10 to 14 μm) times larger than red blood cells but are usually smaller than transitional epithelial cells. White cells shrink in concentrated urine and expand in dilute urine. These cells may occur singly or in clumps. Clumps of white cells alter the number that are counted in the preparation and therefore should be reported. It is sometimes possible to distinguish nuclei, but frequently the nuclei have degenerated. Addition of 2% to 10% acetic acid may enhance the details of nuclei, while destroying red blood cells. Granularity of white cells may be caused by disintegration of the nucleus, phagocytized material and/or granules normally present in the cytoplasm of granulocytes.

White cells may be difficult to differentiate from renal tubular epithelial cells, and distinguishing between polymorphonuclear leukocytes, monocytes/macrophages, lymphocytes, and plasma cells is usually difficult in wet preparations.

Significance
Numbers

Like red blood cells, white cells are rapidly lysed in alkaline or hypotonic urine. The number of white cells may decline as much as 50% within an hour of collection if the sample is kept at room temperature.

Although the normal range of white cells (neutrophils) in urine sediment prepared from a 5 ml aliquot of urine has been reported to be up to three per high power field (40×) in samples collected by cystocentesis, and up to eight per high power field in catheterized or midstream voided samples,[16] several variables should be considered when interpreting the numbers of white cells in urine sediment (Table 11-9).

TABLE 11-8

CONDITIONS ASSOCIATED WITH HEMATURIA

- Strenuous exercise
- Iatrogenic trauma associated with palpation of the kidneys or bladder, cystocentesis, or catheterization of the urinary bladder
- Trauma
- Uroliths in any location
- Renal infarcts due to any cause, including microthrombi related to disseminated intravascular coagulation (associated with white cells, casts, and protein)
- Infection of any portion of the urinary system (also often associated with white cells, proteinuria, and bacteriuria)
- Benign or malignant neoplasms of any portion of the urinary system (or urogenital system in voided samples)
- Chronic passive congestion of the kidneys due to any cause
- Diseases with systemic hemorrhagic tendencies (thrombocytopenia, leptospirosis, warfarin toxicity, hemophilia, etc.)
- Parasites (*Dioctophyma renale*, *Capillaria plica*, *Capillaria felis cati*, microfilaria of *Dirofilaria immitis*, etc.)
- Estrus
- Therapy with cyclophosphamide

TABLE 11-9

FACTORS INFLUENCING NUMBERS OF WHITE CELLS IN URINE SEDIMENT OF DOGS AND CATS WITH BACTERIAL URINARY TRACT INFECTIONS

- Volume of urine produced[a]
- Method of urine collection
- Lysis of cells associated with length of time lapsed between collection and analysis of urine
- Volume of urine centrifuged
- Speed and time of centrifugation
- Volume of urine in which sediment is resuspended
- Magnitude of destruction of cells in alkaline urine
- Clumping of white cells
- Ability to differentiate white cells from urothelial cells
- Suppression of inflammation by endogenous (hyperadrenocorticism) or exogenous glucocorticoids
- Ability of pathogen(s) to induce inflammation
- Suppression of inflammation by concomitant administration of antimicrobial drugs

[a]If the patient does not have pathologic oliguria, this may be inferred by evaluation of urine specific gravity.

Localization

Because white cells are mobile, they can enter the urinary tract at any site. Therefore additional information is needed to localize their source. Localization of leukocyturia usually is based on clinical signs, renal function tests, and radiology/ultrasonography in addition to results of urinalysis.

Detection of white cells in casts localizes their source to at least the renal tubules.

The possibility that pyuria has occurred as a result of passage of urine through the genital tract must be considered in non-catheterized and even catheterized samples of urine. When the origin of pyuria is questionable, a urine sample obtained by cystocentesis may help in localization. Detection of pyuria in urine samples collected by cystocentesis does not exclude the lower urinary tract from involvement in the inflammatory process.

Pathophysiologic Attributes

Substantial numbers of white cells are indicative of active inflammation, a compensatory response to a variety of infectious and noninfectious disorders. The inflammatory response is typically, but not invariably, associated with varying numbers of red blood cells and proteinuria. Detection of a significant number of bacteria in association with pyuria indicates that the inflammatory lesion is active and has been caused or complicated by bacterial infection. However, because bacteria are more difficult to detect than white cells, pyuria may not appear to be associated with bacteria if they are present in

lower numbers (Table 11-10). Therefore the urine of patients with pyuria should routinely be cultured for bacteria.

On occasion, bacterial urinary tract infection occurs without detectable concomitant pyuria. This may occur in patients given glucocorticoids or those that have hyperadrenocorticism or are immunosuppressed. To localize the site of the inflammatory process, additional information is necessary.

Absence of pyuria usually indicates that the urinary tract is not infected. We have occasionally encountered significant asymptomatic bacteriuria without pyuria in dogs and cats, however.

Pyuria (leukocyturia) is a poor index of bacteriuria and therefore is not synonymous with urinary tract infection. Although pyuria should arouse the suspicion of infection, non-septic causes of inflammation (metabolic uroliths, neoplasms, etc.) should be considered.

The leukocyte esterase test strip commonly used to evaluate human urine is an insensitive method to detect pyuria in dogs[95] and a nonspecific method to detect pyuria in cats. Different white cells may have different quantities and types of leukocyte esterases. Lymphocytes do not have leukocyte esterase. Lysed white cells may result in a positive leukocyte esterase strip test but will not be seen in sediment.

Epithelial Cells

Appearance (Plates 9 through 21)

Renal Tubular Cells

Renal tubular epithelial cells originate from the renal tubules (Plates 9 and 10). They are variable in size (10 to 50

TABLE 11-10

CHECKLIST OF POSSIBLE CAUSES OF INFLAMMATION DETECTED BY URINALYSIS BUT UNASSOCIATED WITH MICROSCOPIC BACTERIURIA

- Noninfectious disease of the urinary tract
- Numbers of bacteria in urine too small for consistent detection (bacterial rods <10,000/ml; bacterial cocci <100,000/ml)
- Male dogs with prostatitis
- Infections caused by mycoplasma, ureaplasma, or viruses
- Administration of antimicrobial agents prior to urinalysis

μm) and round and have a large central spherical nucleus and finely granular cytoplasm.

Although proximal tubular cells may be oblong, irregularity of shape and trailing cytoplasm are not pathognomonic features of renal tubular epithelial cells. On occasion, columnar cells with a brush-border (microvilli) may be observed, indicating their origin from proximal renal tubules.

Contrary to often-made statements, small, round cells are not a reliable index of kidney disease (unless they are contained in casts) because they cannot be readily differentiated from white cells or small transitional epithelial cells.

Transitional Epithelial Cells

Transitional epithelial cells (urothelial cells) have a wide variation in size, depending on their depth of origin in transitional epithelium (Plates 11 through 14), and may be two to four times larger (20 to 40 μm) than white cells. The outermost layer of transitional epithelium are large (approximately 40 μm) and flat. Transitional cells from the intermediate layer of urothelium are smaller and more round in appearance. Cells from the basal layer tend to be columnar in shape. If transitional cells absorb water, they may become as large as squamous epithelial cells. In summary, transitional epithelial cells may be pear-shaped, spindle-shaped, caudate, or polygonal and typically have granular cytoplasm. They often exfoliate into urine in large numbers in association with inflammation and may be hyperplastic.

Squamous Epithelial Cells

Squamous epithelial cells are the largest (approximately 50 μm) of the normal cells present in normal urine sediment (Plates 15 through 18). They are typically large, thin, plate-like cells with distinct or irregular outlines and a small, dense nucleus (although they may have larger vesicular nuclei or they may be anucleate). They may occur singly or in sheets. Squamous epithelial cells may have unusual configurations if their edges curl or fold. Squamous epithelial cells folded into a tubular shape may resemble casts.

Neoplastic Cells

Occasionally, neoplastic epithelial cells may be observed in the urine sediment of patients with transitional cell carcinomas, rhabdomyosarcomas, and, less commonly, other types of neoplasms (Plates 19 through 21). Their evaluation is enhanced by examination of freshly collected (or properly preserved) and stained specimens.

Samples collected by catheterization are more likely to yield neoplastic cells than samples collected by cystocentesis. Lavage of the bladder lumen and cytospin preparations may increase the yield of neoplastic cells.

Nuclear and cytoplasmic changes indicative of malignancy are summarized in Table 11-11. It may be difficult to differentiate hyperplastic epithelial cells from neoplastic epithelial cells.

Significance

Cuboidal epithelial cells from the renal tubules, transitional epithelial cells from the renal pelves, ureters, urinary bladder, and urethra, and squamous epithelial cells from the vagina and distal urethra are commonly detected in urine sediment obtained from normal dogs and cats. They are thought to occur as a result of normal attrition and exfoliation of epithelial cells.

Accurate data regarding the number of epithelial cells normally present in the urine of dogs and cats are not available. Although large numbers of cells may exfoliate as a result of disease, there are more reliable methods available that should be used to confirm the presence of urinary lesions.

Characteristics of different types of epithelial cells are described in Table 11-12.

Casts
Theories of Formation

Casts are composed primarily of a matrix of mucoprotein (called Tamm-Horsfall mucoprotein), which by scanning electron microscopy appears as a fibrillar protein meshwork.[12,26] Tamm-Horsfall mucoprotein is locally secreted by epithelial cells that line the loops of Henle, the distal tubules, and the collecting ducts.[18,25,27] Casts are not primarily composed of plasma proteins. Microdissection studies of renal tubules indicate that casts are formed in the loops of Henle, distal tubules, and collecting ducts. Although the mechanism responsible for the precipitation of Tamm-Horsfall mucoprotein into protein fibrils within tubular lumens is not understood, cast formation in these areas of nephrons is thought to be related (at least in part) to the fact that the secretion of Tamm-Horsfall mucoprotein is limited to these sites.[20] The protein fibrils attach to the surface of tubular epithelial cells, which prevents them from being washed away by tubular fluid.

A long-held popular theory is based on the assumption that any material or object present within the lumen of tubules at the time that Tamm-Horsfall mucoprotein forms fibrils will become incorporated into the cast. Entrapment of cells and other structures in the precipitated mucoprotein matrix has been likened to entrapment of fruit and vegetables in gelatin salads. It has also been hypothesized that casts may be formed by conglutination of cells and/or debris within tubular lumens.

TABLE 11-11
CHARACTERISTICS OF MALIGNANT CELLS

Structural Alteration of Cells and Their Nuclei
Nuclear Changes
- Disproportionate enlargement of the nucleus in relation to the cytoplasm
- Increase in chromatin content causing hyperchromasia
- Structural changes such as aberrant chromatin patterns, elongation, irregularity in outline, lobulation and budding, etc.
- Enlargement and/or increase in number of nuclei
- Multinucleated cells, with atypical nuclei
- Increased mitotic activity; abnormal mitotic figures
- Marked thickening of nuclear membrane

Cytoplasmic Changes
- Changes in staining reaction
- Cytoplasmic inclusions such as pigment granules, leukocytes, or cellular debris
- Atypical vacuolization

Whole Cell Changes
- Increase in size
- Aberrant forms

Modification of Cellular Interrelationships
- Irregularity of pattern
- Anisocytosis and anisokaryosis
- Lack of distinct cell boundaries
- Dense crowding of cells and nuclei

Modified from Prall et al.: *Cancer* 29:1087–1089, 1972.

TABLE 11-12
TYPES OF EPITHELIAL CELLS

Renal Tubular Epithelial Cells
- Originate from the renal tubules
- Normally found in urine in relatively small numbers
- Not a reliable index of kidney disease because they are difficult, if not impossible, to differentiate from other types of epithelial cells (unless they are incorporated into casts)

Transitional Epithelial Cells
- Originate from the mucosa lining the renal pelvis, ureters, urinary bladder, and/or proximal urethra
- Normally found in urine in relatively small numbers as a result of maturation and aging
- Exfoliate into urine in large numbers as a result of inflammation or neoplasia (in these instances they may be hyperplastic)

Squamous Epithelial Cells
- Originate from the genital tract
- Commonly present in noncatheterized samples
- Primarily of significance in relation to the fact that they indicate contamination of the urine sample with material from the genital tract
- Vary in morphology when obtained from female dogs, being influenced by the stage of the estrus cycle

Neoplastic Epithelial Cells
- May be observed in patients with transitional cell carcinomas, rhabdomyosarcomas, and, less commonly, other types of neoplasms but are not a consistent finding
- Rarely encountered in patients with renal cell carcinomas
- Often difficult to differentiate from nonneoplastic, hyperplastic transitional epithelial cells

Studies of the surface ultrastructure of casts by scanning electron microscopy indicate that erythrocytes, leukocytes, and renal epithelial cells can also adhere to the surface of a fibrillar network of protein that subsequently surrounds the cells. The results of these structures corroborate the hypothesis that the hyaline cast is the primary structural unit of all casts.[11,15]

Appearance (Figure 11-3 and Plates 22 through 43)
Overview

Casts are cylindrical-shaped structures formed in tubular lumens. Each is literally a cast of the shape of the tubular lumen. They often have parallel sides and may have round, square, irregular, or tapered ends. Because casts are cylinders, they appear thicker in their centers than along their edges.

The shape and length of casts are influenced by the morphology of the tubular lumens in which they formed. Likewise, the width of casts is determined by the diameter of the tubular lumens in which they are formed. Casts formed in loops of Henle or distal tubules are not as wide as those formed in collecting ducts or abnormally dilated tubules. However, even though they vary in length and width, their diameter tends to be uniform throughout their length. They may have the appearance of being compressed from end to end after their formation.

Accurate, precise identification of some casts by light microscopy may be difficult. To avoid misinterpretation, special stains, phase contrast microscopy, and interference contrast microscopy have been advocated by various investigators.

Because casts are retained in renal tubules for a variable time, the cells and other structures they contain often disintegrate. The matrix of casts may also change. For example, hyaline and granular casts may become waxy casts.

Hyaline casts dissolve in neutral urine with a specific gravity of less than 1.003. There is an inverse relationship between the number of intact casts and urine pH. For this reason casts are less commonly observed in alkaline urine. High speed centrifugation and forceful reconstitution of urine may disrupt fragile casts.

Casts are commonly classified on the basis of their morpho-

Transformation of Epithelial, Granular, and Waxy Casts

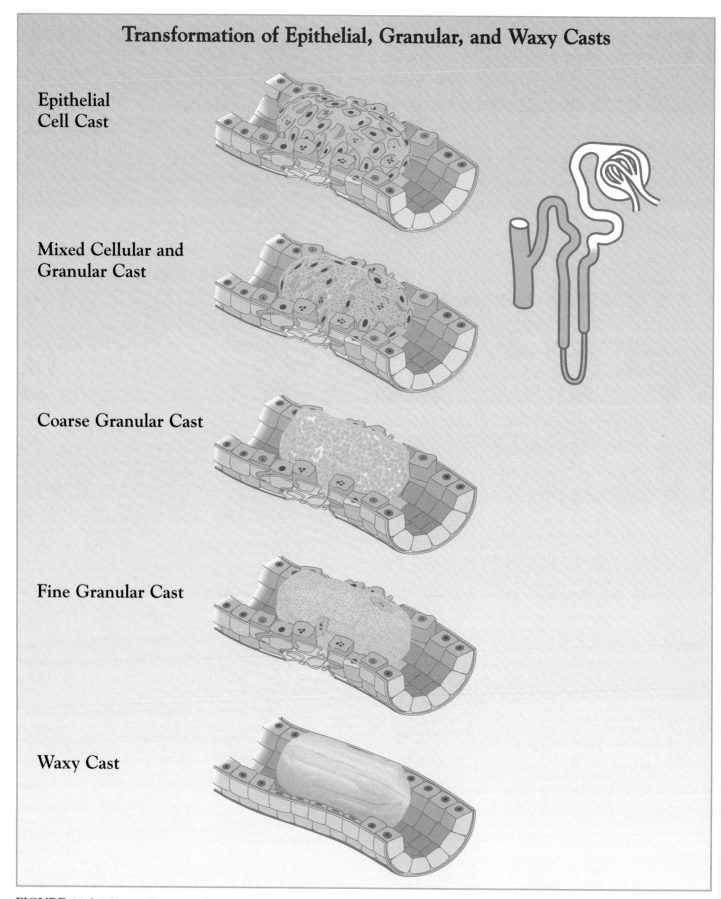

Epithelial
Cell Cast

Mixed Cellular and
Granular Cast

Coarse Granular Cast

Fine Granular Cast

Waxy Cast

FIGURE 11-3 *Schematic illustration of transition between epithelial cell, coarse granular, and waxy casts formed in the loops of Henle, distal tubules, and collecting ducts (shaded area of nephron at upper right). (Adapted from Osborne CA, Stevens JB: Handbook of Canine and Feline Urinalysis. St. Louis, Ralston Purina, 1981, p 103.)*

logic appearance as hyaline, epithelial, granular, waxy, fatty, red blood cell, white cell, hemoglobin, broad, bile-stained, and mixed casts. This classification is often of benefit in providing information about the type of lesion in the renal tubules.

Hyaline Casts (Plates 22 and 23)

Hyaline casts are primarily composed of Tamm-Horsfall mucoprotein; they contain no, or only a few, inclusions.[15,26] Since the refractive index of hyaline casts is similar to that of the surrounding medium, they are usually colorless, homogenous, and semitransparent in unstained sediment. They form in various shapes and sizes and typically have rounded ends. They are best detected in subdued light or following staining. With modified Sternheimer-Malbin stains they appear reddish-pink.

Apparently hyaline casts may also be transformed into waxy casts.

Epithelial Cell, Fatty, Granular, and Waxy Casts (Figure 11-3 and Plates 24 through 39)

Epithelial Cell Casts—A popular, but unproved, hypothesis is that renal tubular epithelial cell, fatty, granular, and waxy casts represent different stages of degeneration of epithelial cells in casts (Figure 11-3). Epithelial cell casts contain varying numbers of highly refractile tubular epithelial cells that have not yet disintegrated (Plate 24). Tubular epithelial cells may be randomly located within the cast matrix, or they may be aligned as they previously were along tubular basement membranes. Scanning electron micrographs have revealed that epithelial cells are attached to a hyaline matrix by fibrin bands. The epithelial cells characteristically have a large, round central nucleus.

Fatty Casts—If lipid accumulates in the cytoplasm of cells prior to desquamation into tubular lumens, highly refractile fat droplets of varying size may be observed. Such casts are sometimes called fatty casts (Plates 25 through 29). Verification of lipid in casts may be achieved by staining with Sudan III or Sudan IV or by examination with polarizing light microscopy.

Granular Casts—Once an epithelial cell cast has formed, its morphologic appearance does not remain static. As a result of being deprived of oxygen and metabolites, epithelial cells degenerate. With time cell margins become indistinct, nuclear material begins to disintegrate, and coarse opaque granules of varying size appear and form a coarse granular cast. As the process of degeneration continues, fine granules are formed and the casts are called fine granular casts. In this scheme of formation, distinction of coarse granular casts from fine granular casts is of no clinical significance (Plates 30 through 36).

Waxy Casts—Further degeneration of the components of the epithelial cell results in the formation of a colorless, homogenous mass with a high refractive index, sharp borders, "broken off" ends, and a dull, waxy appearance. They are called waxy casts (Plates 35 through 39). Waxy casts may contain cracks or fissures.

Other Types of Granular Casts—Granular casts may also occur as a result of precipitation of plasma proteins (that have passed through glomeruli) in Tamm-Horsfall mucoprotein matrix and as a result of degeneration of white cells in casts.

Finely granular casts may also be associated with by-products of protein metabolism excreted by tubular epithelial cells. This observation provides a plausible explanation of why finely granular casts are found in healthy individuals.

It may be impossible to distinguish between degenerated epithelial cells and white cells contained in casts (Plate 24). Casts containing cells whose type cannot be discerned are commonly called cellular casts or cellular-granular casts.

Red Blood Cell Casts (Plates 40 and 41)

Red blood cell casts occur in association with hemorrhage into the renal tubules. They are very fragile. In fresh urine they have a yellow-orange to orange-red color. This color often fades with time, and the red cells may disintegrate. Degeneration and lysis of red cells within a cast that has been retained in a renal tubule may result in a hemoglobin-induced golden-brown color and greater homogeneity.

Hemoglobin and Myoglobin Casts

Hemoglobin casts may be observed following severe intravascular hemolysis and hemoglobinuria. They are yellow to brown in color. Myoglobin casts may be associated with myoglobinuria and resemble hemoglobin casts. They may be homogenous in consistency and have a reddish color or have a granular appearance due to associated tubular cell damage.

White Cell Casts (Plate 42)

White cell casts, composed of white cells and Tamm-Horsfall mucoprotein

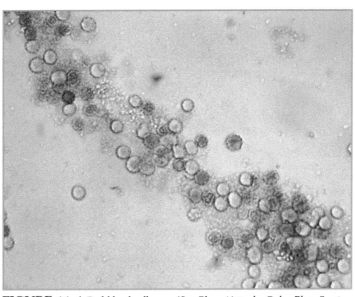

FIGURE 11-4 *Red blood cell cast. (See Plate 41 in the Color Plate Section for more details.)*

> Since the refractive index of hyaline casts is similar to that of the surrounding medium, they are usually colorless, homogenous, and semitransparent in unstained sediment.

matrix, occur when the tubules and interstitium become involved in an inflammatory process. They are difficult to distinguish from renal tubular epithelial cell casts. If the white cells degenerate before they are examined, granular casts may be formed.

Bilirubin Casts

Bilirubin casts are homogeneous and contain yellow or golden brown bilirubin (Plate 43).

Mixed Casts (Plates 30 and 36)

Casts may be composed of a mixture of any of the types just described. For example, casts may contain cells and granular debris (cellular-granular casts) or granular debris and waxy material (granular-waxy casts). One end may appear as a granular cast while the opposite end appears as a hyaline cast.

Broad Casts (Plates 23 and 37)

The term broad cast refers to a wide cast formed in collecting ducts, abnormally dilated loops of Henle or distal tubules, or tubules that have undergone compensatory hypertrophy. Broad casts may be of any type including hyaline, cellular, granular, or waxy in appearance.

Significance
Generalities

Normal urine contains no casts or only a very few. Clinical observations have revealed that a few hyaline or granular casts (less than approximately one or two per low power field in moderately concentrated urine) in the sediment of otherwise normal patients is not a reliable index of significant renal damage. Under these circumstances a few casts are of no apparent diagnostic or prognostic significance. Although casts indicate some pathologic change in the renal tubules, this change may be minor, transitory, and reversible.

Since casts are formed in the loops of Henle, distal tubules, and collecting ducts, detection of significant numbers of casts in urine sediment (so-called cylinduria) indicates tubular involvement in an active pathologic process. Although classification of casts according to their morphologic appearance may provide clues as to the character of the lesion in renal tubules, cast morphology is rarely of specific diagnostic significance.

Absence of casts does not rule out renal tubular disease. Casts may be eliminated in urine immediately after formation or remain within tubules for varying periods while undergoing varying degrees of degeneration.

The number of casts is not a reliable index of the severity, duration, reversibility, or irreversibility of the underlying disease. For example, large or small numbers of casts may occur in patients with acute generalized renal disease because the casts tend to be discharged into the urine in intermittent showers. On the other hand, only a few casts may be observed in the urine of patients with chronic, progressive, generalized nephritis. It is possible for there to be large numbers of casts within the kidneys and very few casts present in urine. Large numbers of casts always indicate active generalized renal disease, which is usually acute but may be reversible or irreversible. Small numbers of casts may occur in patients with acute or chronic generalized renal disease.

Hyaline Casts

There has been a general consensus that hyaline casts are commonly seen in association with renal and extrarenal causes of proteinuria. It has been proposed that albumin and/or other plasma proteins that escape through glomerular capillary walls enhance the precipitation of Tamm-Horsfall mucoprotein.[19] These casts may be associated with mild or severe disease.

Epithelial Cell, Fatty, Granular, and Waxy Casts

These casts may be associated with diseases (infarction, ischemia, nephrotoxins, etc.) that cause degeneration and necrosis of tubular epithelial cells. Since cellular degeneration of epithelial cells in casts occurs after cell death and desquamation, the degree (or stage) of disintegration of epithelial cells does not reflect the microscopic appearance of the tubules but rather the duration of the disease process. Epithelial, fatty, granular, and waxy casts are usually associated with diseases that cause degeneration and necrosis of tubular epithelial cells. Contrary to earlier reports, waxy casts are not a consistent finding in patients with amyloidosis and are not composed of amyloid.

Although all granular casts have a Tamm-Horsfall mucoprotein matrix, the origin of granules varies:

- They may originate from disintegrating tubular epithelial cells.
- They may occur as a result of degeneration of white cells.[26]
- They may arise from precipitation of plasma proteins in Tamm-Horsfall mucoprotein matrix as a result of abnormal permeability of glomeruli.[26]
- Finely granular casts may also be associated with metabolic by-products of protein metabolism excreted by tubular epithelial cells. This provides a plausible explanation of why they are found in healthy individuals.
- Apparently uncommon causes of granules within casts include packed bacteria, bacterial variants, some types of crystals, and precipitated hemoglobin secondary to severe intravascular hemolysis.[5]

Phase contrast or interference contrast microscopy is usually required for accurate identification of different types of granular casts.

Red Blood Cell Casts

Red blood cell casts occur in association with hemorrhage into renal tubules.

> Detection of significant numbers of casts in urine sediment (so-called cylinduria) indicates tubular involvement in an active pathologic process.

Although observation of red blood cells in urine sediment does not specify the site of bleeding, it does indicate involvement of the kidneys. We have rarely encountered them in companion animals, perhaps because they are fragile.

Hemoglobin and Myoglobin Casts

Disorders associated with hemoglobinuria and myoglobinuria may result in formation of hemoglobin and myoglobin casts. Consult Section 5 in Chapter 10 for additional details.

White Cell Casts

White cell casts occur in association with tubulointerstitial inflammation. As for red blood cells, observation of white cells in urine sediment does not indicate the site of inflammation. Detection of these white cell casts indicates renal involvement in the inflammatory process but does not exclude inflammation elsewhere. Absence of white cell casts does not exclude inflammation of the renal tubules.

Bilirubin Casts

Bilirubin casts are associated with bilirubinuria (see the section on bilirubinuria for additional information).

Broad Casts

Broad casts indicate obstruction of more than one nephron if they originate in collecting ducts. At one time, they were called renal failure casts because, when present in large numbers, they were often associated with chronic pyelonephritis. Broad casts may originate in abnormally dilated tubules of nephrons.

Bacteria (Plates 3, 5, 6, and 44 through 51)
Appearance

When present in sufficient numbers, bacterial rods and cocci may be observed in uncentrifuged urine or in urine sediment.[1,13] Proper detection of bacteriuria depends greatly on the skill and experience of the observer.

The sediment must be examined under low light intensity to sharpen contrast and under high dry or oil immersion magnification. Single cocci are more difficult to identify than rods and chains of cocci because they are often mistaken for Brownian movement of amorphous crystals, especially by unskilled observers. Bacteria may be confused with red blood cells because as bacteria go out of focus, they seem to enlarge and rod-shaped bacteria appear to become round.

Bacterial rods (coliforms) can develop in chains, resulting in a filamentous shape in urine that might lead to their misidentification as hyphae (Plate 51). Rod-shaped bacteria may be seen in unstained preparations of urine sediment if more than 10,000 bacteria per milliliter are present, but they may not be consistently detected if their numbers are less.[4] Cocci are difficult to detect in urine sediment if their numbers are less than 100,000 per milliliter.

> ## TABLE 11-13
> ### FACTORS THAT MAY EXPLAIN STERILE BACTERIAL URINE CULTURES WHEN BACTERIA WERE OBSERVED IN URINE SEDIMENT
>
> - Nonviable microbes in urine at time of collection (host defenses; antimicrobial drugs)
> - Urine sample utilized for urinalysis contaminated and improperly preserved following collection
> - Death of fastidious uropathogens between time of sample collection and urine culture
> - Improper or prolonged preservation of urine sample
> - Improper culture technique
> - Misidentification of bacterial look-alikes in urine sediment

When bacteria are detected, they are reported as occasional, few, moderate, or many per high power field. Because bacteria are apparently not affected by centrifugation at 1000 to 3000 rpm for 3 to 5 minutes in the same fashion as cells, crystals, casts, and the like, either centrifuged or uncentrifuged samples may be examined. Centrifugation and examination of urine sediment may facilitate detection of bacteria in the cytoplasm of phagocytic inflammatory cells, however.

Phase contrast microscopy may facilitate detection of bacteria in unstained samples (Plate 44). Gram's stain or new methylene blue stain may aid in detection of bacteriuria and estimation of their numbers and may facilitate selection of antimicrobial drugs (Plates 45 and 47 through 50). It is emphasized that failure to detect bacteria in urine sediment does not exclude their presence.

Significance
Generalities

Microscopic examination of urine for bacteria should be used to complement rather than substitute for qualitative and quantitative urine culture. Although detection of bacteria in urine sediment suggests urinary tract infection, it should be verified by urine culture (Table 11-13). Bacteriuria may or may not be significant, depending on the method of urine collection and the length of time between collection and examination.

Interpretation Versus Collection Method

Normally, urine is sterile until it reaches the midurethra. The urethra of dogs and cats contains a resident population of bacteria that are greatest in number at its distal end. Most of these organisms are gram positive. The significance of bacteria identified in voided or catheterized urine samples should be interpreted with caution, because samples collect-

> **Although detection of bacteria in urine sediment suggests urinary tract infection, it should be verified by urine culture.**

ed by these methods may be contaminated with resident bacteria located in the distal urethral and genital tract. Because bacteria can replicate rapidly in urine, it is best to examine samples soon after they are collected. If timely examination is not possible, the sample should be properly preserved (refer to the section on urine preservation for specific details about methods of preservation).

In general, cystocentesis should be used to collect urine samples for qualitative and quantitative bacterial culture. If dysuria and pollakiuria prevent collection of urine by cystocentesis, it may be necessary to collect urine for culture during voiding or by catheterization. In these situations the external genitalia of males and females must be rinsed with an appropriate cleansing solution before urine is obtained. It may be necessary to clip the hair surrounding the vulva of long-haired female dogs. Only sterilized catheters and collection containers should be used, and the containers should have tight-fitting lids. Sterile containers may be obtained by sterilizing disposable plastic cups in ethylene oxide gas, or they may be purchased from commercial manufacturers. If the results of the quantitative urine culture of noncatheterized midstream or catheterized urine samples are equivocal following serial cultures, collection of urine by cystocentesis should again be considered.

The presence of bacteria in urine aseptically collected by cystocentesis even in low numbers indicates urinary tract infection. However, false-positive results may occur if the needle penetrates a loop during cystocentesis or if the sample is contaminated during transfer to culture media.

Differentiating Bacterial Contaminants and Pathogens

The concept of significant bacteriuria was introduced to allow differentiation between harmless bacterial contaminants of urine and pathogenic organisms causing infectious disease of the urinary system. This concept is based on the observation that a high bacterial count in a properly collected and cultured urine sample indicates the probability of urinary tract infection.

In humans, urine bacterial counts in excess of 100,000 organisms of a single species per milliliter of urine are considered to be significant.[14] Isolation of 10,000 to 100,000 bacteria of a single species per milliliter in catheterized or midstream urine samples is suggestive of bacterial infection. Urine from patients with suspected bacteriuria should be cultured a second time. If the same organism is isolated at a similar or higher concentration, the presence of bacterial infection is confirmed since reproducible results would not be expected as a result of contamination. The presence of less than 10,000 bacteria per milliliter in midstream or catheterized urine samples usually represents contaminants.

Although controlled experiments with statistical analysis have not been performed, clinical studies of quantitative urine culture performed at the University Veterinary Hospital of the University

> Detection of bacteria within the cytoplasm of phagocytes found in urine sediment suggests but does not prove in vivo phagocytosis rather than contamination of urine sample during collection analysis.

of Minnesota and elsewhere[3,6] utilizing the calibrated loop technique for quantitative culture have revealed that noncatheterized midstream urine samples and catheterized urine samples obtained from dogs with clinical, laboratory, and radiographic evidence of urinary tract infection usually contained more than 100,000 bacteria per milliliter. Although urine obtained from most dogs without urinary tract infections was either sterile or contained less than 10,000 bacteria per milliliter of urine (see Table 1-11), counts of 100,000 bacteria per milliliter occurred with sufficient frequency to make this form of urine collection unsatisfactory for routine diagnostic bacterial culture. However, bacterial urinary tract infection may be present in patients with less than 10,000 bacteria per milliliter of urine and should be suspected if patients have characteristic clinical and urinalysis findings. It is noteworthy that bacterial contamination of voided and catheterized samples is more likely to occur in female than male dogs and cats.

The lower limit of numbers of organisms that indicates significant bacteriuria in feline urine cultures has not been determined. However, it may be less than those in humans and dogs because feline urine appears to be less conducive to bacterial growth than urine of dogs or humans (Table 3-16). In addition, other factors may influence results of quantitative culture of urine for bacteria.

Interpretation Versus Length of Time Between Collection and Examination

The significance of detection of bacteria in urine samples allowed to incubate at room temperature prior to examination is unknown. Pathogens and/or contaminants may continue to proliferate, or they may be destroyed. In vitro bacterial growth or destruction is not synonymous with in vivo conditions.

Bacteria contained in urine samples refrigerated for 24 hours or more may not be viable, resulting in false-negative culture results.

Detection of bacteria within the cytoplasm of phagocytes found in urine sediment suggests but does not prove in vivo phagocytosis rather than contamination of the urine sample during collection analysis (see Figure 3-1). Detection of bacteria in improperly preserved samples warrants reexamination of a fresh specimen.

Microscopic Examination Versus Bacterial Numbers

Rod-shaped bacteria may be seen in unstained preparations of urine when numbers are approximately 10,000 per milliliter or greater. Larger numbers (100,000 per milliliter) of cocci may be needed to permit detection. The results of a study in dogs were interpreted to indicate that detection of bacteria in more than one oil immersion microscopic held was an indication of 100,000 bacteria per milliliter or more.

Significant bacteriuria is usually, but not invariably, associated with varying degrees of hematuria, pyuria, and proteinuria (i.e., an inflammatory response). Lack of detection of bacteria in urine sediment does not exclude their presence.

Yeasts and Fungi
Appearance (Plates 52 through 60)

Yeasts consist of oval to round cells with a double refractile wall. They have an ovoid shape, are colorless, and often have characteristic budding forms. They are similar to red blood cells, but are more refractile and more variable in appearance. Unlike red blood cells, they are insoluble in acid and alkali and will not stain with eosin.

Fungi are usually characterized by distinct hyphae (one of the filaments composing the mycelium). Hyphae may be aseptate or segmented (meaning they have cross walls called spetae). Hyphae may be associated with aseptate or septate microconidia. Hyphae must be differentiated from filamentous forms of bacteria (Plate 51).

Occasionally, characteristic forms of deep systemic mycotic agents (blastomycosis, cryptococcosis, etc.) may be detected in urine sediment. Gram's stain or new methylene blue stain can be used to highlight their appearance.

Significance

Yeasts and fungi usually represent contaminants. Infections with *Candida albicans* and *Torulopsis* spp. may occur, especially in patients with resistant urinary tract infections that have been unsuccessfully treated with a variety of antimicrobial agents for prolonged periods.[17] On occasion, fungi (blastomycosis, cryptococcosis, etc.) may be observed in the urine sediment of patients with polysystemic fungal disease involving the urinary system (especially the kidneys).[17,24,28]

Parasites

Eggs of *Dioctophyma renale* are thick-shelled and oval and have characteristic surface mammilations except at their poles (Plates 61 through 63). Ova of *D. renale* may be observed in the urine sediment of animals (usually dogs) infected with this parasite, provided a gravid female is present in the excretory pathway of the urinary system.

Ova of *Capillaria plica* and *Capillaria felis cati* are oval in shape and have bipolar plugs. They are colorless and have a slightly pitted shell (Plate 64). Care must be used to differentiate the ova of *Capillaria* species from those of *Trichuris vulpus* that appear in urine as a result of fecal contamination. Occasionally, adult *Capillaria* may be detected in urine sediment (Figure 11-5).

Microfilaria of *Dirofilaria immitis* occasionally may be observed in the urine sediment of infected dogs, presumably as a result of hemorrhage into the excretory pathway of the urinary system (Plate 65).

Spermatozoa (Plates 65 and 66)

Spermatozoa are a normal finding in the urine of uncastrated male dogs and

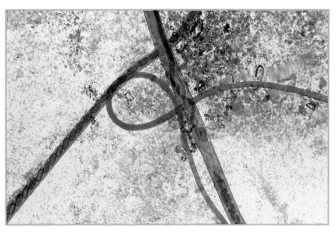

FIGURE 11-5 *Photomicrograph of gravid* Capillaria plica *in the urine sediment of a dog. (×75. Courtesy of Dr. David Senior, Louisiana State University.)*

cats and are readily identified by their characteristic shape. They may be observed in bladder urine obtained by cystocentesis of male dogs and cats, apparently as a result of retrograde ejaculation and/or their motility.[7,9] On occasion, sperm are present as a contaminant in the urine of females following breeding.

Lipiduria
Appearance (Plates 66 and 67)

A layer of white lipid is commonly observed floating on the surface of normal feline urine samples. Under low magnification with subdued light, free lipid droplets appear as black, refractile spheres of variable size. As they float to the undersurface of the coverslip, lipid droplets may move out of the plane of focus of other heavier elements in the sediment located next to the surface of the microscope slide (Plate 66). When stained with Sudan III or IV (Plate 67), triglycerides (neutral fat) have an orange to red color. Lipid droplets that contain cholesterol do not stain with Sudan III or Oil Red-O but typically have a bright Maltese cross light pattern when examined with the aid of polarization light microscopy.

Significance

The origin of fat droplets is often difficult to determine. Fat droplets may originate as a result of physiologic attrition of tubular epithelial cells (especially in cats) and/or as a result of abnormal cytoplasmic degenerative changes in tubular epithelial cells. Lipid-like droplets may occur as a result of contamination of urine with lubricants or the lining of some waterproof paper containers. There is apparently no correlation between lipemia and lipiduria.

Crystals (Table 11-14)
Overview

The advent of effective medical protocols to dissolve and prevent uroliths in dogs and cats has resulted in renewed interest in detection and interpretation of crystalluria. Evaluation of urine crystals may aid in:

> The advent of effective medical protocols to dissolve and prevent uroliths in dogs and cats has resulted in renewed interest in detection and interpretation of crystalluria.

TABLE 11-14

COMMON CHARACTERISTICS OF URINE CRYSTALS

Type of Crystal	Appearance	pH Where Commonly Found		
		Acidic	Neutral	Alkaline
Ammonium urate	Yellow-brown spherulites; thorn apples	+	+	±
Amorphous urates	Amorphous or spheroid yellow-brown structures	+	±	–
Ampicillin	Long, thin needles that are colorless	+	??	??
Bilirubin	Orange-yellow-brown needles or granules	+	–	–
Calcium carbonate	Large yellow-brown spheroids with radial striations or small crystals with spheric ovoid or dumbbell shapes	–	±	+
Calcium oxalate dihydrate	Small colorless envelopes (dipyramidal or octahedral form)	+	+	±
Calcium oxalate monohydrate	Small spindles, "hemp seed," or monohydrate dumbbells	+	+	±
Calcium phosphate	Amorphous, or long, thin prisms	±	+	+
Cholesterol	Flat, colorless rectangular plates with corner notch	+	+	–
Cystine	Flat, colorless hexagonal plates	+	+	±
Hippuric acid	Four- to six-sided colorless elongated plates or prisms with rounded corners	+	+	±
Leucine	Yellow-brown spheroids with radial and concentric laminations	+	–	–
Magnesium ammonium phosphate	Three- to six-sided colorless prisms, sometimes fern-leaf appearnce	±	+	+
Sodium urate	Colorless or yellow-brown needles or slender prisms, sometimes in clusters or sheaves	+	±	–
Sulfa metabolites	Sheaves of needles with central or eccentric binding; shocks of wheat comprised of slender sheaves that grow in such a way as to form two half circles with central binding; sometimes fan-shaped clusters; sometimes globules with striations	+	±	–
Tyrosine	Fine colorless or yellow needles arranged in sheaves or rosettes	+	–	–
Uric acid	Diamond or rhombic rosettes, or oval plates, structures with pointed ends; occasionally, six-sided plates	+	–	–
Xanthine	Amorphous, spheroid, or ovoid structures with a yellow-brown color	+	±	–

+ = crystals commonly occur at this pH; ± = crystals may occur at this pH, but are more common at another pH; – = crystals are uncommon at this pH.

- Detection of disorders predisposing animals to urolith formation
- Estimation of the mineral composition of uroliths
- Evaluation of the effectiveness of medical protocols initiated to dissolve or prevent urolithiasis

Crystals form only in urine that is, or recently has been, oversaturated with crystallogenic substances. Therefore crystalluria represents a risk factor for urolithiasis. However, detection of urine crystals is not synonymous with uroliths and clinical signs associated with them nor are urine crystals irrefutable evidence of a stone-forming tendency. For example, crystalluria that occurs in individuals with anatomically and functionally normal urinary tracts is usually harmless because the crystals are eliminated before they grow to sufficient size to interfere with normal urinary function. In addition, crystals that form following elimination or removal of urine from the patient often are of no clinical importance. Identification of crystals that have formed in vitro does not justify therapy. On the other hand, detection of some types of crystals (e.g., cystine and ammonium urate) in clinically asymptomatic patients, frequent detection of large aggregates of crystals (e.g., calcium oxalate or magnesium ammonium phosphate) in apparently normal individuals, or detection of any form of crystals in fresh urine collected from patients with confirmed urolithiasis may be of diagnostic, prognostic, or therapeutic importance.

In patients with confirmed urolithiasis, microscopic evaluation of urine crystals should not be used as the sole criterion of

TABLE 11-15

IN VITRO AND IN VIVO VARIABLES INFLUENCING CRYSTALLURIA

In Vivo Factors
- Concentration of crystallogenic substances in urine (which in turn is influenced by their rate of excretion and the volume of water in which they are excreted)
- Urine pH (see Table 11-14)
- Solubility
- Excretion of diagnostic agents (such as radiopaque contrast agents) and medications (such as sulfonamides)
- Rate of urine flow

In Vitro Factors
- Temperature
- Evaporation
- pH
- Technique of specimen preparation (e.g., centrifugation versus noncentrifugation and volume of urine examined) and preservation

It is emphasized that in vitro changes that occur following urine collection may enhance formation or dissolution of crystals. Although these changes may be used to enhance detection of certain types of crystals (e.g., acidification to cause precipitation of cystine), in vitro crystal formation may have no clinical relevance to in vivo formation of crystals in urine.

When knowledge of in vivo urine crystal type is especially important, fresh warm specimens should be serially examined. The number, size, and structure of crystals should be evaluated, as well as their tendency to aggregate.

Some clinicians state that in vivo formation of crystals in urine may be a normal phenomenon. However, it is our opinion that in vivo crystalluria represents a risk for urolithiasis by heterogeneous nucleation. However, we agree that detection of crystalluria per se is not a mandate for therapy.

Urine pH

Formation and persistence of several types of crystals are influenced by pH. Therefore it is often useful to consider pH when interpreting crystalluria (Table 11-14).

Different crystals tend to form and persist in certain pH ranges, although there are exceptions. Exceptions may be related to large concentrations of crystallogenic substances in urine or recent in vivo or in vitro changes in urine pH. Some crystals are not affected by the physiologic range of urine pH. Calcium oxalate is one example.

Refrigeration

Refrigeration is an excellent method to preserve many physical, chemical, and morphologic properties of urine sediment. However, it must be used with caution when evaluating crystalluria from qualitative and quantitative standpoints. Although refrigeration of urine samples is likely to enhance formation of various types of crystals, this phenomenon may have no relationship to events occurring in the patient's body.

Diet

Crystalluria may also be influenced by diet (including water intake). Dietary influences on crystalluria would be expected to be more significant during postprandial than fasting states. Dietary influence on crystalluria is of diagnostic importance because urine crystal formation that occurs while patients are consuming hospital diets may be different than crystal formation that occurs when patients are consuming diets fed at home.

the mineral composition of macroliths. Only quantitative urolith analysis can provide definitive information about the mineral composition of the entire stone. However, interpretation of crystalluria in light of other clinical findings often allows tentative identification of the mineral composition of uroliths, especially their outermost layers. Subsequent reduction or elimination of crystalluria by therapy provides a useful index of the efficacy of medical protocols designed to dissolve or prevent uroliths.

Examination of preserved urine samples for crystals may give false results. For example, use of Mucolexx® preservative may result in formation of tyrosine-like crystals (see Plate 107).

Factors Influencing Urine Crystal Formation[21,22,22a,22b]
In Vivo and In Vitro Variables (Table 11-15)

Even though there is not a direct relationship between crystalluria and urolithiasis, detection of crystals in urine is proof that the urine sample is oversaturated with crystallogenic substances. However, oversaturation may occur as a result of in vitro events in addition to, or instead of, in vivo events. Therefore care must be used not to overinterpret the significance of crystalluria. In many instances crystals found in urine sediment were not present when the urine was voided.

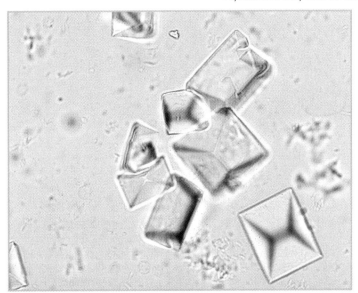

FIGURE 11-6 *Struvite crystals and bacteria. (See Plate 99 in the Color Plate Section for more details.)*

Drugs

Detection of unusual crystals in the urine of patients receiving medications should prompt consideration that the crystals may be drug metabolites.[22a] Drugs associated with crystalluria in dogs and cats include sulfadiazine and its metabolites, ampicillin, and radiopaque contrast agents (Plates 68 through 73, Table 11-14). Other drugs associated with crystalluria in humans include ciprofloxacin, primidone, 5-fluorocytosine, and 6-mercaptopurine.

Combinations of Crystals

Crystals form in a complex environment characterized by constant formation of urine of variable composition that traverses different components of the upper and lower urinary tract. More than one type of crystal may be observed in the same urine sample (Plates 69 and 74).

Observation of a combination of brushite (calcium hydrogen phosphate dihydrate, a mineral precipitated in acid urine) and calcium apatite (calcium phosphate, a mineral precipitated in alkaline urine) crystals in human urine samples supports this hypothesis because brushite would not be expected to form in the alkaline environment required for precipitation of calcium apatite.

Crystals of different composition may also form within the same location. For example, infection-induced magnesium ammonium phosphate crystals may form concomitantly with metabolic crystals (e.g., calcium oxalate, calcium phosphate, cystine, and ammonium urate; Plate 74).

Crystal Habit

Habit is the term commonly used by mineralogists to refer to characteristic shapes of mineral crystals and is commonly used as an index of crystal composition. However, microscopic evaluation of the habits of urine crystals represents only a tentative indicator of their composition because variable conditions associated with their formation, growth, and dissolution may alter their appearance. Therefore definitive identification of crystal composition is dependent on optical crystallography, infrared spectrophotometry, thermal analysis, x-ray diffraction, electron microprobe analysis, or a combination of these.

If confirmation of the composition of microscopic crystalluria is desired, it may be of value to attempt to prepare a large pellet of crystals by centrifugation of an appropriate volume of urine in a conical tip centrifuge tube. Evaluation of the pellet by quantitative methods designed for urolith analysis may provide meaningful information about crystalluria associated with urolithiasis. However, the type of crystals identified by this method may reflect only the outer portions of uroliths.

Bilirubin Crystalluria

Bilirubin may crystallize in urine to form yellow-red or reddish brown needles or granules (Plates 75 and 76). Bilirubin crystals can be observed in highly concentrated urine from normal dogs. When observed in large numbers in serial samples of urine, they should arouse suspicion of an abnormality in bilirubin metabolism.

Calcium Carbonate Crystalluria (Plate 77)

Calcium carbonate crystals have not been detected in canine or feline urine. If dumbbell-shaped crystals are observed in canine or feline urine, they are more likely to be calcium oxalate monohydrate than calcium carbonate.

Calcium Oxalate Crystalluria
Habit

Calcium oxalate dihydrate crystals (weddellite) typically are colorless and have a characteristic dipyramidal, octahedral, or envelope shape (Plates 69, 70, and 78 through 80). Under light microscopy they resemble small or large squares whose corners are connected by intersecting diagonal lines. Scanning electron micrographs reveal them to resemble two pyramids joined at their bases (and thus the name dipyramidal). They vary in size and sometimes occur in aggregates.

Calcium oxalate monohydrate crystals (whewellite) vary in size and may have a spindle, oval (hemp seed), or dumbbell shape (Plates 81 and 85). Calcium oxalate monohydrate crystals with hippuric acid–like morphologic findings have also been observed in dogs, especially those with ethylene glycol toxicity (Plates 82 through 84). They are soluble in hydrochloric acid but insoluble in acetic acid. They may occur in combination with calcium oxalate dihydrate and other types of crystals.

Calcium oxalate crystals have been observed in acidic, neutral, and alkaline urine samples.

Interpretation

Calcium oxalate dihydrate crystals may occur in apparently normal dogs and cats and in dogs and cats with uroliths primarily composed of calcium oxalate. Although they may be observed in dogs intoxicated with ethylene glycol, they are less common than calcium oxalate monohydrate crystals (ethylene glycol toxicity may also occur without crystalluria).

Calcium oxalate monohydrate crystals may occur alone or in combination with calcium oxalate dihydrate or other types of crystals. Large quantities of calcium oxalate monohydrate (or dihydrate) crystals in fresh urine should prompt consideration of hypercalciuric or hyperoxaluric disorders (such as ethylene glycol toxicity), especially if they occur in aggregates or grow to a large size.[33]

Calcium Phosphate Crystalluria
Habit

There are many different types of calcium phosphate crystals. With the exception of brushite, calcium phosphate crystals tend to form in alkaline urine.

> Microscopic evaluation of the habits of urine crystals represents only a tentative indicator of their composition because variable conditions associated with their formation, growth, and dissolution may alter their appearance.

Calcium phosphate crystals are variously described as amorphous phosphates and calcium phosphates. Under light microscopy amorphous phosphates resemble amorphous urate (Plate 86). However, amorphous phosphates typically form in alkaline urine and are soluble in acetic acid. In contrast, amorphous urates often have a yellow granular appearance and are insoluble in acetic acid but are soluble in alkali and at 60°C.

Scanning electron micrographs of amorphous phosphates in human urine revealed that they usually have a spheric habit but may assume doughnut or cast forms. We have recognized the spheric habit of calcium phosphate only in dogs. Calcium phosphates may also form long, thin, colorless prisms, sometimes with one pointed end. These crystals may aggregate into rosettes or appear as needles. Calcium phosphate may also precipitate as elongated, lath-shaped brushite crystals in acidic urine (Plates 87 and 88).

Interpretation

Care must be used in interpretation of amorphous crystals detected by light microscopy since they form from a variety of crystals including calcium phosphate, ammonium urate, and xanthine. In our experience, large numbers of crystals presumed to be composed of calcium phosphate have been observed in apparently normal dogs, dogs with persistently alkaline urine, and dogs with calcium phosphate uroliths composed of a mixture of calcium phosphate and calcium oxalate. Small numbers of calcium phosphate crystals may occur in association with infection-induced struvite crystalluria.

Cholesterol Crystalluria
Habit (Plate 89)

Cholesterol crystals typically appear as large, flat, rectangular plates with a characteristic notch in a corner. By light microscopy, they are colorless and transparent; by polarized light microscopy, a variety of brilliant colors typically are observed.

Interpretation

In humans cholesterol crystals have been reported to be associated with excessive tissue destruction, the nephrotic syndrome, and chyluria. Veterinary experience with them has been too limited to formulate meaningful generalities. However, they have been observed in apparently normal dogs.

Cystine Crystalluria
Habit (Plates 90 through 92)

Cystine crystals are colorless and have a characteristic hexagonal (benzene ring) shape with equal or unequal sides. They may appear singly but commonly aggregate in layers. Their detection may be aided by reduced light intensity because they are thin. Cystine crystals most commonly form in concentrated acidic urine. Formation of markedly alkaline urine as a consequence

of infection or contamination with urease-producing microbes may cause cystine crystals to dissolve.

Addition of glacial acetic acid followed by refrigeration and centrifugation may enhance detection of typical crystals in alkaline urine samples. Cystine crystals are insoluble in acetic acid, alcohol, acetone, ether, and boiling water. They are soluble in ammonia and hydrochloric acid.

Interpretation

Cystine crystalluria is not a normal phenomenon. Cystine uroliths may develop in dogs and cats with the metabolic disorder of cystinuria; however, not all patients with cystinuria develop cystine uroliths (see discussion of magnesium ammonium phosphate and uric acid crystalluria for details about differentiation of cystine crystals from struvite or uric acid crystals).

Drug-Associated Crystalluria[22,22a,22b,23]

Various drugs excreted in urine may form crystals (Plates 68 through 73). Diagnostic and therapeutic drugs may enhance crystalluria in one or a combination of ways, including (1) alteration of urine pH in such fashion as to create an environment that decreases the solubility of some lithogenic substances, (2) alteration of glomerular filtration, tubular reabsorption, and/or tubular secretion of drugs or endogenous substances so as to enhance promoters or impair inhibitors of crystalluria, or (3) precipitation (e.g., drugs or their metabolites) to form crystals (Table 11-16). The prevalence of crystals that contain drugs or their metabolites in dogs, cats, and other animals is unknown. It is probable that crystals containing drugs are often unrecognized because they are not suspected and because of limitations associated with their detection by commonly used methods of quantitative urolith analysis. For this reason, we recommend that the relevant drug history of patients be included along with their urine samples submitted to laboratories for analysis.

Sulfonamide Crystals (Plates 68 through 70)—Perhaps the most commonly recognized drug crystalluria in dogs and cats is that which occurs with sulfonamide administration. Sulfonamides may form different types of crystals, including those described as (1) centrally or eccentrically waisted sheaves (bundles) composed of needle-like crystals (2) needles in fan-shaped configuration, (3) shocks of wheat comprised of slender sheaves that grow in such a way as to form two half circles with central binding, (4) rosettes formed when the two half circles just described finally close, (5) globules with conspicuous radial striations, (6) wedge-shaped crystals with one sharp point and pronounced serrated or "saw tooth" edges on one or both sides, and (7) transparent ovoid crystals with serrations on one or both edges. The lignin test can be used to help identify sulfa-containing (or related) drugs/metabolites in

Large quantities of calcium oxalate crystals in fresh urine should prompt consideration of hypercalciuric or hyperoxaluric disorders, especially if they occur in aggregates or grow to a large size.

urine. This test is based on the reaction of arylamide groups in such drugs with cellulose (such as that contained in newspaper or paper towels) to form a yellow to orange color. To perform a lignin test, add several drops of urine and several drops of hydrochloric acid to newspaper. A yellow-orange color will form almost immediately if a sufficient concentration of sulfa metabolites are present in urine. Uroliths containing varying quantities of sulfonamides have been observed in dogs and cats.

Radiopaque Contrast Agents—We have observed colorless, long, pointed, needle-like crystals in canine urine containing sodium diatrizoate (Hypaque 50[e]; Plate 71) and flat rectangular plates in urine containing diatrizoate meglumine (Renografin[f]; Plate 72). Although ampicillin (Plate 73) and sodium diatrizoate crystals resemble sulfa crystals, urine containing them is negative for the lignin test, which is positive when sulfas are present in urine. The rectangular diatrizoate meglumine crystals resemble cholesterol crystals.

Ampicillin Crystals—We observed wheat sheaf–like crystals presumed to be ampicillin in the urine of a dog when given large doses of ampicillin. Ampicillin crystals appear as long, thin needles or prisms.

Xanthine Crystals—Xanthine crystalluria in dogs usually occurs secondary to therapy with allopurinol (refer to the section on xanthine crystals).

Other Drugs—Other drug-associated forms of crystalluria observed in humans include fluoroquinolones, 5-fluorocytosine, 6-mercaptopurine, methenamine mandelate, nalidixic acid, and theophylline. Methods used to identify crystals suspected of being composed of drugs include infrared spectroscopy, gas or liquid chromatography, and mass spectrometry.[22b]

Hippuric Acid Crystalluria

Hippuric acid crystals are colorless, elongated structures of variable size. They typically have six sides that are connected by rounded corners. They resemble calcium oxalate monohydrate crystals.

True hippuric acid crystals are apparently rare in dogs and cats and therefore are of unknown significance.

Leucine Crystalluria

Leucine crystals typically appear as large yellow or brown spheroids with radial concentric laminations (Plate 93). However, such spheroids may not be pure leucine because it has been reported that pure leucine forms crystals that resemble hexagonal plates.

In humans leucine crystals are indicative of severe liver disease or disorders associated with aminoacidurias. The significance of leucine crystals in dogs has not been well documented. However, we have observed leucine-like crystals in the urine of a 10-month old female Scottish terrier with cystinuria.

> Struvite crystals commonly occur in dogs and occasionally in cats in association with free ammonia produced by microbial urease-induced hydrolysis of urea.

Magnesium Ammonium Phosphate Crystalluria

Habit (Plates 74 and 94 through 105)

Magnesium ammonium phosphate (struvite) crystals typically appear as colorless, orthorhombic (having three unequal axes intersecting at right angles), coffin-like prisms of variable size. Often they have at least three to six sides and oblique ends. Six- to eight-sided struvite crystals in cats are sometimes mistaken for cystine crystals. Unlike cystine crystals, however, they occur in association with other forms of struvite and readily dissolve following acidification with dilute acetic acid.

On occasion, struvite crystals aggregate into fern-like structures. The sharp outlines of struvite crystals characteristically observed in fresh urine may become feather-like or moth eaten as they dissolve.

Interpretation

Struvite crystals commonly occur in dogs and occasionally in cats in association with free ammonia produced by microbial urease-induced hydrolysis of urea. Struvite crystals commonly occur in cats and occasionally in dogs in the absence of detectable urease. In this instance the ammonium component of struvite presumably is generated by renal tubules.

In our experience struvite crystals may be observed in dogs and cats that (1) are apparently normal, (2) have infection-induced struvite uroliths, (3) have sterile struvite uroliths, (4) have nonstruvite uroliths, (5) have uroliths of mixed composition (e.g., a nucleus composed of calcium oxalate and a shell composed of struvite), and (6) have urinary tract disease without uroliths.

Tyrosine Crystalluria

Tyrosine crystals appear as fine, highly refractile, colorless or yellow needles aggregated in sheaves or clusters. In humans they have been reported in association with severe liver dis-

TABLE 11-16

FACTORS PREDISPOSING TO PRECIPITATION OF DRUGS IN URINE

A. Reduced volume of highly concentrated urine
B. Urine stasis
C. High rate of urinary excretion of drugs that are poorly soluble in urine
D. Prolonged treatment with high doses of potentially lithogenic drugs
   1. Sulfonamides
   2. Tetracyclines
   3. Others

TABLE 11-17

COMMON URINARY ARTIFACTS AND CONTAMINANTS

- Air bubbles
- Oil droplets from lubricants
- Coupling gel in samples collected by ultrasound-guided cystocentesis
- Starch granules from surgical gloves
- Glass particles and chips in glass slides
- Hair
- Fecal material
- Parasite ova
- Bacteria, yeasts, and fungi
- Dust
- Fragments of cotton or other fabrics
- Plant spores

ease, or diseases associated with aminoacidurias. However, they have not been a common finding in canine or feline liver disorders (Plates 106 and 107).

Urate Crystalluria
Habit (Plates 108 through 114)

Ammonium urate (also called ammonium biurate) crystals are commonly observed in slightly acidic, neutral, and alkaline urine. They are usually brown or yellow-brown and may form spherulites or spheric bodies with long, irregular protrusions (so-called thorny apple form).

Sodium, potassium, magnesium, and calcium urate salts may precipitate in amorphous form in acidic urine (so-called amorphous urates). They may resemble amorphous phosphates but dissolve in an alkaline environment. As the amorphous crystals grow, they develop a characteristic yellow or yellow-brown color. Sodium urate may also precipitate as colorless or yellowish needles or as slender prisms occurring in sheaves or clusters (Plate 115).

Ammonium urate and amorphous urate crystals are insoluble in acetic acid. However, addition of 10% acetic acid to urine sediment containing these crystals often results in the appearance of uric acid and sometimes sodium urate crystals (see discussion of uric acid crystalluria for details). Addition of acetic acid to amorphous phosphate crystals results in their rapid dissolution, whereas they persist in alkaline urine sediment.

Interpretation

Urate crystals are frequently observed in dogs with portal vascular anomalies with or without concomitant ammonium urate uroliths. They are also commonly detected in dalmatians and English bulldogs. They may be observed in dogs and cats with ammonium urate uroliths caused by disorders other than portal vascular anomalies.

Ammonium urate and amorphous urate may occur in apparently normal dogs and cats, but they are not common.

Uric Acid Crystalluria
Habit (Plates 116 and 117)

Uric acid crystals are often yellow or yellow-brown and may occur in a variety of shapes. The most characteristic forms are diamond or rhombic plates, which may contain concentric rings. They may also appear as rosettes composed of aggregates of many uric acid crystals. Occasionally, uric acid crystals form rhomboid plates with one or more paired protrusions from their sides. Less commonly, they appear as six-sided crystals resembling cystine; however, the six-sided crystals occur in association with typical diamond or rhomboid forms.

Uric acid crystals are soluble in sodium hydroxide but are insoluble in alcohol, hydrochloric acid, and acetic acid.

Interpretation

Although naturally occurring uric acid crystalluria is common in humans, it is uncommon in dogs and cats. When detected, the crystals have the same significance as that described for ammonium and amorphous urates.

Uric acid crystals readily form following the addition of 10% acetic acid to canine or feline urine sediment that contains amorphous urate or ammonium urate crystals. Sodium urate crystals may also appear. Exposure to acetic acid for approximately 20 to 30 minutes is often required before the uric acid crystals become visible. They may grow large if preserved overnight in a covered Petri dish humidified with a sponge soaked in water.

Xanthine Crystalluria[22a,22b]

Xanthine crystals in urine sediment cannot be distinguished from many forms of ammonium urate or amorphous urates by light microscopy (Plate 118). All of these crystals are usually brown or yellow-brown and may form spherules of varying size. Polarizing light microscopy is also an insensitive method to detect xanthine crystalluria. Infrared spectroscopy can be used to confirm that crystals contain xanthine. Xanthinuria may be detected by high pressure liquid chromatography.

Xanthine crystalluria in dogs usually occurs secondary to therapy with excessive dosages of allopurinol in context of the amount of purine precursors in the diet.[5] Allopurinol rapidly binds to and inhibits the action of xanthine oxidase, thereby decreasing conversion of hypoxanthine to xanthine and xanthine to uric acid. The result is a reduction of serum and urine concentrations of uric acid with an increase in serum and urine concentrations of xanthine. The magnitude of allopurinol-induced xanthinuria is influenced by several variables including (1) the dosage of allopurinol, (2) the quantity of purine precursors in the diet, (3) the rate of production of endogenous purine precursors, (4) the rate and completeness of endogenous and exogenous degradation, and (5) the status of hepatic function and its influence on the pharmacokinetics of allopurinol and its metabolites.

We have encountered naturally occurring xanthine crystalluria and xanthine uroliths in cats. Naturally occurring xanthinuria was recently recognized in a family of Cavalier King Charles spaniels in The Netherlands. An autosomal recessive mode inheritance was postulated.[31]

Artifacts and Contaminants

Many exogenous substances may contaminate urine and are a potential source of confusion (Plates 119 through 126). Commonly encountered artifacts and contaminants are listed in Table 11-17.

Starch granules occasionally appear in urine from gloves used during catheterization. They are sometimes confused with fat droplets because they have a Maltese cross pattern when viewed with the aid of polarized light microscopy. However, they are not perfectly round, they are not refractile when viewed by bright light microscopy, they have faceted or scalloped edges, and they typically have an indented center or dimple.

Urine samples collected from table tops, litter trays, or by cystocentesis may be contaminated with feces. Examination of the sediment of contaminated specimens may reveal partly digested muscle fibers, plant cells, and different types of bacteria. When in doubt as to the origin of structures in urine sediment, it is best to reexamine a fresh sample known not to be contaminated with fecal material.

---

[a]Hycor Biomedical, Garden Grove, CA.
[b]Clay Adams, Division of Becton Dickinson & Co., Parsippany, NJ.
[c]In the United States, manufactured for IDEXX by Bayer. Petstix is a trademark of Bayer Corporation; used under license by IDEXX Laboratories, Inc. Available in Canada from Bayer, Inc.
[d]Available from Lerner Laboratories, Pittsburgh, PA.
[e]Winthrop Laboratories, New York, NY.
[f]Bristol-Myers Squibb, New Brunswick, NJ.

REFERENCES AND SUGGESTED READINGS

1. Allen TA, Jones RL, Purvance J: Microbiologic evaluation of canine urine: Direct microscopic examination and preservation of specimen quality for culture. JAVMA 190:1289–1291, 1987.
2. Bartges JW, Osborne CA, Felice LJ: Canine xanthine uroliths: Risk factor management, in Kirk RW, Bonagura JD (eds): Current Veterinary Therapy XI. Philadelphia, WB Saunders, 1992, pp 900–905.
3. Barsanti JA, Blue J, Edmunds J: Urinary tract infections due to indwelling bladder catheters in dogs and cats. JAVMA 187:384–388, 1985.
4. Bradley M, Schumann GB, Ward PCJ: Examination of urine, in Henry JB (ed): Clinical Diagnosis and Management by Laboratory Methods, ed 16, vol 1. Philadelphia, WB Saunders, 1979, pp 559–634.
5. Chew DJ: Urinalysis, in Bovee KC (ed): Canine Nephrology. Media, PA, Harwal Publishing, 1984.
6. Chew DJ, DiBartola SP: Diagnosis and pathophysiology of renal disease, in Ettinger SJ (ed): Textbook of Veterinary Internal Medicine, ed 3, vol 2. Philadelphia, WB Saunders, 1989, pp 1893–1961.
7. Dooley MP, Pineda MH, Hooper JG, Hsu WH: Retrograde flow of semen caused by electroejaculation in the domestic cat. 10th International Congress Animal & Artificial Insemination, Urbana, IL, Jun 10–14, 1981, p 363.
8. Fairley KF, Birch DF: A simple method for identifying glomerular bleeding. Kidney Int 21:105–108, 1982.
9. Ferguson JM, Renton JP: Observation on the presence of spermatozoa in canine urine. J Small Anim Pract 29:691–694, 1988.
10. Gadeholt H: Quantitative examination of urinary sediment with special regard to sources of error. Br Med J 1:1547, 1964.
11. Haber MH, Lindner LE: The surface ultrastructure of urinary casts. Am Clin Path 68:547–552, 1977.
12. Hoyer JR, Seiler MW: Pathophysiology of Tamm-Horsfall protein. Kidney Int 16:279–289, 1979.
13. Jenkins RD, Fenn JP, Matsen JM: Review of urine microscopy for bacteria. JAMA 255:3397–3404, 1986.
14. Kass EM: The role of asymptomatic bacteriuria in the pathogenesis of pyelonephritis, in Quinn EL, Kass EM (eds): Biology of Pyelonephritis. Boston, MA, Little Brown, 1960.
15. Lindner LE, Haber MH: Hyaline casts in the urine: Mechanism of formation and morphologic transformations. Am J Clin Path 80:347–352, 1983.
16. Ling GV, Kaneka JJ: Microscopic examination of canine urine sediment. Calif Vet 30:14, 1976.
17. Lulich JP, Osborne CA: Fungal urinary tract infections, in Kirk RW, Bonagura JD (eds): Current Veterinary Therapy XI. Philadelphia, WB Saunders, 1992, pp 914–919, 1992.
18. McKenzie JK, McQueen EG: Immunofluorescent localization of Tamm-Horsfall mucoprotein in human kidney. J Clin Pathol 22:334, 1969.
19. McQueen EG: The nature of urinary casts. J Clin Pathol 15:367–373, 1962.
20. McQueen EG, Engel GB: Factors determining the aggregation of urinary protein. J Clin Pathol 19:392–396, 1966.
21. Osborne CA, Davis LS, Sanna J, et al: Identification and interpretation of crystalluria in domestic animals: A light and scanning electron microscopic study. Vet Med 85:18–37, 1990.
22. Osborne CA, O'Brien TD, Ghobrial HK, et al: Crystalluria: Observations, interpretations, and misinterpretations. Vet Clin North Am 16:45–65, 1986.
22a. Osborne CA, Lulich JB, Bartges JW, et al: Drug-induced urolithiasis. Vet Clin North Am Small Anim Pract 29:251–266, 1999.
22b. Osborne CA, Lulich JP, Ulrich LK, et al: Pharmacologic treatment and uroliths—Cause or cure. Proceedings of the 16th Annual Veterinary Medical Forum, San Diego, pp 650–651, 1998.
23. Osborne CA, Stevens JB: Handbook of Canine and Feline Urinalysis. St. Louis, Ralston Purina, 1981.
24. Pollak VE, Arbel C: The distribution of Tamm-Horsfall mucoprotein (Uromucoid) in the human nephron. Nephron 6:667, 1969.
25. Rutecki GJ, Goldsmith C, Schreiner GE: Characterization of proteins in urinary casts: Fluorescent antibody identification of Tamm-Horsfall mucoprotein in matrix and serum proteins in granules. N Engl J Med 284:1049–1052, 1979.
26. Schenk EA, Schwartz RH, Lewis RA: Tamm-Horsfall mucoprotein. I. Localization in the kidney. Lab Invest 25:92–95, 1971.
27. Shull RM, Hayden DW, Johnston GR: Urogenital blastomycosis in a dog. JAVMA 171:730–735, 1977.
28. Strasinger SK: Urinalysis and Body Fluids, ed 3. Philadelphia, FA Davis, 1994.
29. Thai SM, DeBellis CC, Iverson SA, Schumana GB: Comparison of dysmorphic erythrocytes with other urinary sediment parameters of renal bleeding. Am J Clin Path 86:784–787, 1986.
30. vanZuilen CD, Nickel RF, VanDijk TH, et al: Xanthinuria in a family of Cavalier King Charles spaniels. Vet Q 19:172–174, 1997.

The smart antimicrobial for urinary infections.

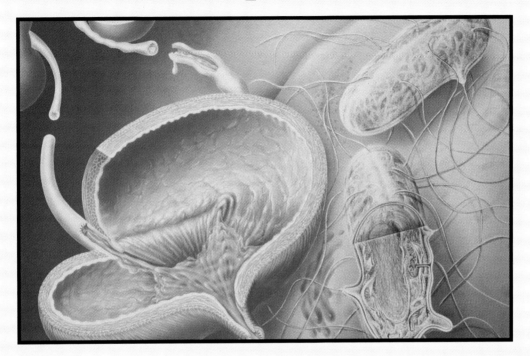

- Broad spectrum of activity against urinary pathogens

- Achieves high concentrations in urogenital system

- Excellent renal tolerance

- Phagocytic accumulation augments Baytril concentration in infected tissue

- Rapidly bactericidal

- Once-daily dosing simplifies pet owner compliance

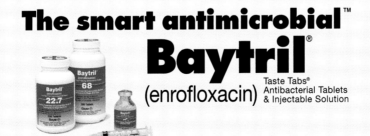
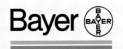

Baytril® (enrofloxacin)

22.7 mg and 68 mg Antibacterial Tablets and Injectable Solution

CAUTION:

Federal (U.S.A.) law restricts this drug to use by or on the order of a licensed veterinarian.

DESCRIPTION:

Enrofloxacin is a synthetic chemotherapeutic agent from the class of the quinolone carboxylic acid derivatives. It has antibacterial activity against a broad spectrum of Gram negative and Gram positive bacteria (See Tables I and II). It is rapidly absorbed from the digestive tract, penetrating into all measured body tissues and fluids (See Table III).

Tablets are available in two sizes (22.7 and 68.0 mg enrofloxacin). Each mL of injectable solution contains: enrofloxacin 22.7 mg, n-butyl alcohol 30 mg, potassium hydroxide for pH adjustment and water for injection, q.s.

CHEMICAL NOMENCLATURE AND STRUCTURAL FORMULA:

1-cyclopropyl-7-(4-ethyl-1-piperazinyl)-6-fluoro-1,4-dihydro-4-oxo-3-quinolinecarboxylic acid.

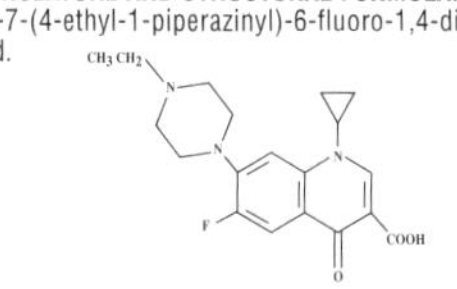

ACTIONS:

Microbiology: Quinolone carboxylic acid derivatives are classified as DNA gyrase inhibitors. The mechanism of action of these compounds is very complex and not yet fully understood. The site of action is bacterial gyrase, a synthesis promoting enzyme. The effect on *Escherichia coli* is the inhibition of DNA synthesis through prevention of DNA supercoiling. Among other things, such compounds lead to the cessation of cell respiration and division. They may also interrupt bacterial membrane integrity.[1]

Enrofloxacin is bactericidal, with activity against both Gram negative and Gram positive bacteria. The minimum inhibitory concentrations (MICs) were determined for a series of 39 isolates representing 9 genera of bacteria from natural infections in dogs and cats, selected principally because of resistance to one or more of the following antibiotics: ampicillin, cephalothin, colistin, chloramphenicol, erythromycin, gentamicin, kanamycin, penicillin, streptomycin, tetracycline, triple sulfa and sulfa/trimethoprim. The MIC values for enrofloxacin against these isolates are presented in Table I. Most strains of these organisms were found to be susceptible to enrofloxacin *in vitro* but the clinical significance has not been determined for some of the isolates.

The susceptibility of organisms to enrofloxacin should be determined using enrofloxacin 5 mcg disks. Specimens for susceptibility testing should be collected prior to the initiation of enrofloxacin therapy.

TABLE I – MIC Values for Enrofloxacin Against Canine and Feline Pathogens (Diagnostic laboratory isolates, 1984)

Organisms	Isolates	MIC Range (mcg/mL)
Bacteroides spp.	2	2
Bordetella bronchiseptica	3	0.125-0.5
Brucella canis	2	0.125-0.25
Clostridium perfringens	1	0.5
Escherichia coli	5*	≤0.016-0.031
Klebsiella spp.	11*	0.031-0.5
Proteus mirabilis	6	0.062-0.125
Pseudomonas aeruginosa	4	0.5-8
Staphylococcus spp.	5	0.125

*Includes feline isolates.

The inhibitory activity on 120 isolates of seven canine urinary pathogens was also investigated and is listed in Table II.

TABLE II – MIC Values for Enrofloxacin Against Canine Urinary Pathogens (Diagnostic laboratory isolates, 1985)

Organisms	Isolates	MIC Range (mcg/mL)
E. coli	30	0.06-2.0
P. mirabilis	20	0.125-2.0
K. pneumoniae	20	0.06-0.5
P. aeruginosa	10	1.0-8.0
Enterobacter spp.	10	0.06-1.0
Staph. (coag. +)	20	0.125-0.5
Strep. (alpha hemol.)	10	0.5-8.0

Distribution in the Body: Enrofloxacin penetrates into all canine and feline tissues and body fluids. Concentrations of drug equal to or greater than the MIC for many pathogens (See Tables I, II and III) are reached in most tissues by two hours after dosing at 2.5 mg/kg and are maintained for 8-12 hours after dosing. Particularly high levels of enrofloxacin are found in urine. A summary of the body fluid/tissue drug levels at 2 to 12 hours after dosing at 2.5 mg/kg is given in Table III.

TABLE III – Body Fluid/Tissue Distribution of Enrofloxacin in Dogs and Cats Single Oral Dose = 2.5 mg/kg (1.13 mg/lb)

	Post-treatment Enrofloxacin Levels			
	Canine (n = 2)		Feline (n = 4)	
Body Fluids (mcg/mL)	**2 Hr.**	**8 Hr.**	**2 Hr.**	**12 Hr.**
Bile	–	–	2.13	1.97
Cerebrospinal Fluid	–	–	0.37	0.10
Urine	43.05	55.35	12.81	26.41
Eye Fluids	0.53	0.66	0.45	0.65
Whole Blood	1.01	0.36	–	–
Plasma	0.67	0.33	–	–
Serum	–	–	0.48	0.18
Tissues (mcg/g)				
Hematopoietic System				
Liver	3.02	1.36	1.84	0.37
Spleen	1.45	0.85	1.33	0.52
Bone Marrow	2.10	1.22	1.68	0.64
Lymph Node	1.32	0.91	0.49	0.21
Urogenital System				
Kidney	1.87	0.99	1.43	0.37
Bladder Wall	1.36	0.98	1.16	0.55
Testes	1.36	1.10	1.01	0.28
Prostate	1.36	2.20	1.88	0.55
Ovaries	–	–	0.78	0.56
Uterine Wall	1.59	0.29	0.81	1.05
Gastrointestinal and Cardiopulmonary Systems				
Lung	1.34	0.82	0.91	0.33
Heart	1.88	0.78	0.84	0.32
Stomach	3.24	2.16	3.26	0.27
Small Intestine	2.10	1.11	2.72	0.40
Large Intestine	–	–	0.94	1.10
Other				
Fat	0.52	0.40	0.24	0.11
Skin	0.66	0.48	0.46	0.17
Muscle	1.62	0.77	0.53	0.29
Brain	0.25	0.24	0.22	0.12
Mammary Gland	0.45	0.21	0.36	0.30
Feces	1.65	9.97	0.37	4.18

Pharmacokinetics:

In dogs, the absorption and elimination characteristics of the oral formulation are linear (plasma concentrations increase proportionally with dose) when enrofloxacin is administered at up to 11.5 mg/kg, twice daily.[2] Approximately 80% of the orally administered dose enters the systemic circulation unchanged. The eliminating organs, based on the drug's body clearance time, can readily remove the drug with no indication that the eliminating mechanisms are saturated. The primary route of excretion is via the urine. The absorption and elimination characteristics beyond this point are unknown. In cats, no oral absorption information is available at other than 2.5 mg/kg, administered orally as a single dose. Saturable absorption and/or elimination processes may occur at greater doses. When saturation of the absorption process occurs, the plasma concentration of the active moiety will be less than predicted, based on the concept of dose proportionality.

Following an oral dose in dogs of 2.5 mg/kg (1.13 mg/lb) enrofloxacin reached 50% of its maximum serum concentration in 15 minutes and peak serum level was reached in one hour. The elimination half-life in dogs is approximately 2½-3 hours at that dose, while in cats, it is greater than 4 hours. In a study comparing dogs and cats, the peak concentration and the time to peak concentration were not different. A graph indicating the mean serum levels following a dose of 2.5 mg/kg (1.13 mg/lb) in dogs (oral and intramuscular) and cats (oral) is shown in Figure 1.

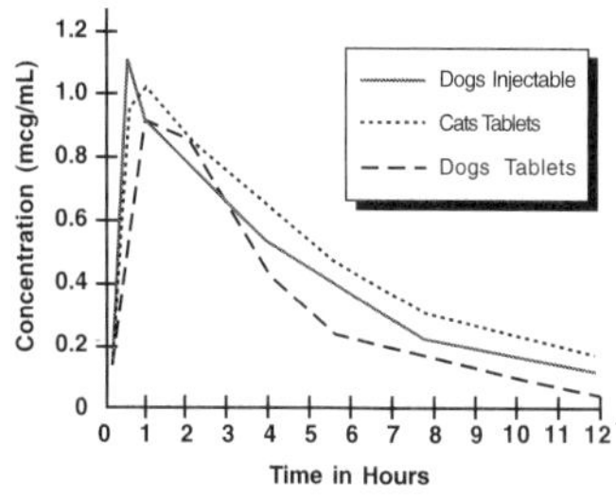

Figure 1 - Serum Concentrations of Enrofloxacin Following a Single Oral or Intramuscular Dose at 2.5 mg/kg in Dogs and a Single Oral Dose at 2.5 mg/kg in Cats.

The lower limit of the dose range was based on efficacy studies in dogs and cats where enrofloxacin was administered at 2.5 mg/kg twice daily. Target animal safety and toxicology studies were used to establish the upper limit of the dose range and treatment duration.

Breakpoint:

Based on pharmacokinetic studies of enrofloxacin in dogs and cats after a single oral administration of 2.5 mg enrofloxacin/kg BW (i.e. half of the lowest-end single daily dose range) and the data listed in Tables I and II, the following breakpoints are recommended for canine and feline isolates.

Zone Diameter (mm)	MIC (µg/mL)	Interpretation
≥ 21	≤ 0.5	Susceptible(S)
18 - 20	1	Intermediate (I)
≤ 17	≥ 2	Resistant (R)

A report of "Susceptible" indicates that the pathogen is likely to be inhibited by generally achievable plasma levels. A report of "Intermediate" is a technical buffer and isolates falling into this category should be retested. Alternatively the organism may be successfully treated if the infection is in a body site where drug is physiologically concentrated. A report of "Resistant" indicates that the achievable drug concentrations are unlikely to be inhibitory and other therapy should be selected.

Standardized procedures require the use of laboratory control organisms for both standardized disk diffusion assays and standardized dilution assays. The 5 µg enrofloxacin disk should give the following zone diameters and enrofloxacin powder should provide the following MIC values for reference strains.

QC strain	MIC (µg/mL)	Zone Diameter (mm)
E. coli ATCC 25922	0.008 - 0.03	32 - 40
P. aeruginosa ATCC 27853	1 - 4	15 - 19
S. aureus ATCC 25923		27 - 31
S. aureus ATCC 29213	0.03 - 0.12	

INDICATIONS:

Dogs & Cats: Baytril® (brand of enrofloxacin) Antibacterial Tablets and Injectable Solution are indicated for the management of diseases in dogs and cats associated with bacteria susceptible to enrofloxacin.

EFFICACY CONFIRMATION:

Dogs: Clinical efficacy was established in dermal infections (wounds and abscesses) associated with susceptible strains of *Escherichia coli, Klebsiella pneumoniae, Proteus mirabilis*, and *Staphylococcus intermedius*; respiratory infections (pneumonia, tonsillitis, rhinitis) associated with susceptible strains of *Escherichia coli* and *Staphylococcus aureus*; and urinary cystitis associated with susceptible strains of *Escherichia coli, Proteus mirabilis*, and *Staphylococcus aureus*.

Cats: Clinical efficacy was established in dermal infections (wounds and abscesses) associated with susceptible strains of *Pasturella multocida, Staphylococcus aureus*, and *Staphylococcus epidermidis*.

CONTRAINDICATIONS:

Enrofloxacin is contraindicated in dogs and cats known to be hypersensitive to quinolones.

Dogs: Based on the studies discussed under the section on Animal Toxicology, the use of enrofloxacin is contraindicated in small and medium breeds of dogs during the rapid growth phase (between 2 and 8 months of age). The safe use of enrofloxacin has not been established in large and giant breeds during the rapid growth phase. Large breeds may be in this phase for up to one year of age and the giant breeds for up to 18 months. In clinical field trials utilizing a daily oral dose of 5.0 mg/kg, there were no reports of lameness or joint problems in any breed. However, controlled studies with histological examination of the articular cartilage have not been conducted in the large or giant breeds.

ADVERSE REACTIONS:

Dogs: Two of the 270 (0.7%) dogs treated with Baytril® (brand of enrofloxacin) Tablets at 5.0 mg/kg per day in the clinical field studies exhibited side effects, which were apparently drug related. These two cases of vomition were self-limiting.

No drug related side effects were reported in 122 clinical cases treated with Baytril® (enrofloxacin) Injectable Solution followed by Baytril Tablets at 5.0 mg/kg per day.

Cats: No drug-related side effects were reported in 124 cats treated with Baytril® (Brand of Enrofloxacin) Tablets at 5.0 mg/kg per day for 10 days, in clinical field studies.

ANIMAL TOXICOLOGY:

Dogs: Adult dogs receiving enrofloxacin orally at a daily dosage rate of 52 mg/kg for 13 weeks had only isolated incidences of vomition and inappetence. Adult dogs receiving the tablet formulation for 30 consecutive days at a daily treatment of 25 mg/kg did not exhibit significant clinical signs nor were there effects upon the clinical chemistry, hematological or histological parameters. Daily doses of 125 mg/kg for up to 11 days induced vomition, inappetence, depression, difficult locomotion and death while adult dogs receiving 50 mg/kg/day for 14 days had clinical signs of vomition and inappetence.

Adult dogs dosed intramuscularly for three treatments at 12.5 mg/kg, followed by 57 oral treatments at 12.5 mg/kg all at 12 hour intervals, did not exhibit either significant clinical signs or effects upon the clinical chemistry, hematological or histological parameters.

Oral treatment of 15 to 28 week old growing puppies with daily dosage rates of 25 mg/kg has induced abnormal carriage of the carpal joint and weakness in the hindquarters. Significant improvement of clinical signs is observed following drug withdrawal. Microscopic studies have identified lesions of the articular cartilage following 30 day treatments at either 5, 15 or 25 mg/kg in this age group. Clinical signs of difficult ambulation or associated cartilage lesions have not been observed in 29 to 34 week old puppies following daily treatments of 25 mg/kg for 30 consecutive days nor in 2 week old puppies with the same treatment schedule.

Tests indicated no effect on circulating microfilariae or adult heartworms (*Dirofilaria immitis*) when dogs were treated at a daily dosage rate of 15 mg/kg for 30 days. No effect on cholinesterase values was observed.

No adverse effects were observed on reproductive parameters when male dogs received 10 consecutive daily treatments of 15 mg/kg/day at 3 intervals (90, 45 and 14 days) prior to breeding or when female dogs received 10 consecutive daily treatments of 15 mg/kg/day at 4 intervals: between 30 and 0 days prior to breeding, early pregnancy (between 10th & 30th days), late pregnancy (between 40th & 60th days), and during lactation (the first 28 days).

Cats: Cats in age ranges of 3 to 4 months and 7 to 10 months received daily treatments of 25 mg/kg for 30 consecutive days with no adverse effects upon the clinical chemistry, hematological or histological parameters. In cats 7-10 months of age treated daily for 30 consecutive days, 2 of 4 receiving 5 mg/kg, 3 of 4 receiving 15 mg/kg, 2 of 4 receiving 25 mg/kg and 1 of 4 nontreated controls experienced occasional vomition. Five to 7 month old cats had no side effects with daily treatments of 15 mg/kg for 30 days, but 2 of 4 animals had articular cartilage lesions when administered 25 mg/kg/day for 30 days.

Doses of 125 mg/kg for 5 consecutive days to adult cats induced vomition, depression, incoordination and death while those receiving 50 mg/kg for 6 days had clinical signs of vomition, inappetence, incoordination and convulsions, but they returned to normal.

DRUG INTERACTIONS:

Compounds that contain metal cations (e.g., aluminum, calcium, iron, magnesium) may reduce the absorption of some quinolone-class drugs from the intestinal tract. Concomitant therapy with other drugs that are metabolized in the liver may reduce the clearance rates of the quinolone and the other drug.

Dogs: Enrofloxacin has been administered to dogs at a daily dosage rate of 10 mg/kg concurrently with a wide variety of other health products including anthelmintics (praziquantel, febantel, sodium disophenol), insecticides (fenthion, pyrethrins), heartworm preventatives (diethylcarbamazine) and other antibiotics (ampicillin, gentamicin sulfate, penicillin, dihydrostreptomycin). No incompatibilities with other drugs are known at this time.

Cats: Enrofloxacin was administered at a daily dosage rate of 5 mg/kg concurrently with anthelmintics (praziquantel, febantel), an insecticide (propoxur) and another antibacterial (ampicillin). No incompatibilities with other drugs are known at this time.

PRECAUTION:

Quinolone-class drugs should be used with caution in animals with known or suspected Central Nervous System (CNS) disorders. In such animals, quinolones have, in rare instances, been associated with CNS stimulation which may lead to convulsive seizures.

Quinolone-class drugs have been associated with cartilage erosions in weight-bearing joints and other forms of arthropathy in immature animals of various species.

Safety in breeding or pregnant cats has not been established.

HUMAN WARNINGS:

For Use in Animals Only. Keep Out of Reach of Children.

Avoid contact with eyes. In case of contact, immediately flush eyes with copious amounts of water for 15 minutes. In case of dermal contact, wash skin with soap and water. Consult a physician if irritation persists following ocular or dermal exposure. Individuals with a history of hypersensitivity to quinolones should avoid this product. In humans, there is a risk of user photosensitization within a few hours after excessive exposure to quinolones. If excessive accidental exposure occurs, avoid direct sunlight.

To report adverse reactions or to obtain a copy of the Material Safety Data Sheet, call 1-800-633-8405.

DOSAGE AND ADMINISTRATION:

The dose range of Baytril (brand of enrofloxacin) Tablets in dogs and cats is 5 to 20 mg/kg (2.27-9.07 mg/lb) of body weight, either as a single dose or divided into two (2) equal daily doses administered at twelve (12) hour intervals. Selection of a dose within this range should be based on clinical experience, the severity of disease, and susceptibility of the pathogen.

Animals which receive doses in the upper-end of the dose range should be carefully monitored for clinical signs that may include inappetence, depression, and vomition. For dogs, Baytril Injectable Solution may be used initially as a single intramuscular dose at 2.5 mg/kg.

TABLETS:

Dogs & Cats: The duration of treatment should be selected based on clinical evidence. Generally, administration of Baytril Tablets should continue for at least 2-3 days beyond cessation of clinical signs. For severe and/or complicated infections, more prolonged therapy, up to 30 days, may be required. If no improvement is seen within five days, the diagnosis should be reevaluated and a different course of therapy considered.

INJECTABLE SOLUTION:

Dogs Only: Baytril Injectable Solution may be used as the initial dose at 2.5 mg/kg. It should be administered intramuscularly (IM) as a single dose, followed by initiation of Baytril Tablet therapy.

Baytril Tablets and Injectable Solution may be administered as follows:

Weight of Animal	Baytril Injectable Solution* (Dogs Only) 2.5mg/kg	Baytril Tablet (Dogs and Cats) **Once Daily Dosing Chart**			
		5.0 mg/kg	10.0 mg/kg	15.0 mg/kg	20.0 mg/kg
9.1 kg (20 lb)	1.00 mL	2 x 22.7 mg tablets	1 x 22.7 mg plus 1 x 68 mg tablets	2 x 68 mg tablets	2 x 22.7 mg plus 2 x 68 mg tablets
27.2 kg (60lb)	3.00 mL	2 x 68 mg tablets	4 x 68 mg tablets	6 x 68 mg tablets	8 x 68 mg tablets

* The initial Baytril Injectable administration should be followed 12 hours later by initiation of Baytril Tablet therapy.

The 22.7 mg tablet and the 68 mg tablet are double scored for accurate dosing.

The lower limit of the dose range was based on efficacy studies in dogs and cats where enrofloxacin was administered at 2.5 mg/kg twice daily. Target animal safety and toxicology studies were used to establish the upper limit of the dose range and treatment duration.

STORAGE:

Protect injectable from direct sunlight. Do not freeze.

HOW SUPPLIED:

Code Number	Baytril Injectable Solution 22.7 mg/mL Vial Size
1865	20 mL

Baytril Tablets

Taste Tabs® Code Number	Film-Coated Tablet Size	Tablet Size	Tablets/Bottle
0387	1868	22.7 mg	100 Double Scored
0388	1881	22.7 mg	500 Double Scored
0389	1869	68.0 mg	50 Double Scored
0390	1882	68.0 mg	250 Double Scored

U.S. Patent No. 4,670,444

REFERENCES:

[1] Dougherty, T.J. and Saukkonen, J.J. Membrane Permeability Changes Associated with DNA Gyrase Inhibitors in *Escherichia coli* Antimicrob. Agents and Chemoth., V. 28, Aug. 1985, 200-206.

[2] Walker, R.D. *et al*, Pharmacokinetic Evaluation of Enrofloxacin Administered Orally to Healthy Dogs. Am. J. Res. V. 53, No. 12, Dec. 1992; 2315-2319.

Bayer Corporation
Agriculture Division, Animal Health,
Shawnee Mission, Kansas 66201, U.S.A.

NADA 140-441, Approved by FDA
NADA 140-913, Approved by FDA

71018820, R.9

January, 1999

Bayer

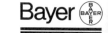

Color Plates

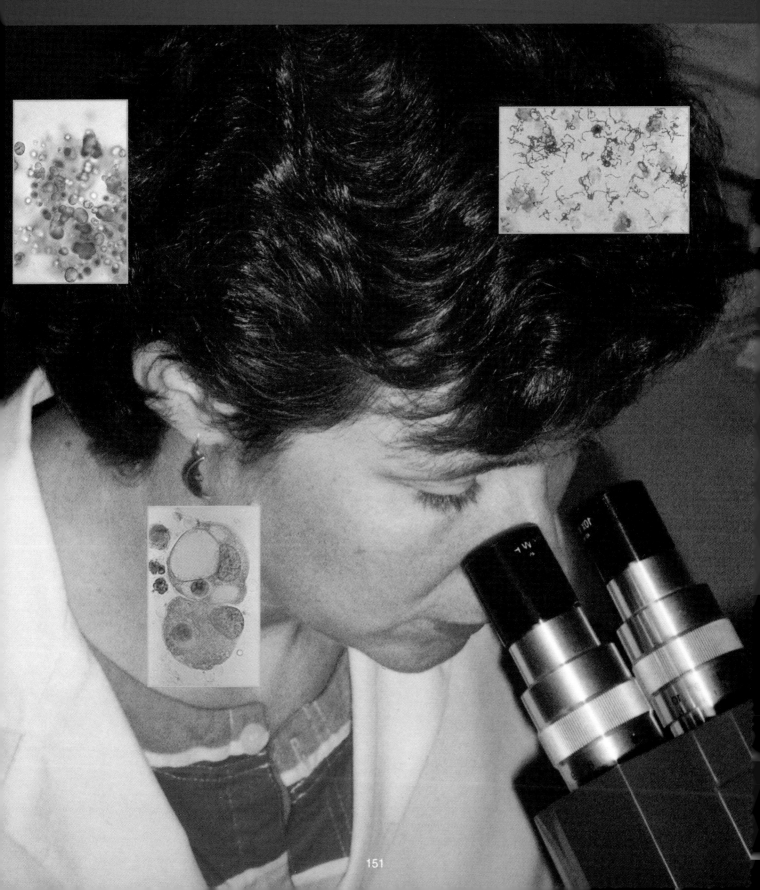

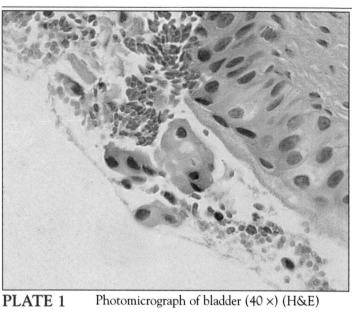

PLATE 1   Photomicrograph of bladder (40 ×) (H&E)

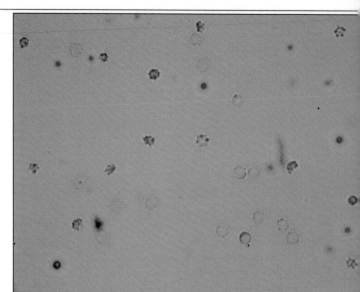

PLATE 4   Crenated red blood cells in urine (160×) (Unstained)

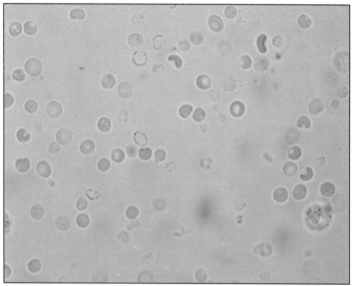

PLATE 2   Red blood cells in urine (160×) (Unstained)

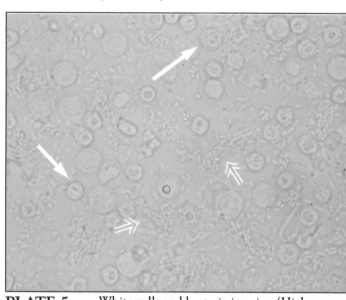

PLATE 5   White cells and bacteria in urine (High power magnification) (Unstained)

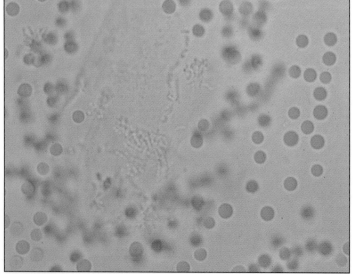

PLATE 3   Red blood cells and cornified epithelial cell in urine (160×) (Unstained)

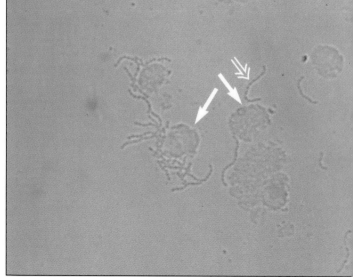

PLATE 6   White cells and bacterial cocci in urine (High power magnification) (Unstained)

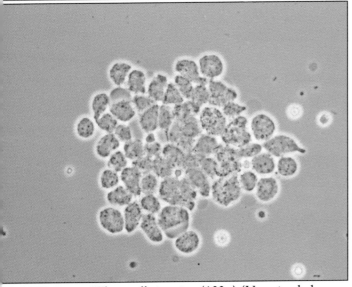

PLATE 7   White cells in urine (100×) (Unstained phase microscopy)

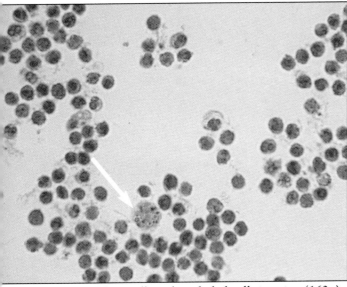

PLATE 8   White cells and epithelial cells in urine (160×) (Sternheimer-Malbin stain)

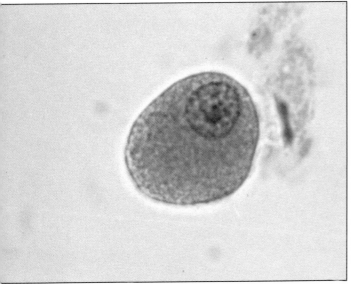

PLATE 9   Epithelial cell in dog urine (High power magnification) (Sedistain)

PLATE 1
Photomicrograph of a section of luminal surface of urinary bladder obtained from a 6-year-old neutered domestic shorthair cat with cystitis. Note red blood cells and transitional epithelial cells on the mucosal surface of the bladder.

PLATE 2
Red blood cells in urine of a dog. Specific gravity was 1.029. An occasional white cell is also present.

PLATE 3
Red blood cells surrounding a cornified epithelial cell in the urine of a dog. Note bacteria adhered to the surface of the epithelial cell.

PLATE 4
Crenated red blood cells in the urine sediment from a dog.

PLATE 5
White cells (*closed arrow*) and bacteria (*open arrow*) in the urine sediment of a dog.

PLATE 6
White cells (*closed arrows*) and bacterial cocci (*open arrow*) in the urine sediment of a dog.

PLATE 7
Cluster of white cells in urine.

PLATE 8
Numerous white cells and an occasional epithelial cell (*arrow*).

PLATE 9
Epithelial cell in the urine sediment of a dog. The eccentrically located nucleus is consistent with renal tubular origin.

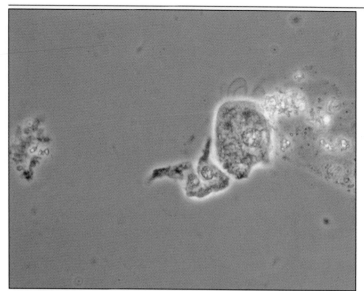

PLATE 10   Caudate epithelial cell (160×) (Phase contrast microscopy)

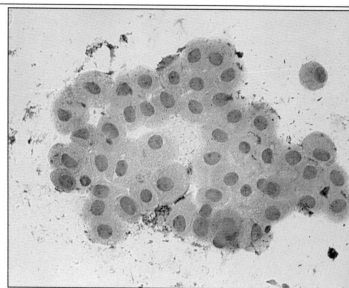

PLATE 13   Transitional epithelial cells (40×) (New methylene blue stain)

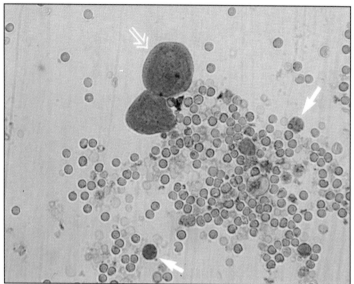

PLATE 11   Epithelial cells, red blood cells, and white cells (100×) (Sedistain)

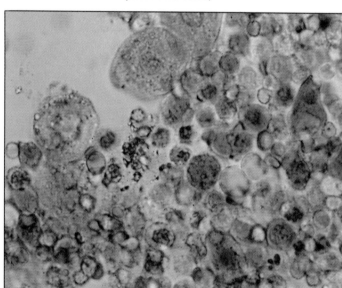

PLATE 14   Epithelial cells, red blood cells, white cells, and cells of uncertain origin (160×) (Sedistain)

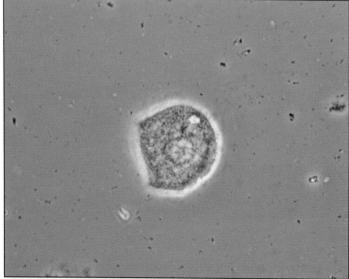

PLATE 12   Epithelial cell (160×) (Unstained phase contrast microscopy)

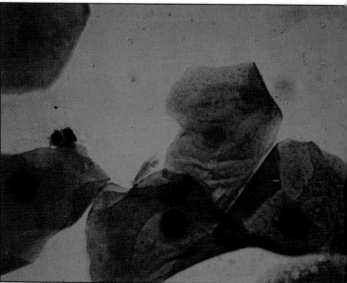

PLATE 15   Cornified squamous epithelial cells (400×) (Unstained)

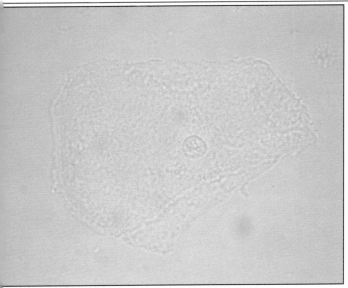

PLATE 16   Squamous epithelial cells (100×) (Unstained)

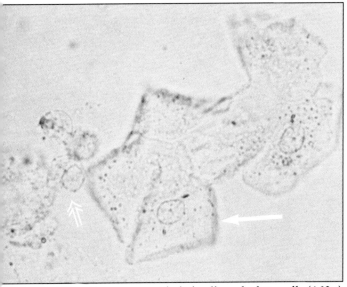

PLATE 17   Squamous epithelial cells and white cells (160×)
(Unstained)

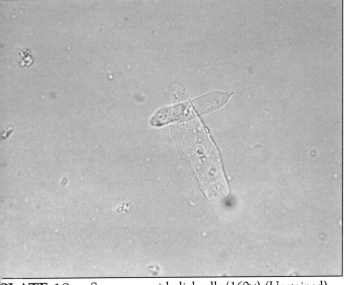

PLATE 18   Squamous epithelial cells (160×) (Unstained)

PLATE 10
Caudate epithelial cell with trailing cytoplasm.

PLATE 11
Transitional epithelial cells (*open arrow*), red blood cells (*closed long arrow*), and occasional white cells (*closed short arrows*) in urine sediment.

PLATE 12
Transitional epithelial cell in urine sediment.

PLATE 13
Clump of transitional epithelial cells in the urine sediment of a 12-year-old neutered female miniature schnauzer with calcium oxalate urocystoliths.

PLATE 14
Nucleated epithelial cells surrounded by red blood cells, stained and unstained white cells, and cells of uncertain origin.

PLATE 15
Cornified squamous epithelial cells.

PLATE 16
Squamous epithelial cells in urine sediment from a voided urine sample.

PLATE 17
Squamous epithelial cells (*closed arrow*) and occasional white cells (*open arrow*).

PLATE 18
Squamous epithelial cells resembling casts.

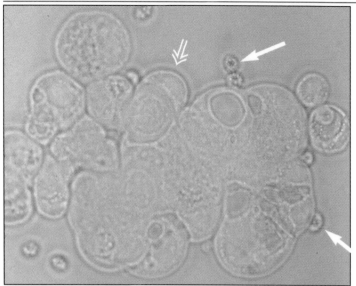

PLATE 19   Neoplastic transitional cells and red cells (160×)
(Unstained)

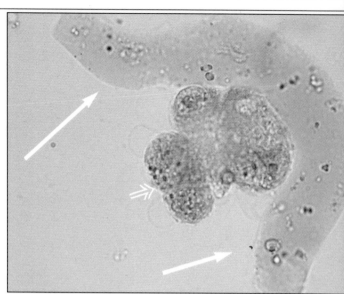

PLATE 22   Hyaline cast and epithelial cell (High power
magnification) (Sedistain)

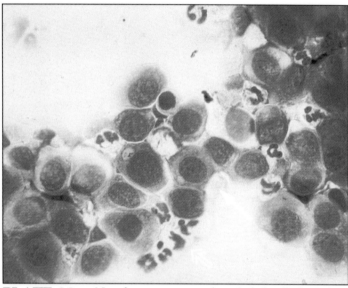

PLATE 20   Neoplastic transitional epithelial cells (400×)
(New methylene blue)

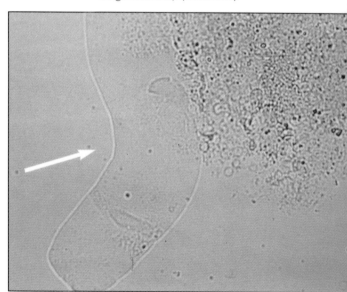

PLATE 23   Broad hyaline cast (160 ×) (Unstained)

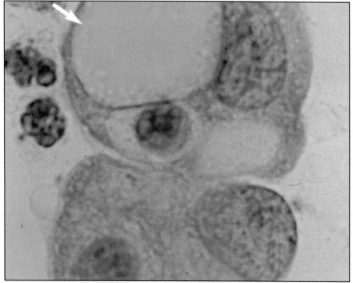

PLATE 21   Neoplastic transitional epithelial cells and white
cells (400×) (New methylene blue)

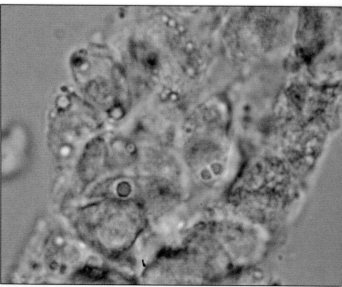

PLATE 24   Cellular cast (250×) (Unstained)

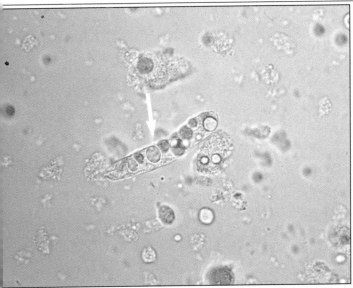

PLATE 25   Fatty cast in feline urine (160×) (Unstained)

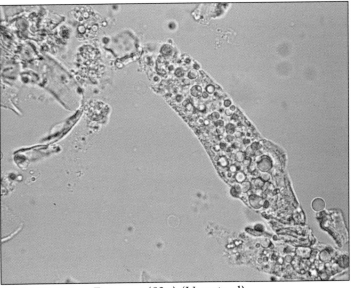

PLATE 26   Fatty cast (82×) (Unstained)

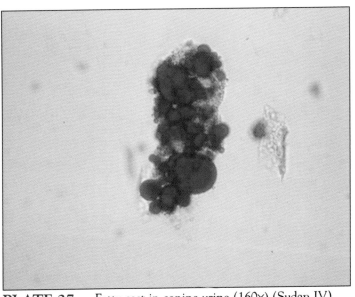

PLATE 27   Fatty cast in canine urine (160×) (Sudan IV)

PLATE 19
Clump of transitional cells (*open arrow*) and adjacent red cells (*closed arrows*) in the urine sediment of a dog with a transitional cell carcinoma of the urinary bladder.

PLATE 20
Neoplastic transitional epithelial cells illustrating nuclear enlargement (*closed arrow*), hyperchromasia, enlargement of nucleoli, and increased cell size (compare to size of leukocytes [*open arrow*]).

PLATE 21
Neoplastic transitional epithelial cells and white cells in the urine sediment of a dog. Note the cytoplasmic inclusion in the epithelial cell cytoplasm (*arrow*).

PLATE 22
Hyaline cast (*arrow*) and epithelial cell (*open arrow*) in the urine sediment of a dog.

PLATE 23
Broad hyaline cast (*arrow*) adjacent to unidentified amorphous debris.

PLATE 24
Cellular cast in canine urine sediment.

PLATE 25
Feline urine sediment containing a fatty cast (*arrow*) surrounded by disintegrating cells, occasional fat droplets, and amorphous debris.

PLATE 26
Fatty cast.

PLATE 27
Urine sediment from a 14-year-old neutered male pug containing a fatty cast with numerous orange staining fat droplets.

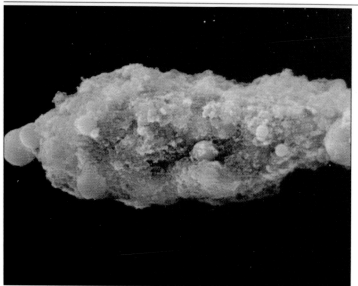

PLATE 28   Scanning electron micrograph of fatty cast

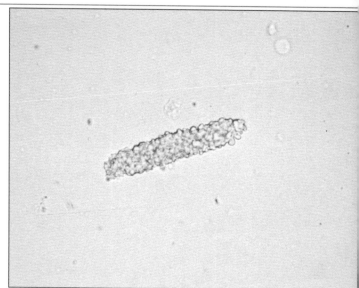

PLATE 31   Granular cast (100×) (Unstained)

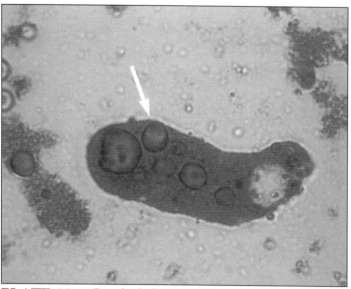

PLATE 29   Renal tubular cast (100×)

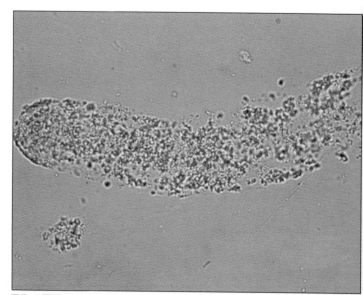

PLATE 32   Granular cast (160×) (Unstained)

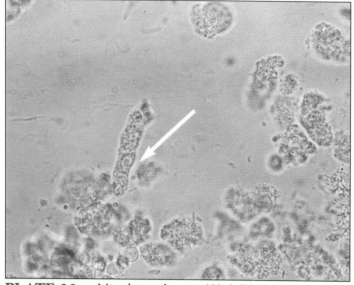

PLATE 30   Mixed granular cast (82×) (Unstained)

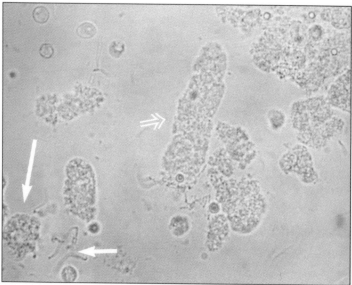

PLATE 33   Granular cast and various cells (160×)
(Unstained)

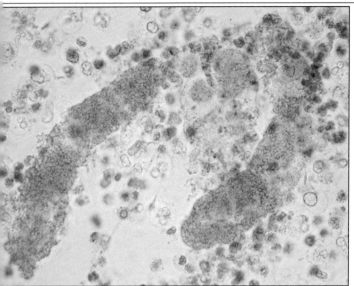

PLATE 34   Granular cast and cells (High power
             magnification) (Sedistain)

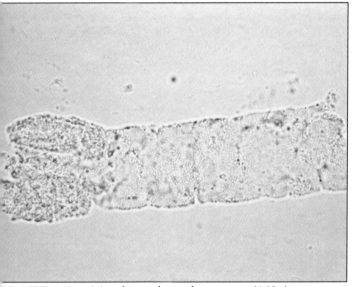

PLATE 35   Mixed granular and waxy cast (160×)
             (Unstained)

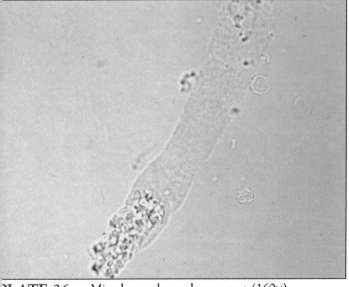

PLATE 36   Mixed granular and waxy cast (160×)
             (Unstained)

PLATE 28
Scanning electron micrograph of fatty casts of the
type described in Plate 27.

PLATE 29
Renal tubular cast observed in urine sediment
obtained from an adult male domestic shorthair cat.
Note the droplets of fat (Sudan IV) (*arrow*)
trapped in the hyaline proteinaceous matrix (new
methylene blue).

PLATE 30
Mixed granular cast containing what appears to be a
cell (*arrow*) and surrounding granular epithelial
cells.

PLATE 31
Granular cast in canine urine sediment.

PLATE 32
Granular cast.

PLATE 33
Granular casts (*open arrow*), granular disintegrating
epithelial cells (*long closed arrow*), bacteria (*short
closed arrow*), and occasional white blood cells.

PLATE 34
Granular casts surrounded by numerous white
cells, occasional red blood cells, and occasional
epithelial cells.

PLATE 35
Mixed granular and waxy cast.

PLATE 36
Mixed granular and waxy cast in canine urine
sediment.

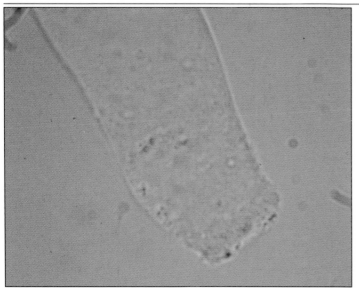

PLATE 37   Waxy broad cast (250×) (Unstained)

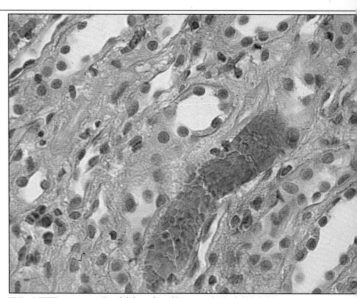

PLATE 40   Red blood cell cast (40×)(H&E)

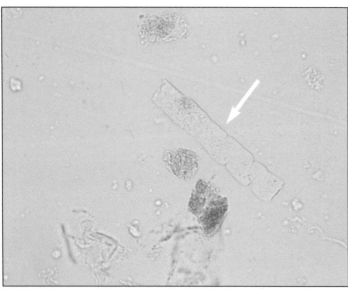

PLATE 38   Waxy cast and cells (High power magnification) (Unstained)

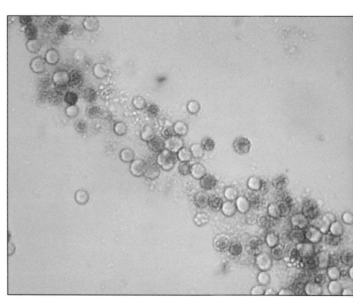

PLATE 41   Red blood cell cast (40×) (Sedistain)

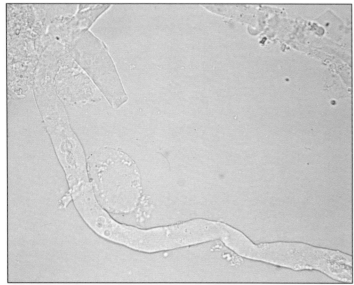

PLATE 39   Elongated waxy cast (High power magnification) (Unstained)

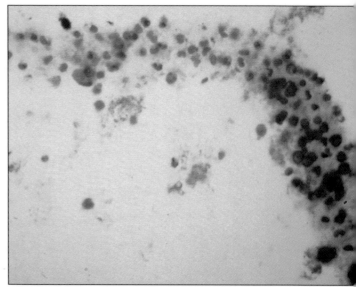

PLATE 42   White cell cast (104×) (Sedistain)

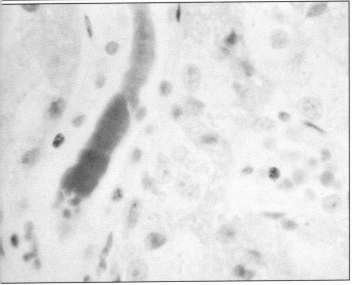

PLATE 43 Bilirubin cast (400×) (H&E)

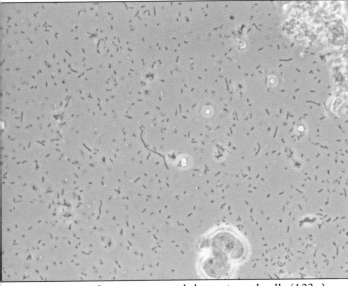

PLATE 44 Canine urine with bacteria and cells (102×)
(Unstained phase microscopy)

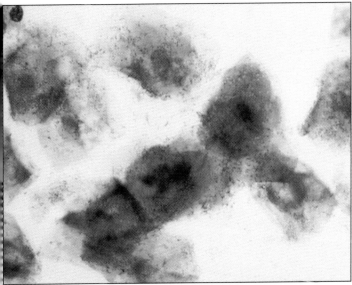

PLATE 45 Squamous epithelial cells and bacteria (High
power magnification) (Wright's stain)

PLATE 37
Waxy broad cast in canine urine sediment.

PLATE 38
Waxy cast (*arrow*) with adjacent disintegrating
cells.

PLATE 39
Elongated waxy cast.

PLATE 40
Photomicrograph of a red blood cell cast in a
tubular lumen contained in a section of kidney
removed from an 8-year-old neutered female
domestic shorthair cat.

PLATE 41
Red blood cell cast. (Courtesy of Dr. Richard Scott,
Animal Medical Center, New York, NY.)

PLATE 42
White cell cast. (Courtesy of Dr. Richard Scott,
Animal Medical Center, New York, NY.)

PLATE 43
Photomicrograph of a bilirubin cast in a section of
canine kidney.

PLATE 44
Canine urine sediment containing numerous
bacteria and an occasional cell.

PLATE 45
Bacteria adhered to squamous epithelial cells.
(Courtesy of Dr. Shirley Johnston, University of
Minnesota.)

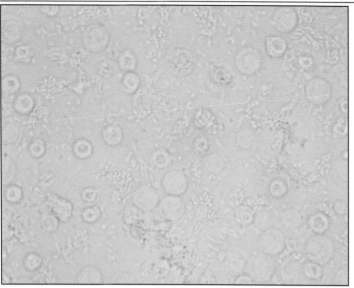

PLATE 46   Bacteria and white cells (High power magnification) (Unstained)

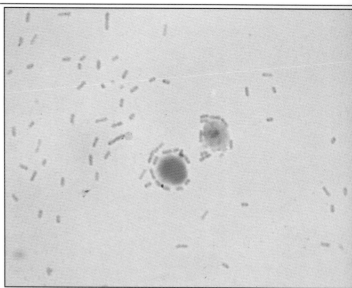

PLATE 49   Bacteria and degenerating white cells (High power magnification) (Gram's stain)

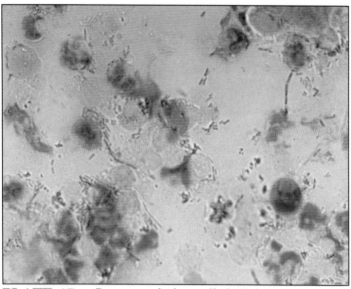

PLATE 47   Bacteria and white cells (160×) (New methylene blue)

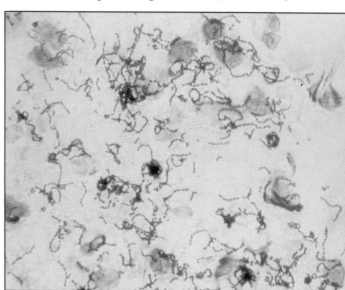

PLATE 50   Bacteria and degenerating white cells (250×) (Gram's stain)

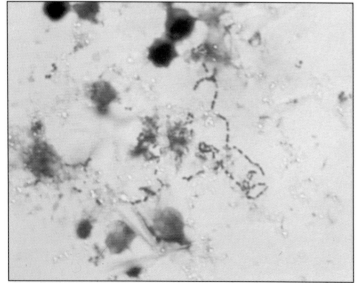

PLATE 48   Bacteria and disintegrating cells (High power magnification) (Diff-Quik®)

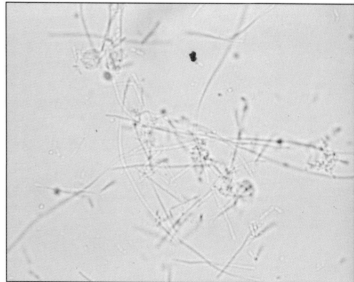

PLATE 51   *Escherichia coli* in urine (High power magnification) (Unstained)

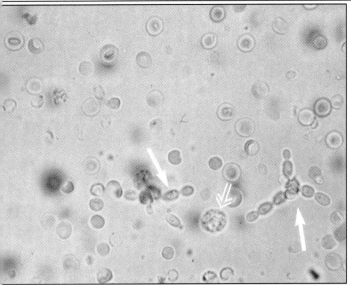

PLATE 52 Budding yeast and red blood cells (160×) (Unstained)

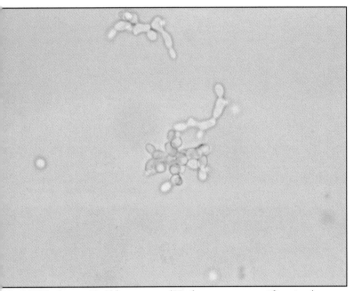

PLATE 53 Budding yeast (High power magnification) (Unstained)

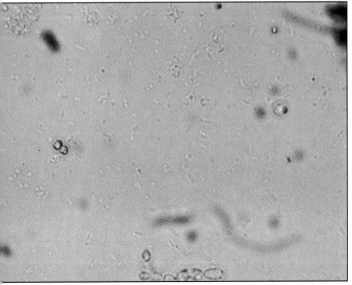

PLATE 54 Budding yeast (High power magnification) (Unstained)

PLATE 46
Numerous bacteria and white cells in canine urine sediment.

PLATE 47
Numerous bacteria and degenerating white cells in canine urine sediment.

PLATE 48
Chains of bacteria and disintegrating cells in canine urine sediment.

PLATE 49
Gram-negative bacteria surrounding unidentified cells in canine urine sediment.

PLATE 50
Numerous gram-positive chains of bacteria and degenerating white cells in canine urine sediment.

PLATE 51
Chains of *Escherichia coli* forming filaments that resemble fungal hyphae.

PLATE 52
Budding yeast (*closed arrows*) in urine sediment of a cat, surrounded primarily by red blood cells. An occasional white cell is also present (*open arrow*).

PLATE 53
Budding yeast cells in canine urine sediment. Absence of inflammatory cells suggests that they are contaminants.

PLATE 54
Budding yeast cells (*Torulopsis* spp.) in the urine sediment of a 2-year-old male English bulldog with cystitis.

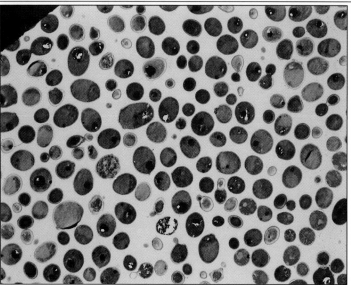

PLATE 55   Yeast cells (Transmission electron micrograph 2070×)

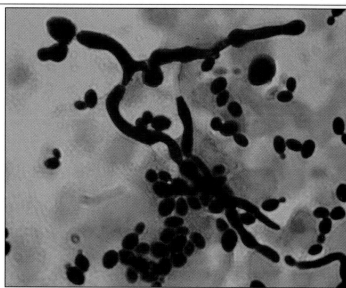

PLATE 58   Budding yeast and hyphae (250×) (Gram's stain)

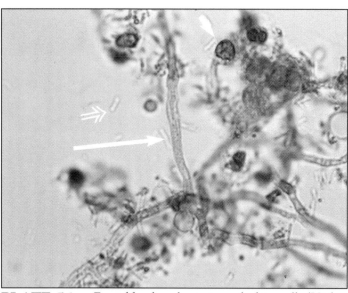

PLATE 56   Fungal hyphae, bacteria, and white cells (High power magnification) (Sedistain)

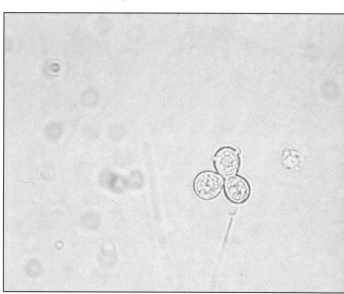

PLATE 59   Budding yeast (High power magnification) (Unstained)

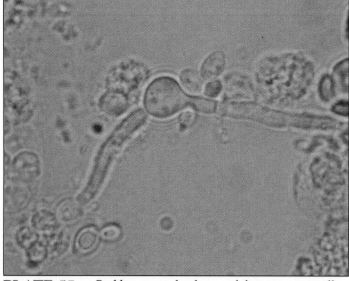

PLATE 57   Budding yeast, hyphae, and disintegrating cells (250×) (Unstained)

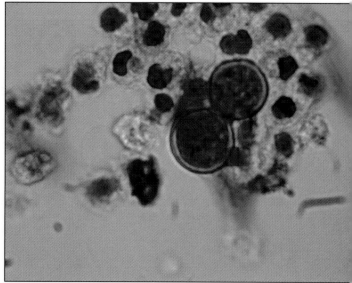

PLATE 60   Budding yeast form of blastomycosis and white cells (250×) (New methylene blue)

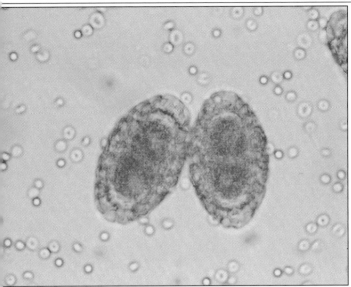

PLATE 61 *Dioctophyma renale* ova (50×) (Unstained)

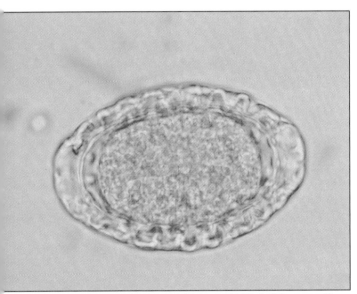

PLATE 62 *Dioctophyma renale* ovum (100×) (Unstained)

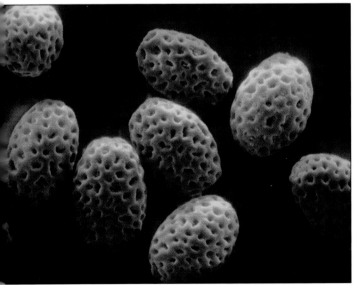

PLATE 63 *Dioctophyma renale* ova (Transmission election micrograph 648×)

PLATE 55
Transmission electron micrograph of the yeast cells described in Plate 54.

PLATE 56
Fungal hyphae (*long closed arrow*), bacteria (*open arrow*), and white cells (*short closed arrow*) in canine urine sediment.

PLATE 57
Budding yeast cells and hyphae surrounded by disintegrating cells in the urine sediment of a dog.

PLATE 58
Budding yeast cells and hyphae in urine sediment of the dog described in Plate 57.

PLATE 59
Budding yeast form of blastomycosis in canine urine sediment.

PLATE 60
Budding yeast form of blastomycosis and adjacent white cells in canine urine sediment.

PLATE 61
Dioctophyma renale ova in urine sediment of a 14-month-old female mixed breed dog.

PLATE 62
Higher magnification of *Dioctophyma renale* ovum in the urine sediment of the dog described in Plate 61.

PLATE 63
Scanning electron micrograph of *Dioctophyma renale* ova in the urine sediment of the dog described in Plate 61.

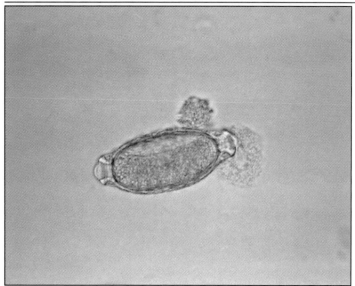

PLATE 64   *Capillaria plica* ovum (160×) (Unstained)

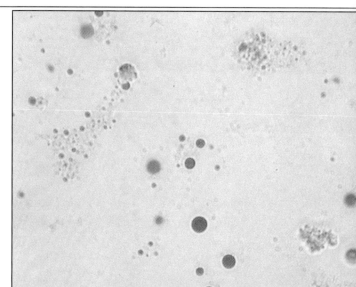

PLATE 67   Lipid droplets (40×) (Sudan IV)

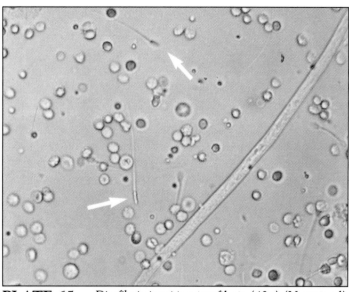

PLATE 65   *Dirofilaria immitis* microfilaria (40×) (Unstained)

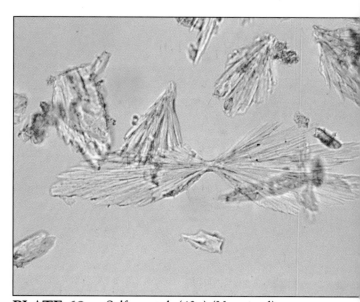

PLATE 68   Sulfa crystals (40×) (Unstained)

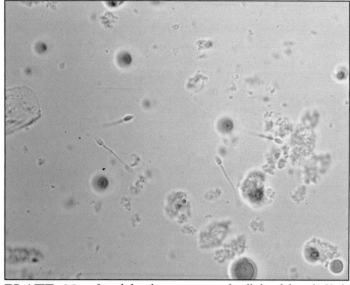

PLATE 66   Lipid droplets, sperm, and cellular debris (160×) (Unstained)

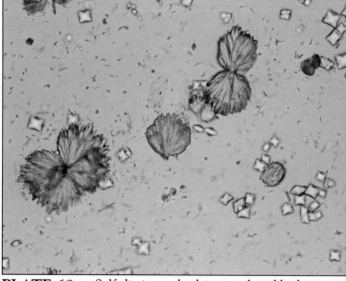

PLATE 69   Sulfadiazine and calcium oxalate dihydrate crystals (50×) (Unstained)

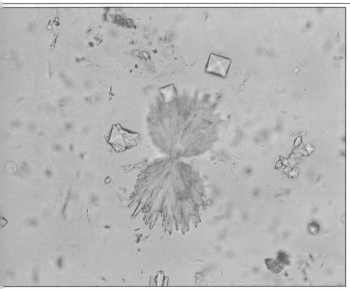

PLATE 70   Sulfadiazine and calcium oxalate dihydrate crystals (100×) (Unstained)

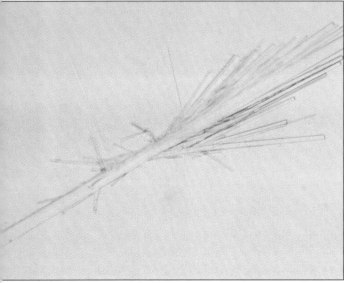

PLATE 71   Hypaque® radiographic contrast agent crystals (12.5×) (Unstained)

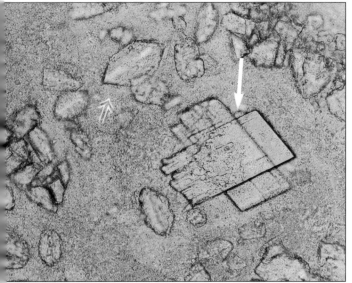

LATE 72   Renografin crystals (50×) (Unstained)

PLATE 64
Capillaria plica ovum in the urine sediment of a dog.

PLATE 65
Microfilaria of *Dirofilaria immitis* in the urine sediment of a dog surrounded by red blood cells, white cells, spermatozoa (*arrows*), and occasional epithelial cells.

PLATE 66
Lipid droplets, sperm, and cellular debris in the urine sediment of a cat.

PLATE 67
Lipid droplets in feline urine sediment.

PLATE 68
Photomicrograph of sulfa crystals in the urine sediment of an adult male dog given sulfadiazine-trimethoprim orally.

PLATE 69
Sulfadiazine and calcium oxalate dihydrate crystals in the urine sediment of an adult male Bichon Frise.

PLATE 70
Sulfadiazine and calcium oxalate dihydrate crystals in urine sediment of dog described in Plate 69.

PLATE 71
Hypaque® radiographic contrast agent crystals in the urine sediment of a dog.

PLATE 72
Crystals (*closed arrow*) in urine sediment of a 4-year-old male pug collected soon after retrograde positive contrast urethrocystography. The positive contrast agent used for the study was diatrizoate meglumine (Renografin). The crystals are surrounded by red blood cells. Note the similarity to cholesterol crystals (Plate 89). Some struvite crystals are also present (*open arrow*).

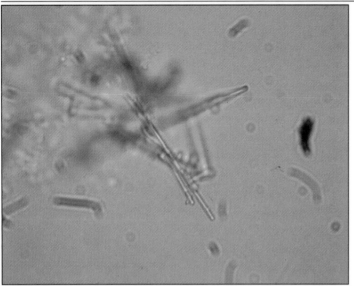

PLATE 73   Crystals in dog treated with ampicillin (250×) (Unstained)

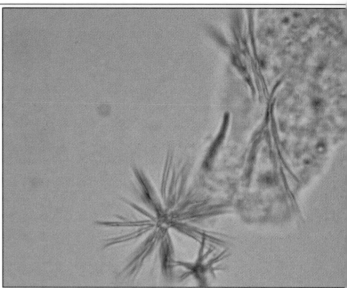

PLATE 76   Bilirubin crystals and unidentified cell (250×) (Unstained)

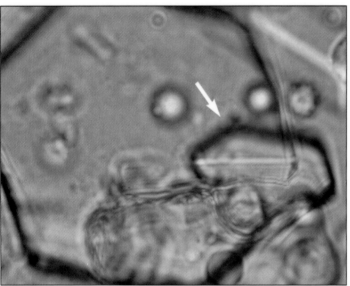

PLATE 74   Cystine and magnesium ammonium phosphate crystals and red blood cells (250×) (Unstained)

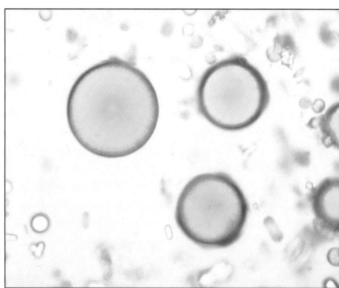

PLATE 77   Calcium carbonate crystals in equine urine (40×) (Unstained)

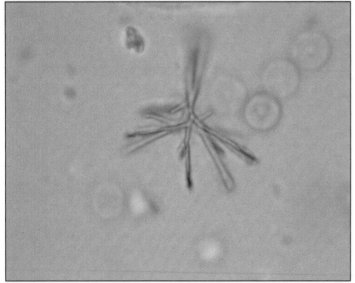

PLATE 75   Bilirubin crystal, red blood cells, and white cells (400×) (Unstained)

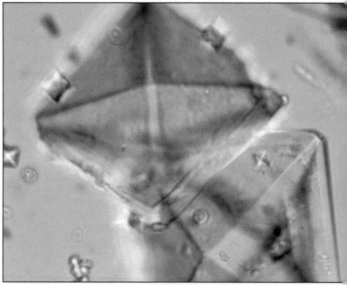

PLATE 78   Calcium oxalate dihydrate crystals (160×) (Unstained)

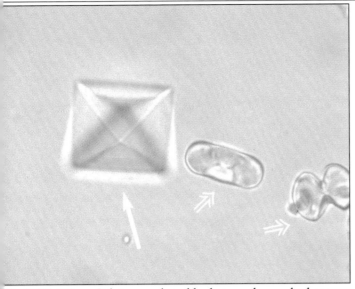

PLATE 79 Calcium oxalate dihydrate and monohydrate crystals (100×) (Unstained)

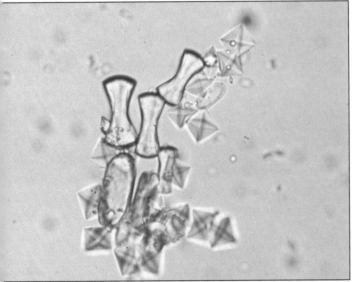

PLATE 80 Calcium oxalate dihydrate and monohydrate crystals (40×) (Unstained)

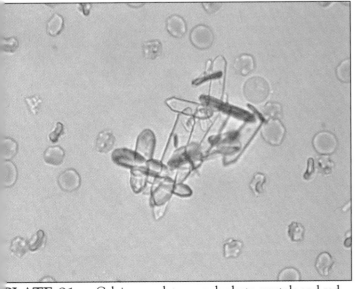

PLATE 81 Calcium oxalate monohydrate crystals and red blood cells (High power magnification) (Unstained)

PLATE 73
Needle-shaped crystals in the urine sediment of an adult female beagle dog being treated with ampicillin.

PLATE 74
Cystine crystals, magnesium ammonium phosphate crystals (*arrow*), and red blood cells in the urine sediment of a 6-year-old neutered English bulldog.

PLATE 75
Bilirubin crystal, red blood cells, white cells, and a squamous epithelial cell in the urine sediment of a dog.

PLATE 76
Bilirubin crystals and an unidentified cell in the urine sediment of a dog.

PLATE 77
Calcium carbonate crystals in the urine sediment of a horse.

PLATE 78
Variable sizes of calcium oxalate dihydrate crystals in the urine sediment of a dog.

PLATE 79
Calcium oxalate dihydrate (*closed arrow*) and calcium oxalate monohydrate crystals (*open arrows*) in the urine sediment of a dog with calcium oxalate uroliths. (From Osborne CA et al: Identification and interpretation of crystalluria in domestic animals: A light and electron microscopic study. *Vet Med* 85:18–37, 1990.)

PLATE 80
Calcium oxalate dihydrate and calcium oxalate monohydrate crystals in the urine sediment of a cat.

PLATE 81
Calcium oxalate monohydrate crystals and red blood cells in the urine sediment of a dog.

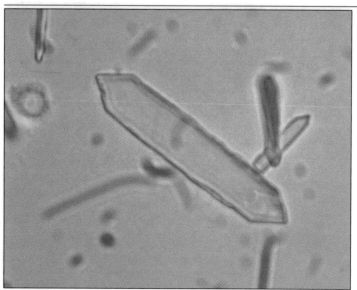

PLATE 82   Calcium oxalate monohydrate crystals (100×) (Unstained)

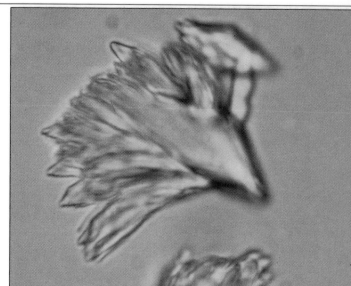

PLATE 85   Calcium oxalate monohydrate crystal aggregate (250×) (Unstained)

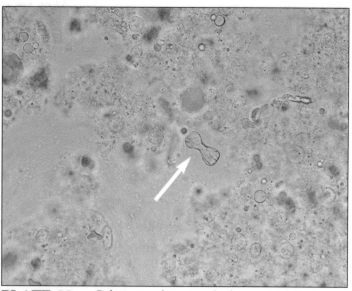

PLATE 83   Calcium oxalate monohydrate crystal (100×) (Unstained)

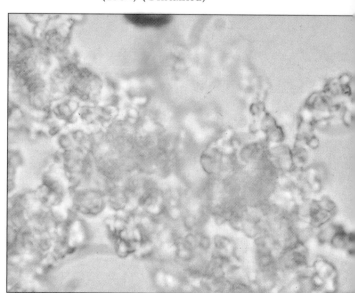

PLATE 86   Amorphous calcium phosphate crystals (250×) (Unstained)

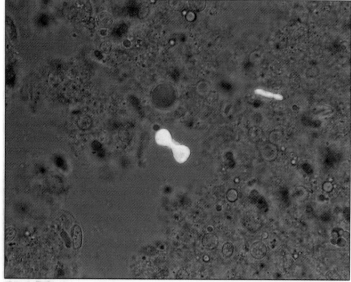

PLATE 84   Calcium oxalate monohydrate crystal (100×) (Unstained phase contrast microscopy)

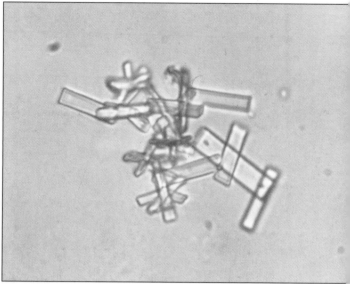

PLATE 87   Brushite crystals (250×) (Unstained)

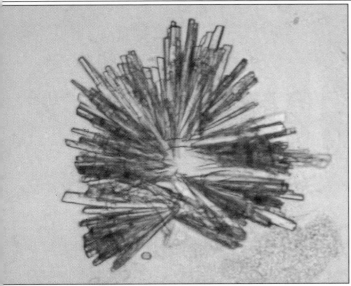

PLATE 88   Aggregate of brushite crystals in pig urine (16×) (Unstained)

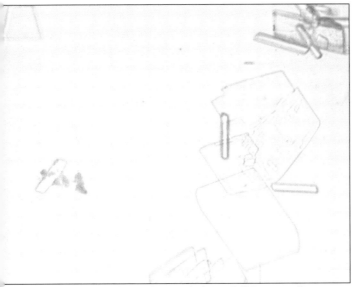

PLATE 89   Cholesterol crystals (100×) (Unstained)

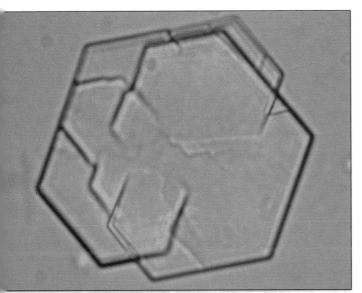

PLATE 90   Cystine crystals (250×) (Unstained)

PLATE 82
Calcium oxalate monohydrate crystals in the urine sediment of a dog with ethylene glycol toxicity.

PLATE 83
Calcium oxalate monohydrate crystal (*arrow*) in urine sediment of a uremic dog that had ingested ethylene glycol.

PLATE 84
Calcium oxalate monohydrate crystal in urine sediment of the uremic dog described in Plate 83.

PLATE 85
Aggregate of calcium oxalate monohydrate crystals in the urine sediment of a 7-year-old castrated male miniature schnauzer with calcium oxalate urocystoliths. (From Osborne CA et al: Identification and interpretation of crystalluria in domestic animals: A light and electron microscopic study. *Vet Med* 85:18–37, 1990.)

PLATE 86
Amorphous calcium phosphate crystals in the urine sediment of a 3-year-old male Lhasa Apso dog.

PLATE 87
Brushite crystals in the urine sediment of a dog.

PLATE 88
Aggregate of calcium hydrogen phosphate dihydrate (brushite) crystals in the urine sediment of a pig.

PLATE 89
Cholesterol crystals in canine urine sediment (see Plate 72).

PLATE 90
Cystine crystals in the urine sediment of a 2-year-old neutered male English bulldog with cystine uroliths.

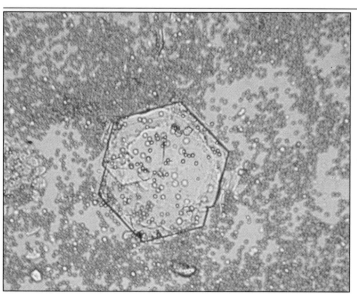

PLATE 91   Cystine crystals and red blood cells (25×) (Unstained)

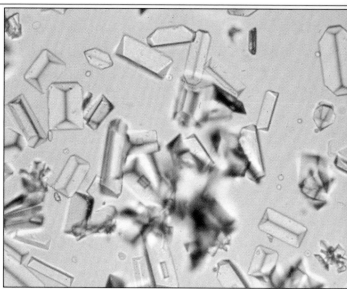

PLATE 94   Magnesium ammonium phosphate crystals (20×) (Unstained)

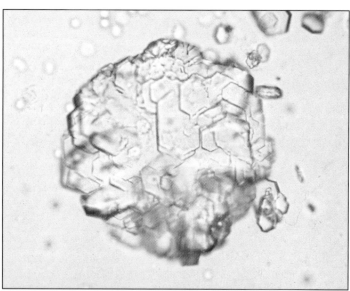

PLATE 92   Cystine crystal aggregate and red blood cells (40×) (Unstained)

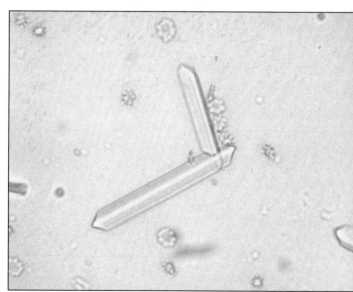

PLATE 95   Struvite crystals and crenated red blood cells (160×) (Unstained)

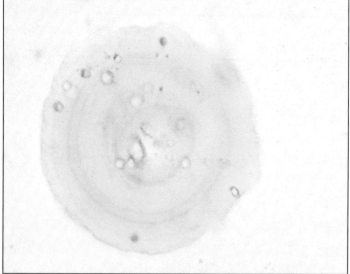

PLATE 93   Crystal with morphologic characteristics similar to those of leucine (160×) (Unstained)

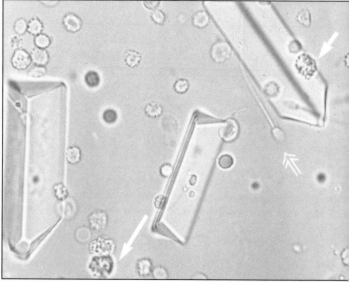

PLATE 96   Struvite crystals. crenated red blood cells, white cells, and spermatozoa (100×) (Unstained)

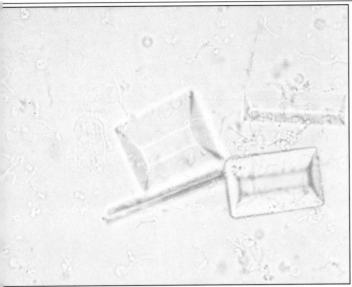

PLATE 97 Struvite crystals, white cells, and bacteria (100×) (Unstained)

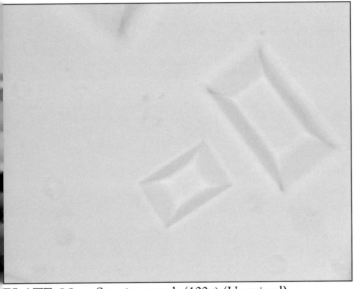

PLATE 98 Struvite crystals (100×) (Unstained)

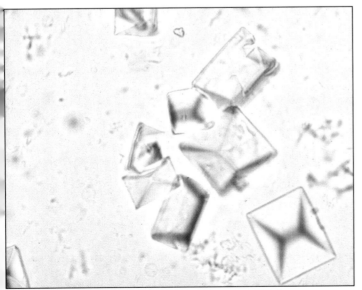

PLATE 99 Struvite crystals and bacteria (High power magnification) (Unstained)

PLATE 91
Cystine crystals and numerous red blood cells in the urine sediment of a dog.

PLATE 92
Aggregate of cystine crystals and red blood cells in the urine sediment of a 2-year-old female domestic shorthair cat.

PLATE 93
Photomicrograph of crystal with morphologic characteristics similar to those of leucine, which formed in the urine sediment of an 11-year-old male mixed-breed dog. (From Osborne CA et al: Identification and interpretation of crystalluria in domestic animals: A light and electron microscopic study. *Vet Med* 85:18–37, 1990.)

PLATE 94
Magnesium ammonium phosphate crystals in the urine sediment of a 6-year-old neutered female miniature schnauzer.

PLATE 95
Struvite crystals and crenated red blood cells in the urine sediment of a 9-year-old neutered male domestic shorthair cat with urethral obstruction.

PLATE 96
Struvite crystals surrounded by crenated red blood cells, an occasional white cell (*closed arrow*), and occasional spermatozoa (*open arrow*).

PLATE 97
Struvite crystals, white cells, and bacteria in the urine sediment of a dog.

PLATE 98
Struvite crystals in the urine sediment a dog.

PLATE 99
Struvite crystals and bacteria in the urine sediment of a dog.

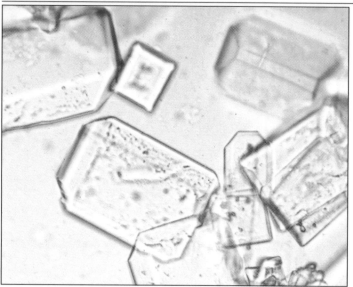

PLATE 100   Struvite crystals (High power magnification) (Unstained)

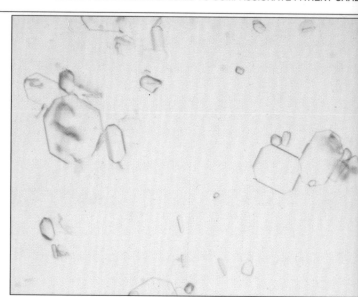

PLATE 103   Magnesium ammonium phosphate crystals (40×) (Unstained)

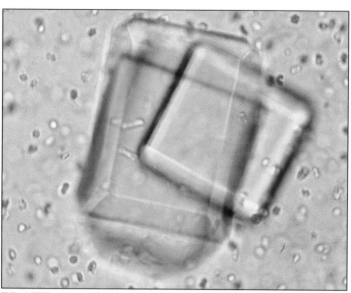

PLATE 101   Struvite crystals and red blood cells (40×) (Unstained)

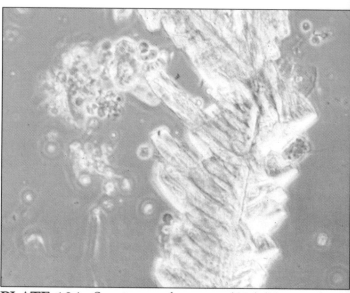

PLATE 104   Struvite crystal aggregate (64×) (Unstained phase microscopy)

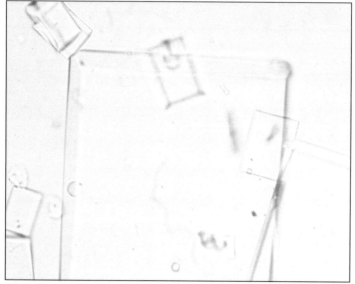

PLATE 102   Struvite crystals (40×) (Unstained)

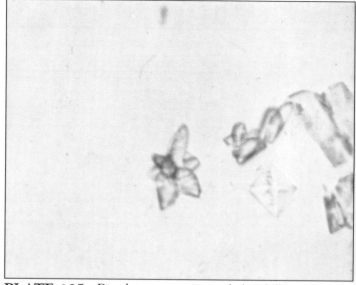

PLATE 105   Dissolving struvite crystals (40×) (Unstained)

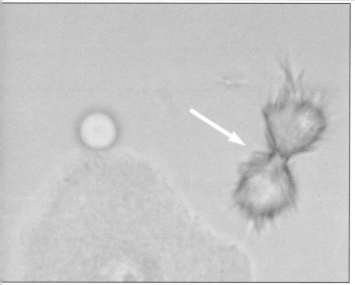

PLATE 106 Tyrosine-like crystal and epithelial cell (High power magnification) (Unstained)

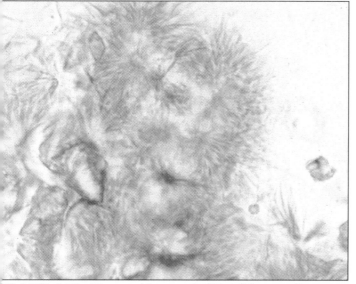

PLATE 107 Tyrosine-like crystals (50×) (Unstained)

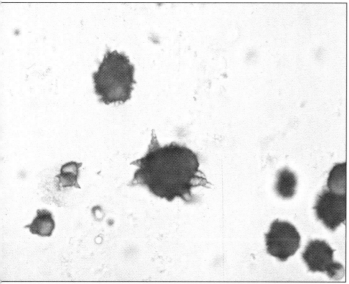

PLATE 108 Thorn-apple ammonium urate crystals (40×) (Unstained)

PLATE 100
Struvite crystals in the urine sediment of a cat.

PLATE 101
Struvite crystals and red blood cells in the urine sediment of a cat.

PLATE 102
Variable sizes of struvite crystals in the urine sediment of a cat.

PLATE 103
Magnesium ammonium phosphate crystals in the urine sediment of a 2-year-old castrated male domestic shorthair cat. (From Osborne CA et al: Identification and interpretation of crystalluria in domestic animals: A light and electron microscopic study. *Vet Med* 85:18–37, 1990.)

PLATE 104
Aggregate of struvite crystals in the urine sediment of a dog.

PLATE 105
Dissolving struvite crystals in the urine sediment of a dog.

PLATE 106
Tyrosine-like crystal (*arrow*) and an epithelial cell in canine urine sediment.

PLATE 107
Tyrosine-like crystals in a canine urine sample preserved with Mucolexx®.

PLATE 108
Thorn-apple ammonium urate crystals in the urine sediment of a dog.

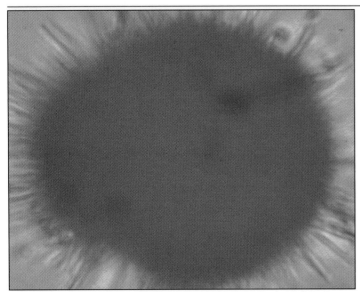

PLATE 109   Thorn-apple ammonium urate crystal (40×)
(Unstained)

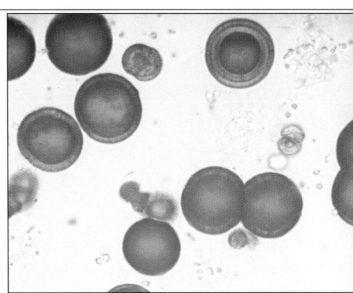

PLATE 112   Ammonium urate crystals (40×) (Unstained)

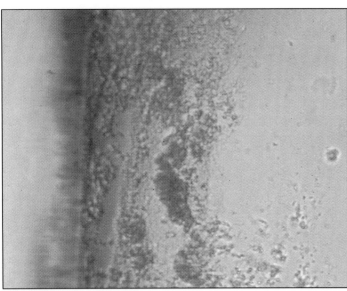

PLATE 110   Amorphous urate crystals (25×) (Unstained)

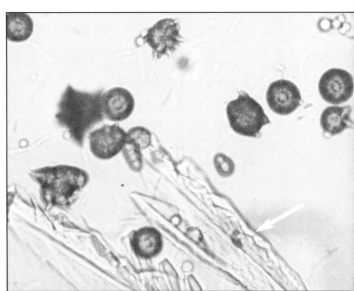

PLATE 113   Ammonium urate crystals and dissolving
struvite crystals (40×) (Unstained)

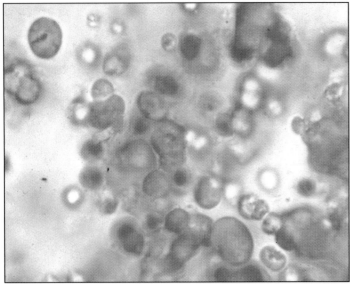

PLATE 111   Ammonium urate crystals (250×) (Unstained)

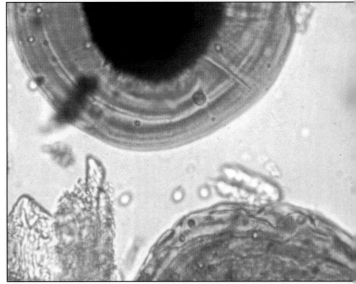

PLATE 114   Ammonium urate crystals and dissolving crystals
(40×) (Unstained)

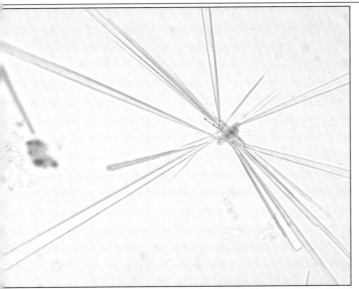

PLATE 115 Sodium urate crystals (128×) (Unstained)

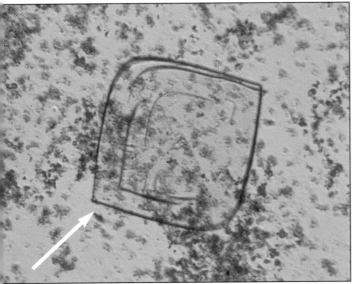

PLATE 116 Uric acid and amorphous urate crystals (25×) (Unstained)

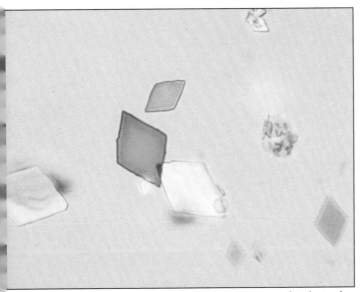

PLATE 117 Uric acid crystals (250×) (Unstained polarized light microscopy)

PLATE 109
Thorn-apple form of ammonium urate crystal in the urine of a dog.

PLATE 110
Amorphous urate crystals in the urine sediment of a 4-year-old male English bulldog. The crystals have accumulated at the edge of the coverslip.

PLATE 111
Ammonium urate crystals in the urine sediment of a cat.

PLATE 112
Ammonium urate crystals in the urine sediment of an adult male Dalmatian.

PLATE 113
Ammonium urate crystals and dissolving struvite crystals (*arrow*) in the urine sediment of a dog.

PLATE 114
Ammonium urate crystals and dissolving crystals in the urine sediment of a dog.

PLATE 115
Sodium urate crystals in the urine sediment of a dog.

PLATE 116
Uric acid crystals (*arrow*) surrounded by amorphous urate crystals in the urine sediment of an adult male Dalmatian.

PLATE 117
Uric acid crystals in the urine sediment of a 7-month-old Yorkshire terrier with a portovascular anomaly.

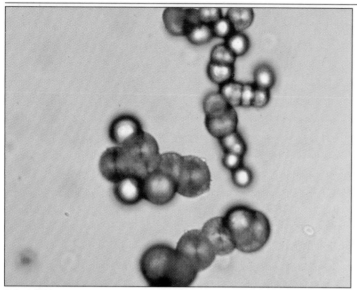

PLATE 118   Xanthine crystals (40×) (Unstained)

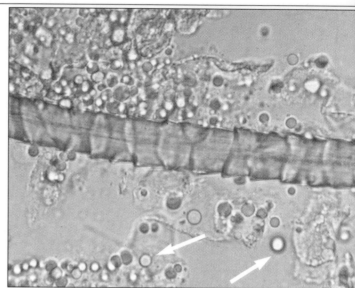

PLATE 121   Hair shaft, lipid droplets, and debris (Low power magnification) (Unstained)

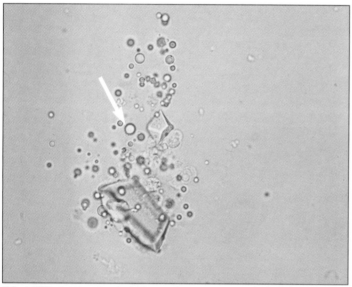

PLATE 119   Air bubbles and struvite crystals (High power magnification) (Unstained)

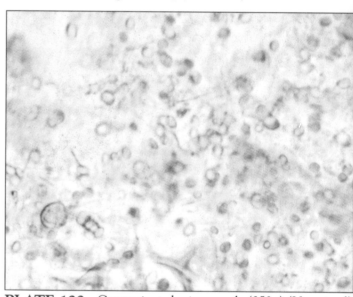

PLATE 122   Contaminated urine sample (250×) (Unstained)

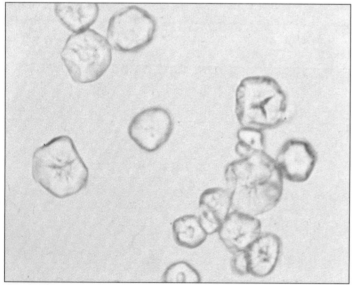

PLATE 120   Starch granules (64×) (Unstained)

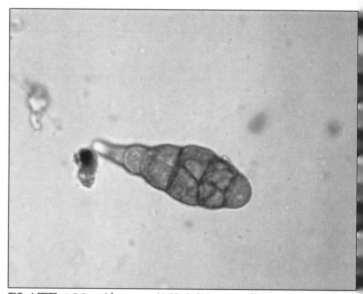

PLATE 123   *Alternaria* (160×) (Unstained)

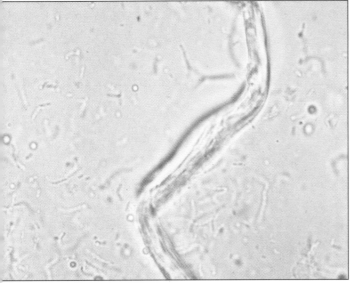

PLATE 124 Cotton fiber and bacteria (High power magnification) (Unstained)

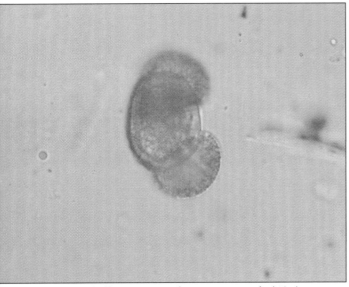

PLATE 125 Pollen grains and struvite crystals (40×) (Unstained)

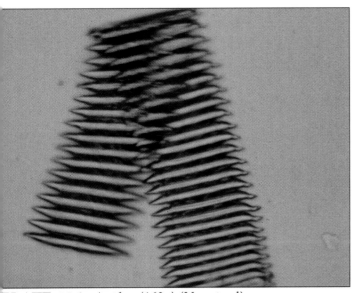

PLATE 126 Artifact (160×) (Unstained)

PLATE 118
Xanthine crystals in the urine sediment of a dog being treated with allopurinol.

PLATE 119
Air bubbles (*arrow*) and struvite crystals in the urine sediment of a dog.

PLATE 120
Starch granules in urine sediment.

PLATE 121
Hair shaft surrounded by lipid droplets (*arrow*) and debris.

PLATE 122
Urine sample contaminated with fecal material during cystocentesis. The contaminants resemble yeast-like cells and cell walls of plant origin.

PLATE 123
Alternaria, a yeast contaminant of urine sediment.

PLATE 124
Cotton fiber surrounded by numerous bacteria.

PLATE 125
Pollen grains and struvite crystals in the urine sediment of a cat.

PLATE 126
Artifact from collection container, transfer pipette, microscope slide, or coverslip in the urine sediment of a dog.

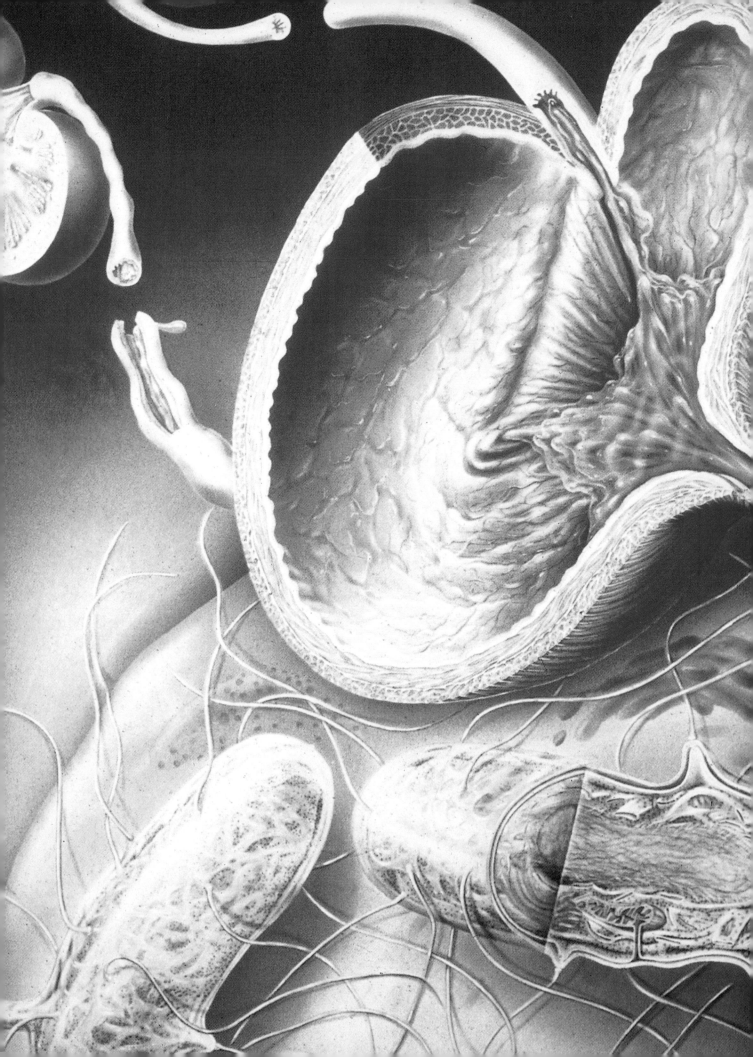

Appendix A

Teach me to feel another's distress, to sooth the pain I see.
Teach me the power of compassion, to live my life for we,
not me.

C.A.O.

Interpretation of Clinical Cases

CASE 1: Consider the following results obtained by analysis of a fresh urine sample obtained by cystocentesis from a 5-year-old spayed miniature schnauzer.

Color	Yellow	Protein	2+
Turbidity	Cloudy	RBC	Numerous/hpf
Specific gravity	1.035	White cells	Numerous/hpf
Glucose	Negative	Casts	None
pH	8.0	Epithelial cells	Many
Bilirubin	Negative	Bacteria	Many cocci
Acetone	Negative	Crystals	Moderate struvite
Occult blood	4+		

The best interpretation of the results of this urinalysis is that the patient:
   a. Has an inflammatory process somewhere along the urinary tract caused by bacterial infection.
   b. Has an inflammatory process somewhere along the genitourinary tract caused by bacterial infection.
   c. Has an inflammatory process somewhere along the urinary tract caused or complicated by bacterial infection.
   d. Is normal, and the sample was contaminated during the process of analysis.
   e. Has struvite uroliths associated with urinary tract infection.

The best answer = c

Comments
   a. The results do not permit differentiation between bacterial infection as a cause or complication of urinary tract infection. Most bacterial urinary tract infections develop secondary to abnormality in host defense mechanisms.
   b. Although this answer is not totally incorrect, it is an overstatement to definitely conclude that the genital tract is involved in a sample obtained by cystocentesis.
   c. In light of comments for a and b, this appears to be the best interpretation.
   d. The results are definitely abnormal and would not be expected to be caused by contamination.
   e. Although magnesium ammonium phosphate uroliths may be present, struvite crystalluria is not by itself a reliable index of their occurrence.

CASE 2: A 5-year-old female mixed breed dog is admitted as an emergency to your hospital in the late hours of the evening because of severe vomiting. The owner has no information about the dog's urination habits. Physical examination reveals that the dog is dehydrated (9% loss of body weight due to fluid loss); an appropriate quantity of lactated Ringer's solution is administered parenterally to correct the dehydration. The next morning samples of blood and voided urine are collected for analysis. Consider the following results:

Urinalysis			
Color	Light yellow	Protein	Negative
Turbidity	Clear	RBC	Occasional/hpf
Specific gravity	1.014	White cells	Occasional/hpf
Glucose	Negative	Casts	None
pH	5.5	Epithelial cells	Many
Acetone	Negative	Bacteria	Negative
Bilirubin	Negative	Crystals	Few amorphous crystals

Blood urea nitrogen = 60 mg/100 ml
Serum amylase = Two times normal value

Hemogram
PCV = 49%
White cells = 24,000/cmm
Total neutrophils = 80% (75% mature; 5% immature)
Lymphocytes = 10%
Monocytes = 10%
Platelets = Adequate
Total protein = 7.8 g/dl

(continued on page 182)

CASE 2 (continued)

The best interpretation of these findings is that:
a. The dog has prerenal azotemia caused by fluid loss due to vomiting.
b. The dog has primary renal failure associated with an impaired ability to concentrate urine, azotemia, vomiting, and dehydration.
c. The dog has hypoadrenocorticism associated with vomiting, impaired renal conservation of sodium and water, and prerenal azotemia.
d. The dog has azotemia, but no inference about cause can be established with these data.
e. The dog has acute pancreatitis associated with concomitant primary renal failure.

The best answer = d

Comments
a. Although a prerenal cause of azotemia is possible, failure to collect a urine sample prior to parenteral fluid administration precludes determination of whether the low urine specific gravity was induced by diuresis or impaired ability of the kidneys to concentrate urine.
b. This situation is possible but cannot be confirmed because parenteral fluids were given prior to collection of a urine sample (see a).
c. See comments for a and b.
d. See comments for a and b. However, since the dog is dehydrated, at least a portion of the azotemia is prerenal in origin.
e. See comments for a and b.

CASE 3: Consider the following results obtained by analysis of a voided urine sample collected from a 5-year-old intact female shih tzu.

Color	Yellow	Protein	2+
Turbidity	Cloudy	RBC	50–60/hpf
Specific gravity	1.019	White cells	Numerous/hpf
Glucose	Negative	Casts	Occasional hyaline/lpf
pH	6.0	Epithelial cells	Many
Bilirubin	Negative	Bacteria	None
Acetone	Negative	Crystals	None
Occult blood	2+		

The best interpretation of the results of this urinalysis is that the patient has:
a. Infection somewhere in the urinary tract.
b. Infection somewhere in the genitourinary system.
c. Inflammation somewhere in the urinary tract.
d. Inflammation somewhere in the genitourinary system.
e. Inflammation involving the renal tubules.

The best answer = d

Comments
a. The fact that the inflammatory response has been caused or complicated by an infection has not been established. In vitro culture of urine for significant bacteriuria is warranted.
b. See comments for a.
c. Collection of a voided urine sample does not exclude the genital tract from consideration.
d. The inflammatory components in this sample could have originated in the urinary and/or genital system.
e. This information is not sufficiently specific to localize the inflammatory process to the renal tubules. Hyaline cysts are not an index of renal tubular inflammation.

CASE 4: Consider the following results obtained by analysis of a voided urine sample obtained from a 12-year-old spayed female Boston terrier.

Color	Light yellow	Protein	2+
Turbidity	Slightly cloudy	RBC	20–30/hpf
Specific gravity	1.013	White cells	60–70/hpf
Glucose	Negative	Casts	Occasional White cells/lpf
pH	6.0	Epithelial cells	Moderate
Bilirubin	Negative	Bacteria	Rods
Acetone	Negative	Crystals	None
Occult blood	2+		

The best interpretation of this urinalysis is that the patient has an infectious inflammatory disease involving at least the:
   a. Urinary tract.
   b. Urinary bladder.
   c. Renal tubules.
   d. Glomeruli.
   e. Renal vessels.

The best answer = c

Comments
   a. Detection of white cell casts that are formed in the distal tubules and collecting ducts allows localization of the disease to a specific location within the urinary tract.
   b. See comments for a.
   c. Detection of white cell casts is reliable evidence of tubular involvement in the infectious inflammatory process. However, concurrent involvement of other portions of the urinary tract cannot be excluded
   d. Available data do not permit confirmation or elimination of glomerular involvement.
   e. Available data do not permit confirmation or elimination of renal vascular involvement.

CASE 5: A 7-year-old male miniature schnauzer has dysuria of 4 weeks' duration. Hematuria has been noted throughout urination. Physical examination reveals 7% clinical dehydration and thickening of the bladder wall. Urinalysis of a sample collected by cystocentesis revealed the following:

Color	Yellow	Protein	2+
Turbidity	Cloudy	RBC	Too numerous to count/hpf
Specific gravity	1.017	White cells	80–100/hpf
Glucose	Negative	Casts	2 to 4 granular/hpf
pH	7.0	Epithelial cells	Many
Bilirubin	Negative	Bacteria	None
Acetone	Negative	Crystals	Many calcium oxalate and struvite
Occult blood	4+		

The best interpretation of these clinical results is:
   a. The dog has bacterial cystitis and pyelonephritis.
   b. The dog has bacterial cystitis.
   c. The dog has inflammatory disease of the upper and lower urinary tract.
   d. The dog has metabolic uroliths and secondary urinary tract infection.
   e. The dog has a bleeding disorder and is hemorrhaging into the urinary tract.

The best answer = c.

Comments
   a. A urine culture validating significant bacteriuria would be required to validate bacterial infection. Dysuria and thickening of the bladder wall indicate the lower urinary tract is involved, while inappropriate urine concentration associated with clinical dehydration and granular casts indicates bilateral renal involvement.

(continued on page 184)

b. See comments for a.
c. The combination of pyuria, hematuria, and proteinuria is consistent with inflammation. As described in a, the upper and lower urinary tract are involved. The underlying cause of the inflammation requires further diagnostic study.
d. Detection of crystalluria is not synonymous with urolithiasis, and detection of inflammation is not synonymous with bacterial infection. However, older male miniature schnauzers have increased risk for calcium oxalate uroliths. Calcium oxalate uroliths may predispose to bacterial urinary tract infections. Infections caused by urease-producing bacteria such as staphylococci or *Proteus* spp. may result in struvite crystalluria. Further evaluation would be required to prove these possibilities.
e. The hematuria is associated with inflammation.

Bacterial culture of the urine sample collected by cystocentesis revealed greater than 100,000 CFU/ml of *Escherichia coli* that were susceptible to amoxicillin–clavulanic acid, cephalexin, chloramphenicol, enrofloxacin, gentamicin, and trimethoprim/sulfa. Considering that both the upper and lower urinary tract are involved in the infectious inflammatory process, which antimicrobial agent would you choose?

The best answer = enrofloxacin

- Enrofloxacin has good tissue penetration of the kidneys and prostate gland.
- Enrofloxacin attains high urine concentrations that are sustained for extended periods. Urine concentration may exceed minimum inhibitory concentrations in patients with renal failure.
- Enrofloxacin is not nephrotoxic and has a wide safety margin.
- Enrofloxacin has an extended spectrum of activity.
- Enrofloxacin is often effective against resistant bacteria.
- Enrofloxacin is not affected by plasmid-mediated resistance.

CASE 6: Consider the following results obtained by analysis of a voided urine sample from a 9-year-old male miniature poodle:

Color	Yellow	Protein	1+
Turbidity	Cloudy	RBC	5–10/hpf
Specific gravity	1.040	White cells	5–10/hpf
Glucose	Negative	Casts	Many granular/lpf
pH	6.0	Epithelial cells	Moderate
Bilirubin	Negative	Crystals	Occasional calcium oxalate
Acetone	Negative	Bacteria	None
Occult blood	1+		

The best interpretation of the results of this urinalysis is that the patient:
a. Has acute primary renal failure.
b. Has chronic primary renal failure.
c. Has acute renal disease.
d. Has chronic renal disease.
e. Is normal.

The best answer = c

Comments
a. Concentration of urine to this degree indicates that an adequate population of nephrons are functional to prevent primary renal failure. The small quantity of protein and high specific gravity indicate that primary renal failure and glomerulotubular imbalance are improbable.
b. See comments for a.
c. Detection of many granular casts is indicative of renal disease, even though urine concentration indicates that the disease is not of sufficient magnitude to cause renal failure. The large number of casts suggests (but does not prove) that the disorder is acute. The acute renal disease is associated with an inflammatory response.
d. This answer is possible, although c is more probable. Additional information would be required to prove or disprove either answer.
e. The findings are definitely abnormal.

Appendix B

Compassionate doctors recognize that overtreatment of their patients is the antithesis of compassion.

C.A.O.

Recommendations for the Treatment of Renal Failure

SPECIFIC THERAPY (Tables B-1 and B-2)

Specific therapy of generalized renal disease associated with renal failure involves retarding or resolving the development of renal lesions by eliminating or controlling the causes of the lesions. Examples of specific treatment include correcting hypercalcemia that has resulted in calcium nephropathy, administering antibiotics to eliminate bacterial infections, removing lesions that are causing obstructive uropathy (e.g., tumors or uroliths), and correcting abnormal renal perfusion responsible for ischemic renal lesions.

TABLE B-1

SEVEN PRINCIPLES GUIDING THE TREATMENT OF RENAL FAILURE

1. No therapy will eliminate renal lesions; they must heal spontaneously. The polysystemic metabolic and biochemical disorders caused by generalized renal lesions can, however, be modified or eliminated by appropriate therapy.
2. Reversible nonrenal disorders that may have precipitated or aggravated a uremic crisis should be detected and eliminated.
3. The potential reversibility of renal disease and renal dysfunction should be evaluated with the knowledge that adequate renal function is not synonymous with total renal function.
4. Specific therapy to eliminate or control the underlying causes of failure should be formulated with the objective of preventing further renal destruction.
5. Supportive and symptomatic therapeutic protocols that minimize alterations in fluid, electrolyte, acid-base, endocrine, and nutrient balance should be initiated to promote the sustenance of life until the processes of regeneration, repair, and compensatory adaptation allow the kidneys to regain adequate function to reestablish homeostasis. Such therapy should be formulated according to whether the patient has oliguric or nonoliguric primary renal failure.
6. Drugs should be administered to patients with renal failure only after considering the routes and rates of metabolism and elimination and the potential to induce adverse reactions in the uremic environment.
7. Overtreatment must be avoided.

185

TABLE B-2

SOME TREATABLE CAUSES OF AZOTEMIA IN PATIENTS WITH PRIMARY RENAL FAILURE

I. **Specific Treatment Available**
   A. Prerenal causes
      1. Decreased Renal Perfusion
         a. Dehydration
         b. Cardiovascular dysfunction
         c. Severe hypoalbuminemia
         d. Hypoadrenocorticism
      2. Increased Urea Metabolism
         a. Gastrointestinal hemorrhage
         b. Extensive tissue necrosis
         c. High protein diet
         d. Catabolic drugs
            — Glucocorticoids
            — Antineoplastic agents
            — Tetracyclines (antianabolic?)
            — Excessive thyroid supplementation
   B. Postrenal causes
      1. Rent in excretory pathway
      2. Urinary tract obstruction
         a. Uroliths
         b. Operable neoplasms
         c. Herniated urinary bladder
         d. Blood clots
         e. Spay granuloma
         f. Others
   C. Primary renal causes
      1. Acute tubular necrosis
         a. Ischemia
            — Prolonged hypovolemia
            — Nonsteroidal antiinflammatory drug toxicity
            — Thromboembolic disorders
         b. Nephrotoxins, including:
            — Aminoglycoside antibiotics
            — Ethylene glycol
            — Heme pigments
            — Amphotericin B
            — Cis-platinum
      2. Hypercalcemic nephropathy
      3. Bacterial and fungal urinary tract infections
      4. Some glomerulonephropathies
      5. Immune disorders
      6. Adverse drug reactions
      7. Heat stroke

II. **No Specific Treatment Available**
   A. Inherited and congenital diseases
   B. Polycystic disease and presence of perirenal pseudocysts
   C. Amyloidosis
   D. Feline infectious peritonitis
   E. Neoplasia
   F. Periarteritis nodosa
   G. Idiopathic disease

TABLE B-3

SUMMARY OF POTENTIALLY LIFE-THREATENING CLINICAL FINDINGS ASSOCIATED WITH RENAL FAILURE

I. **Alterations That May Be Immediately Life Threatening**
   A. Severe dehydration
   B. Severe acidosis
   C. Severe hypokalemia or hyperkalemia
   D. Severe hypocalcemia

II. **Alterations That Are Usually Not An Immediate Threat to Life**
   A. Severe azotemia
   B. Severe hyperphosphatemia
   C. Moderate anemia
   D. Moderate hypercalcemia

TABLE B-4

SOME COMMON DRUGS THAT SHOULD GENERALLY BE AVOIDED IN PATIENTS WITH RENAL FAILURE

I. **Prophylactic Antibiotics (unless there is need for urinary tract catheterization)**

II. **Catabolic Drugs**
   A. Glucocorticoids
   B. Antineoplastic agents
   C. Tetracycline (?)

III. **Nonsteroidal Antiinflammatory Agents (especially if volume depleted)**

IV. **Urine Acidifiers**
   A. Ammonium chloride
   B. Methionine
   C. Others

V. **Urinary Antiseptics**
   A. Methenamine mandelate
   B. Nalidixic acid

VI. **Magnesium- and Phosphorus-Containing Antacids**

VII. **Nephrotoxic Drugs**
   A. Aminoglycoside antibiotics
   B. Amphotericin B
   C. Cis-platinum

Although determining the initiating cause of the disease process in dogs and cats with renal failure is frequently difficult, the value of formulating specific therapy based on etiologic/pathologic diagnosis is emphasized. In patients with an acute onset of renal failure, elimination of the primary cause is associated with the possibility of recovering adequate renal function to maintain a normal life style and life span. Because the lesions responsible for chronic renal failure are irreversible, they cannot be completely eliminated or partially reversed by initiating specific therapy. Regardless, progression of renal lesions and thus renal failure may be retarded or resolved by therapy designed to eliminate active renal diseases. Therefore, diagnostic plans directed especially at detecting reversible renal diseases should be performed before plans for conservative medical management are formulated. Nonrenal conditions that precipitate or contribute to uremic crises should also be sought and corrected.

SUPPORTIVE THERAPY (Tables B-3, B-4, B-5, B-6, and B-7)

Conservative medical management of renal failure consists of supportive and symptomatic therapy designed to correct deficits and excesses in fluid, electrolyte, acid-base, endocrine, and nutritional balance. The goal is to minimize the clinical and pathophysiologic consequences of reduced renal function. Supportive and symptomatic treatment should not be expected to halt, reverse, or eliminate renal lesions responsible for chronic renal failure. Supportive or symptomatic treatment is most beneficial when combined with specific therapy directed at correcting the primary cause of renal disease.

Caveat

The choice of therapy for renal failure should encompass

TABLE B-5

RISK FACTORS THAT MAY PREDISPOSE GERIATRIC PATIENTS TO ADVERSE DRUG EVENTS

A. Decline in function of various organs and systems associated with aging
B. Increased likelihood of multiple diseases affecting more than one organ or body system
C. Altered absorption, distribution, biotransformation, and excretion of drugs
  1. Reduced renal clearance
  2. Potential for reduced hepatic biotransformation and clearance
  3. Decreased binding of some drugs to protein
  4. Altered distribution of drugs associated with:
    a. Reduced total body water
     — Reduced thirst
     — Impaired urine concentration
    b. Reduced muscle mass and increased body fat
D. Greater likelihood of exposure to:
  1. Multiple drugs
  2. Nephrotoxic drugs

Modified from Aucoin DP: Drug therapy in the geriatric animal. *Vet Clin North Am* 19:41–47, 1989. Modified with permission.

---

knowledge of the patient's previous history of adverse drug events (e.g., rash, tremors, anorexia, vomiting, diarrhea). To minimize adverse drug reactions, it is best to avoid unnecessary use of multiple combinations of drugs.

TABLE B-6

CHECKLIST OF FACTORS THAT MAY MINIMIZE UREMIC ANOREXIA

I. Correct Underlying Abnormalities by Minimizing Deficits and Excesses
A. Fluid balance
B. Serum concentrations of nitrogenous wastes
C. Serum electrolyte concentrations
  1. Potassium
  2. Sodium
  3. Calcium
  4. Phosphorus
D. Serum hydrogen ion concentration
E. Serum concentrations of hormones
  1. Parathyroid hormone
  2. Erythropoietin
  3. Vitamin D

  4. Angiotensin
  5. Renin
F. Others

II. Enhance Palatability of Diet
A. When changing diet:
  1. Switch foods gradually
  2. Maintain texture and flavor similar to usual diet
B. Try flavoring agents
  1. Clam juice
  2. Tuna juice
  3. Chicken broth
  4. Water
  5. Liquid elemental diets
    — Feline Renal Care™ᵃ
    — Impact™ᵇ with taurine added

    — Ensure®ᶜ with taurine added
  6. Garlic
  7. Brewers yeast
  8. Carnitine?
C. Warm to body temperature

III. Modify Feeding Patterns
A. Emphasize frequent small meals
B. Offer rewards
  1. Favorite foods
  2. Maintenance foods
C. Hand feed
D. Avoid adverse associations with eating
  1. Medications
  2. Injections
  3. Others
(continued on page 188)

TABLE B-6 (continued)

E. Prevent food aversion
1. Do not offer diets designed for long-term management of renal failure during periods of nausea and vomiting.
2. Do not adversely alter taste of food by mixing it with medications

IV. Minimize Vomiting
A. Correct underlying abnormalities (see I.)
B. Pharmacologic antiemetics
1. Metoclopramide (0.2–0.5 mg/kg every 12 hours)
2. Cimetidine (2.5–5 mg/kg every 12 hours)

V. Implement Pharmacologic Appetite Stimulation
A. Diazepam (0.2–0.3 mg/kg every 12 hours)
B. Oxazepam (0.2–0.4 mg/kg every 24 hours)
C. Cyproheptadine? (2–4 mg/kg every 24 hours)
D. Propofol
E. B vitamins
F. Anabolic agents?

VI. Enteral Feeding
A. Hand feeding
B. Nasogastric tube feeding

---

[a]Pet-Ag.   [b]Sandoz Nutrition.
[c]Ross Laboratories.

TABLE B-7

THERAPEUTIC OPTIONS FOR MANAGEMENT OF POLYURIC RENAL FAILURE

Treatable Abnormality	Clinical Correlates	Therapeutic Options[a]
Negative fluid balance	Dehydration Vomiting/diarrhea Polyuria/nocturia Adipsia Hypernatremia Hyperproteinemia	Unlimited access to water If vomiting or unwilling to drink, consider parenteral fluid administration
Undernutrition	Weight loss due to tissue loss Anemia Hypoalbuminemia Proteinuria Leukopenia	Provide balanced diet to minimize deficits and excesses in fluid, acid-base, electrolyte, calorie, and endocrine balance and to minimize production of metabolic wastes Minimize anorexia

Metabolic acidosis	Reduced serum concentrations of total CO_2 or HCO_3
	Decreased blood pH
		Dietary protein reduction
		    Renal failure diets
		    Home-made diets (caution)
		Avoid diets producing acidic urine
		Sodium bicarbonate (10 mg/kg q8–12h)[b]
		Potassium citrate (40–60 mg/kg q12h)[b]
		    (Caution: may enhance intestinal absorption of aluminum, resulting in toxicity)

Hyperphosphatemia	Elevated serum phosphorus concentration
	Extraosseous mineralization
	Increased serum parathyroid hormone concentration
	Increased urinary fractional excretion of phosphorus
	Renal osteodystrophy
		Correct dehydration
		Dietary protein reduction
		    Renal failure diets
		    Home-made diets (caution)
		Intestinal phosphate binding agents
		    Aluminum carbonate (30–90 mg/kg/day)[b]
		        (Caution: concomitant use of citrate salts may enhance intestinal absorption of aluminum, resulting in toxicity)
		    $CaCO_3$, Ca acetate (100 mg/kg/day)[b]
		    Others

Hypoproliferative anemia	Typically normocytic, normochromic anemia Pale mucous membranes	Minimize blood sampling Erythropoietin replacement Consider if Hct below ±18%

(continued on page 159)

Treatable Abnormality	Clinical Correlates	Therapeutic Options[a]
Hypoproliferative anemia (continued)	Anorexia Weakness Depression	Epogen[c] (50–100 U/kg 3 times a week); increase dose interval when Hct > ±35% Ferrous sulfate: 50–100 mg/day PO Androgen therapy (?) Decanandrolin (1–1.5 mg/kg/week); double dose if no response in 3 months
Systemic hypertension	Increased arterial blood pressure Retinal lesions (hemorrhage, detachment, others)	Gradual dietary sodium reduction Enalapril (0.25 mg/kg q12–24h)[b] Diltiazem (7.5 mg q8–12h)[b] Amlodipine (0.625 mg PO q24h—cats)[b] Combinations

Hypokalemia	Anorexia
	Muscle weakness
	Ventral neck flexion
	Decreased serum K+ concentration
		Oral potassium supplementation
		    Potassium gluconate (2–4 mEq q8–12 h)[b]
		    Potassium citrate (40–60 mg/kg q12h)[b]
		Parenteral potassium supplementation

Hypernatremia	Elevated serum sodium concentration Dehydration Depression	Correct dehydration Proper use of sodium-containing medications
Hyperkalemia	Oliguria/anuria Weakness Muscle trembling EKG abnormalities	Correct dehydration with polyionic fluids containing reduced quantities of potassium Promote polyuria Avoid potassium supplementation
Hypocalcemia	Decreased serum calcium concentration Muscle twitching	Verify absolute hypocalcemia First correct hyperphosphatemia Oral calcium supplementation[b] Vitamin D therapy (calcitriol [1.5–3.5 ng/kg/day])[b]
Hypercalcemia	Increased serum calcium concentration Polydipsia/polyuria Weakness, anorexia	Correction dehydration Correct hyperphosphatemia Others
Urinary tract infection	Microburia Pyuria, hematuria, proteinuria Positive urine culture	Appropriate antimicrobial therapy Avoid nephrotoxic drugs Adjust dosage according to route of elimination and degree of renal dysfunction

Progression of renal failure	Progressive decrease in creatinine clearance
	Progressive increase of serum creatinine concentration
	Progressive increase in the magnitude of proteinuria
		Eliminate underlying causes of renal failure
		Correct reversible components of renal failure
		    Prerenal azotemia
		    Postrenal azotemia
		Minimize iatrogenic renal damage
		    Avoid nephrotoxic drugs
		    Avoid unnecessary urinary catheterization
		    Avoid unnecessary surgery on urinary system
		    Avoid unnecessary contrast radiography
		Dietary modification
		    Provide only necessary quantities of high biologic value protein
		    Minimize phosphorus
		    Gradual calorie reduction
		    Gradual sodium reduction
		    Avoid saturated lipids
		    Others
		Avoid diets producing acidic urine
		Minimize hypokalemia
		Control hypertension

[a]Management options should be instituted sequentially and only if necessary.

[b]Values represent starting dose, which should be adjusted on the basis of laboratory and clinical response. Calcitriol should be considered only if the patient's serum concentration of calcium and phosphorus can be serially monitored.

[c]Amgen Inc., Thousand Oaks, CA

Appendix C

Treatment of Bacterial Urinary Tract Infections: Basic Concepts and Their Application

I. **Prevention of Bacterial Urinary Tract Infections**

II. **Correction of Predisposing Cause(s)**

III. **Antimicrobial Therapy**
   A. Terminology
   B. Use and Misuse of Antimicrobial Drugs
   C. Antimicrobial Susceptibility Tests
      1. Indications
      2. Disk Diffusion Susceptibility Tests
      3. Antibiotic Dilution Susceptibility Tests
      4. In Vitro Verus In Vivo Susceptibility
      5. Multiple Isolates
   D. Empirical Choice of Antimicrobial Drugs
      1. Empiricism Defined
      2. Empirical Treatment of Bacterial UTI
   E. Serum Versus Urine Concentrations of Drugs
   F. Bacteriostatic Versus Bactericidal Drugs
   G. Drug Combinations
   H. Drug Dosages and Maintenance Schedules for Nonazotemic Patients
   I. Modification of Drugs, Dosage, and

   Maintenance Schedules for Patients With Intrarenal Azotemia
   J. Duration of Antimicrobial Therapy
   K. Fostering Client Compliance With Treatment Recommendations
   L. Monitoring Response to Therapy
   M. Management of Recurrent UTIs
      1. Relapses
      2. Reinfections
      3. Recurrences Attributable to Bacterial Infections of the Prostate
   N. Prevention of Frequent Reinfections
   O. Adverse Drug Reactions

IV. **Step-By-Step Checklists of Therapeutic Protocols for Uncomplicated and Complicated Bacterial UTIs**
   A. Initial Episode of Untreated Lower UTI
   B. Infrequent Renfections
   C. Relapses
   D. Frequent Reinfections
   E. Prevention of Frequent Reinfections
   F. Prevention and Treatment of Catheter-Induced UTI

PREVENTION OF BACTERIAL URINARY TRACT INFECTIONS

Systemic and local host defenses are designed to be effective barriers to infections caused by microbes (see Chapter 3). Normal host defense mechanisms, however, may be damaged or overwhelmed if large quantities of bacteria are introduced into the urinary tract during diagnostic and therapeutic maneuvers in patients with infectious or noninfectious urinary disorders or patients with nonurinary disorders.

The best cure is prevention. To prevent iatrogenic UTI, indiscriminate use of urinary catheters should be avoided. As an alternative, practitioners can consider collecting samples by cystocentesis or midstream samples during voiding (see Chapter 6).

CORRECTION OF PREDISPOSING CAUSE(S)

Urinary tract infections associated with transient reversible abnormalities in local host defenses are usually classified as uncomplicated or simple UTIs. In this setting, self-repair of damaged host defenses may result in spontaneous resolution of the infection.

> CAUTION: Remission of clinical signs is not necessarily synonymous with eradication of urinary tract infection.

You may recall that dysfunction of host defense mechanisms is an extremely important predisposition to UTIs (Chapter 3, Tables 3-8 and 3-9). Because bacteria can best colonize and multiply in tissues of the urinary tract when host defenses are inadequate, permanent elimination of pathogens is most likely to occur if predisposing dysfunction of host defenses are recognized and corrected (Chapter 3, Table 3-9, and Table C-1).

Therapy of recurrent bacterial UTIs should not be considered to be effective solely on the basis of amelioration of clinical signs but should be verified by serial evaluation of urine cultures and urinalyses at appropriate intervals. Equally important is anticipation, prevention, and treatment of symptomatic or asymptomatic recurrences of UTIs because if untreated, they may result in irreversible and even progressive disease.

ANTIMICROBIAL THERAPY
Terminology

If the term "antibiotic" is valid, is the term "antimicrobic" valid or should we use the term "antimicrobial?" *Webster's Unabridged Dictionary* defines "-ial" as an adjective-forming suffix (as in antimicrobial drug), whereas "-ic" is a suffix used to form nouns (as in antimicrobic). But if the term antimicrobial is valid, is the term "antibiotial" valid? The English language can be confusing, which explains why when after we have "filled in" an antimicrobial susceptibility test request form, we have "filled it out."

Use and Misuse of Antimicrobial Drugs

Antimicrobial agents are the cornerstone of therapy for bacterial UTIs. However, they should not be given without considering the risks and desired benefits or without implementing plans for appropriate follow-up evaluations. Compassion for the well-being of our patients will guide us to avoid overtreating with antimicrobial drugs. Although they can be life saving when properly used, antimicobial drugs are not to be viewed as the proverbial pill for every ill.

Administration of antimicrobial agents for treatment of signs of upper or lower urinary tract disease that are not caused by bacterial infection persists as a common cause of overtreatment (Chapter 3, Table 3-4). Cats with self-limiting abacterial idiopathic lower urinary tract disease (LUTD) are a well-documented illustration of this point. Despite the fact that only a small percentage of these patients have bacterial UTIs,

in our experience they are still commonly treated with antibiotics. Although the clinical signs of idiopathic feline LUTD typically resolve in 3 to 7 days with or without antimicrobial treatment, when antimicrobial agents are prescribed, they usually receive the credit for the cure.

Antimicrobial Susceptibility Tests
Indications

Evaluation of the susceptibility of infecting bacteria to antimicrobial drugs is advisable as a general guide for selecting therapeutic agents because different bacterial pathogens isolated from dogs and cats with UTIs may vary widely in their susceptibility to specific antimicrobial agents (Tables C-2 and C-2A). Culture and antimicrobial susceptibility tests should be the standard of practice for symptomatic patients recently treated with antimicrobial drugs. Examples of urinary pathogens associated with polyresistant strains include *Pseudomonas aeruginosa* and *Klebsiella* spp., as well as *Enterobacter* spp., *Escherichia coli*, and *Proteus* spp. are. There are conflicting reports about whether or not staphylococci are becoming more resistant to commonly used antimicrobial agents.[1,2]

If patients develop frequently recurrent infections, follow-up evaluation of the susceptibility of infecting bacteria to antimicrobial drugs is indicated to determine whether changes in susceptibility have occurred. We emphasize the importance of this therapeutic test for patients recently treated with antimicrobial drugs (Chapter 3, Tables 3-10 and 3-11). In this setting, the susceptibility of bacterial pathogens is unpredictable and therefore cannot be obtained from tables generated from data derived from untreated patients (Tables C-2 and C-2A).

Disk Diffusion Susceptibility Tests

Two main types of antimicrobial susceptibility tests are currently in common use. The agar diffusion (Kirby-Bauer) method consists of Mueller-Hinton agar plates that have been inoculated with a standardized suspension of a single uropathogen (pure culture). Paper discs impregnated with different antimicrobial drugs are then placed on the plate. After incubation for 18 hours at 37°C, antimicrobial susceptibility is estimated by measuring the zones of inhibition of bacterial growth surrounding each disk. Zones of inhibition are then interpreted in light of established standards and recorded as resistant, susceptible, or intermediate. Because of differences in the ability of various antibiotics to diffuse through agar, the antibiotic disk surrounded by the largest zone of inhibition of bacterial growth is not necessarily the drug most likely to be effective.

The disk diffusion test of antimicrobic susceptibility was primarily designed to treat infections based on knowledge of serum concentrations of the antimicrobial drug. Therefore the concentration of antimicrobics (except nitrofurantoin) in the paper disks is comparable to typical serum concentrations of drugs. Many drugs, however, attain concentrations in urine that are 10 to 100 times greater than those observed in serum. If the pathogen isolated from urine is reported to be susceptible to a drug on the disk diffusion panel, that drug is likely to be effective in vitro if it is excreted in urine and the patient does not have primary renal failure. If the results of the disk diffusion test

TABLE C-1

OBJECTIVES FOR TREATMENT OF BACTERIAL URINARY TRACT INFECTIONS

1. A prerequisite for effective and safe treatment is an accurate diagnosis.
2. Objectives of urinalysis.
   a. Urinalysis should be used to screen the patient for evidence of UTI.
   b. Microscopic evaluation of urine sediment is an insensitive method of detecting bacteria. Since bacteria are more difficult to detect than white cells, pyuria may appear to be unassociated with low numbers of bacteria. Quantitative cultures should be evaluated if significant pyuria is observed.
   c. Microscopic evaluation of urine sediment is a nonspecific method of detecting bacteria. Inexperienced observers often misinterpret Brownian movement of amorphous material as bacteria.
3. Objectives of collecting urine samples for diagnostic bacterial culture.
   a. Obtain quantitative (number of bacteria per ml of urine) in addition to qualitative (identification of bacteria) cultures.
   b. Collect samples prior to administration of diagnostic radiopaque contrast agents or therapeutic agents, especially antimicrobial drugs.
   c. If antimicrobial therapy was initiated without confirmation by urine culture and subsequent events dictate need for diagnostic bacterial culture, discontinue antimicrobial therapy for 3 to 5 days before collecting urine for culture.
   d. Consider the collection method when interpreting results of urine culture.
   e. Samples collected by cystocentesis are most reliable for bacterial culture because bacterial contamination from the lower genitourinary tract is eliminated. Cystocentesis also eliminates catheter-induced trauma and UTI.
   f. The urinary bladders of patients with cystitis may be too small to safely collect urine by cystocentesis. Urine formation may be enhanced with parenteral fluids or furosemide. Inducing diuresis is not suitable for diagnostic urinalysis; it is acceptable to facilitate diagnostic culture of urine collected by cystocentesis. However, diuresis will reduce quantitative culture counts.
   g. Voided urine samples are unreliable for diagnostic urine culture. If circumstances mandate collection of a voided sample, collect urine in a sterilized container. Interpret results in conjunction with urinalysis. Greater than 100,000 colony-forming units per milliliter in a minimally contaminated urine sample is probably significant.
4. Objective of preserving urine for diagnostic bacterial culture.
   a. Do not incubate urine samples prior to bacterial culture; in vitro bacterial growth will interfere with interpretation of quantitative results.
   b. Bacteria that contaminate urine during collection and transport to the laboratory can rapidly multiply unless the sample is properly preserved. When more than 30 minutes is expected to elapse between the time of urine collection and the time of analysis or culture, refrigerate (do not freeze) the sample to minimize in vitro bacterial growth.

   This step is especially important for samples contaminated during collection by voiding or catheterization.
   c. The most reliable culture results are obtained if refrigerated samples are evaluated within 6 hours; results are often unreliable in samples refrigerated more than 12 hours.
5. Interpretation of results of diagnostic urine culture.
   a. Results should be interpreted in conjunction with results of urinalysis. Isolation of bacteria in absence of an inflammatory response suggests contamination of the sample.
   b. Confirmation that a significant number of bacteria are associated with pyuria indicates that the inflammatory lesion is active and has been caused or complicated by bacterial infection.
   c. 80% to 85% of bacterial UTI are caused by a single species of bacteria; 15% to 20% are caused by more than one bacterial species. Detection of multiple bacterial species suggests sample contamination, especially in samples collected by voiding or catheterization.
6. Because healthy animals are innately resistant to bacterial UTI, confirmation of UTI should prompt a search for predisposing abnormalities in host defenses so that they may be eliminated or controlled.
7. Absence of bacterial infection prior to diagnostic or therapeutic techniques does not mean it will not develop subsequently. If gross hematuria and dysuria develops or persists after transurethral catheterization, cystoscopy, or urethral surgery, evaluate the patient for bacterial UTI.
8. Antimicrobics should be selected on the basis of antimicrobial susceptibility tests of causative pathogens. Choose drugs eliminated in high concentration in urine. Pending the availability of bacterial culture and antimicrobial susceptibility results, select antimicrobics to treat patients suspected of having UTI on the basis of Gram stain–facilitated identification of bacteria in urine sediment.
9. Aggressive treatment with appropriate dosages of antimicrobics is indicated. Choose drugs that are likely to attain high urine concentrations.
10. Urine should be recultured 3 to 5 days following the initiation of therapy to check the efficacy of the antimicrobic in sterilizing the urine (so-called test of efficacy or TOE). Cystocentesis is the collection method of choice for culture of urine for bacteria after initiating antimicrobic therapy.
11. Antimicrobial therapy is continued until there is clinical and laboratory evidence of response. For uncomplicated bacterial UTI a 10 to 14 day interval is usually effective. For infections associated with some other abnormality, duration of therapy is dependent on the underlying cause(s). For best results, the patient's response should be monitored by bacterial culture and urinalysis.
12. Because symptomatic or asymptomatic recurrences (reinfections or relapses) may be associated with progressive and potentially irreversible disease, they should be anticipated, prevented, and, when necessary, treated.

are interpreted to indicate that the pathogen is resistant to the drug, the drug may or may not still be effective if its urine concentration is substantially higher than its serum concentration. Examples of some drugs that are excreted in high concentration in urine include ampicillin, cephalexin, chloramphenicol, enrofloxacin, oxytetracycline, penicillin G, and trimethoprim.

Agar diffusion antimicrobial susceptibility tests may be useful for patients with renal infections and acute bacterial prostatitis because renal and prostate tissue concentrations of antibiotics are more likely to correspond to serum concentrations of antibiotics.

Antibiotic Dilution Susceptibility Tests

The second type of commonly used susceptibility test is the antibiotic dilution susceptibility test. It is designed to determine the minimum concentration of the antimicrobial drug that can inhibit the growth of uropathogens. After inoculation and incubation of uropathogens into wells containing serial twofold dilutions of antimicrobial drugs at concentrations achievable in tissues and urine of patients given usual drug dosages, the minimum inhibitory concentration (MIC) is determined. The MIC is defined as the lowest antimicrobial concentration (or the highest dilution) without visible bacterial growth. The MIC is several dilutions lower than the minimum bactericidal concentration (MBC) of drugs. The MIC is then compared to antimicrobial concentrations expected to be present in urine after administration of therapeutic doses of a drug. Thus, rather than report absolute susceptibility or resistance, the concentration of drugs that will inhibit the growth of the bacteria is determined. In general, the antimicrobial agent is likely to be effective in vivo if it can achieve a concentration four times the MIC (Table C-3).

> **KEY POINT:** The MIC of an antimicrobial drug varies with each type of infecting pathogen. In addition, the MIC for the same type of pathogen may vary with different episodes of relapsing infections.

In Vitro Versus In Vivo Susceptibility

Although in vitro susceptibility tests are valuable, clinical and laboratory evidence of response to an antimicrobial drug is the ultimate parameter of success. Factors other than in vitro susceptibility may affect in vivo effectiveness of antimicrobial drugs. The integrity of natural host defense mechanisms and the likelihood that antimicrobial drugs can reach therapeutic concentrations at the site(s) of infection should also be considered.

Multiple Isolates

If a UTI associated with more than one pathogen is identified and the organisms do not have similar antimicrobial sensitivities, initial treatment of the predominant pathogen with an effective drug is recommended. Urine should then be recultured during therapy. If the second pathgen can still be isolated, a therapeutic approach for it should be devised.

Empirical Choice of Antimicrobial Drugs
Empiricism Defined

Webster's Dictionary defines an empirical remedy as one cho-

sen on the basis of practical (uncontrolled) experience without reference to scientific principle. In context of bacterial UTI, empirical treatment consists of selecting an antibacterial drug without knowledge of the susceptibility of bacteria for which the drug is being given to eliminate.

Empirical (uncontrolled) observations based on experience can be valuable. However, when choices based on experience are viewed in retrospect as mistakes, experience has the reputation of being a tough teacher. In this setting, she gives the test first and the lesson afterward.

Because of our biases we often misinterpret our experiences. For example, when a desired clinical response occurs coincidently with administration of a drug, many practitioners interpret the outcome as a cause-and-effect relationship. How often have we said, "I treated the pet with an antibiotic and it responded?" In reality, just because a patient gets better does not necessarily mean that it did so in response to treatment.

What about those patients that do not respond to empirical treatment with antimicroial drugs? Can we assume that they did not have bacterial UTI? The answer is no. Just because a patient with urinary tract signs thought to be associated with bacterial UTI fails to respond to treatment with antibiotics does not mean the diagnosis and approach to treatment were wrong. Persistent signs of urinary disease may be caused in part by an abnormality predisposing to UTI such as a calcium oxalate urolith or a neoplasm (Chapter 3, Table 3-9).

Empirical Treatment of Bacterial UTI

Experience has shown that patients with acute onset of uncomplicated bacterial UTI often "respond" to empirical antimicrobial treatment selected in the absence of results of antimicrobial susceptibility tests. In this situation, making an empirical but educated "guess" of the proper antibiotic is an accepted standard of practice provided patients do not have a history of frequently reccurent clinical signs and have not been given antibacterial drugs to treat signs of urinary tract disease in the past 3 to 6 weeks. In this situation, the choice of drug should be based on known properties of antimicrobial agents in combating UTIs caused by commonly isolated organisms (Chapter 3, Table 3-12, and Tables C-2 and C-2A) and knowledge that the drug can attain a high concentration in urine (Table C-3). The following results of studies of the in vitro susceptibility of common urinary tract pathogens (obtained from previously untreated patients) to selected oral antimicrobial agents may be helpful in selecting the proper drug[3,4]:

> **CAUTION:** The following data were generated more than 15 years ago. There is evidence that susceptibility patterns of some bacteria are changing.[1,2]

- Almost 100% of the staphylococci and streptococci/enterococci are expected to respond to penicillin (50,000 IU/lb divided three times daily) or ampicillin (35 mg/lb divided three times daily). Conversely, only 56% of *Escherichia coli*, 33% of *Klebsiella*, and 0% of *Pseudomonas* responded to oral ampicillin.
- Almost 80% of the *E. coli* are likely to respond to trimethoprim-sulfadiazine (12 mg/lb divided twice daily). This drug

TABLE C-2
GUESSTIMATED SUSCEPTIBILITY OF URINARY BACTERIAL PATHOGENS TO SOME COMMONLY USED ANTIMICROBIAL DRUGS

Pathogens (listed alphabetically)	Antimicrobials[a] With ≥90% Efficacy (listed alphabetically)	Antimicrobials[a] With 70%–90% Efficacy (listed alphabetically)
Enterobacter spp.	Enrofloxacin Trimethoprim-sulfadiazine	Cephalosporins (1st and 2nd gen.)
Escherichia coli	Cefoxitin Enrofloxacin	Amoxicillin-clavulanate Cephalosporins (1st, 2nd, and 3rd gen.) Trimethoprim-sulfadiazine
Klebsiella spp.	Cephalosporins (1st gen.) Enrofloxacin	Cephalosporins (2nd and 3rd gen.) Trimethoprim-sulfadiazine
Proteus spp.	Amoxicillin-clavulanate Cefoxitin Enrofloxacin	Amoxicillin Ampicillin Cephalosporins (1st, 2nd, and 3rd gen.) Trimethoprim-sulfadiazine
Pseudomonas aeruginosa	Amikacin Enrofloxacin Imipenem	
Staphylococcus intermedius	Amoxicillin-clavulanate Cephalexin Enrofloxacin	Amoxicillin Chloramphenicol Trimethoprim-sulfadiazine
Streptococcus-Enterococcus	Ampicillin Amoxicillin Amoxicillin-clavulanate	Nitrofurantoin Trimethoprim-sulfadiazine

[a]Prior treatment with antimicrobics may alter the susceptibility of bacterial pathogens to these drugs.

The following table emphasizes the importance of knowledge of urine concentrations vs. plasma concentrations when interpreting susceptibility data.

TABLE C-2A
IN VITRO SUSCEPTIBILITY OF SOME CANINE AND FELINE UROPATHOGENS TO ENROFLOXACIN[a]

Pathogen	Number of Isolates		% Susceptibility Based on Plasma Concentrations of 2 µg/ml[a]						Predicted % in Vivo Susceptibility if Urine Concentration Is ~200 µg/ml[a]
			Susceptible		Intermediate		Resistant		
	Dog	Cat	Dog	Cat	Dog	Cat	Dog	Cat	
Escherichia coli	235	104	94	98	0	0	6	2	≥99
Enterococcus spp.	26	18	39	39	27	28	34	33	~70
Klebsiella pneumoniae	12	3	100	100	0	0	0	0	≥99
Proteus mirabilis	61	4	98	100	0	0	2	0	≥99
Pseudomonas aeruginosa	16	2	31	50	25	50	44	0	≥99
Staphylococcus intermedius	49	8	98	63	2	0	0	37	≥99
Streptococcus—beta hemolytic	23	0	83	0	17	0	0	0	≥99

[a]Data based on antimicrobial dilution assay and generated for year 1998 by Cynthia Lindeman, University of Minnesota Veterinary Diagnostic Laboratory.

TABLE C-3

AVERAGE CANINE URINE CONCENTRATIONS OF ANTIMICROBIAL AGENTS[a]

Drug	Dose[b] (mg/kg)	Route of Administration	Mean Urine Concentration (±SD)
Amikacin	5 mg/kg every 8 hours	Subcutaneous	342 (±143) µg/ml
Amoxicillin	11 mg/kg every 8 hours	Oral	202 (±93) µg/ml
Ampicillin	26 mg/kg every 8 hours	Oral	309 (±55) µg/ml
Cephalexin	18 mg/kg every 8 hours	Oral	500 µg/ml
Chloramphenicol	33 mg/kg every 8 hours	Oral	123.8 (±39.7) µg/ml
Enrofloxacin	5 mg/kg every 24 hours	Oral	200 (±10) µg/ml
Gentamicin	2 mg/kg every 8 hours	Subcutaneous	107.4 (±33.0) µg/ml
Hetacillin	26 mg/kg every 8 hours	Oral	300.3 (±156.1) µg/ml
Kanamycin	4 mg/kg every 12 hours	Subcutaneous	529.6 (±150.5) µg/ml
Nitrofurantoin	5 mg/kg every 8 hours	Oral	100 µg/ml
Penicillin G	36,700 U/kg every 8 hours[c]	Oral	294.9 (±210.7) U/ml
Penicillin V	26 mg/kg every 8 hours	Oral	148.3 (±98.5) µg/ml
Sulfisoxazole	22 mg/kg every 8 hours	Oral	1466.3 (±832.4) µg/ml
Tetracycline	18 mg/kg every 8 hours	Oral	137.9 (±64.6) µg/ml
Trimethoprim-sulfadiazine	13 mg/kg every 12 hours	Oral	55.0 (±19.2) µg/ml
Tobramycin	1 mg/kg every 8 hours	Subcutaneous	66.0 (±39.0) µg/ml

[a]Data courtesy of Dr. Gerald V. Ling, University of California Davis.
[b]Frequency of administration of drugs should be based on manufacturer recommendations and the ability of clients to comply with recommendations.
[c]Dosage of penicillin G expressed in units per kg.

was also highly effective (100%) against staphylococci. Conversely, approximately 70% of *Proteus* and 50% of *Streptococcus* or *Enterococcus* and *Enterobacter* responded to trimethoprim-sulfadiazine.

■ About 80% of *Proteus mirabilis* respond to oral penicillin or ampicillin at the same doses and maintenance intervals suggested for streptococci or staphylococci.

■ About 90% of *Pseudomonas aeruginosa* respond to oral tetracycline (25 mg/lb divided three times daily).[5] (Note—In our recent experience, most *Pseudomonas* isolates are resistant to tetracycline).

■ More than 90% of *Klebsiella pneumoniae* were susceptible to cephalexin (50 mg/lb divided three times daily).[5]

Serum Versus Urine Concentrations of Drugs

Rigid generalities about the relative importance of tissue, urine, and serum concentrations of antimicrobial agents used to treat UTIs are difficult to formulate. We emphasize that serum or urine concentrations of antimicrobial agents do not necessarily reflect their tissue concentrations. With these limitations in mind, we make the following recommendations:

■ Select agents that have high urine concentrations (at least four times the MIC) for treating lower UTIs. Refer to the section on antimicrobial susceptibility tests for additional informtion.

■ To treat acute bacterial infections of the prostate (Tables C-4 and C-5) or kidney, select antimicrobial agents that attain high concentrations in serum and (if possible) urine.

Bacteriostatic Versus Bactericidal Drugs

Urinary tract pathogens often respond satisfactorily to bacteriostatic (those that inhibit multiplication) and bactericidal (those that kill) antimicrobial agents (Table C-6). The use of bactericidal agents, however, appears to be superior if persistent impairment in the patient's natural defense mechanism exists. Keep in mind that whether a drug ultimately has bactericidal or bacteriostatic activity may depend on the concentration of each drug to which pathogenic bacteria are exposed. Bactericidal drugs may become nonbactericidal if concentrations below the minimum bactericidal concentration are not reached or sustained for a sufficient period at the site(s) of infection.

Drug Combinations

Simultaneous administration of combinations of different antimicrobial drugs may result in a variety of effects that can be antagonistic, additive, or synergistic. Although drugs with the same mechanism of action are often additive when used in combination, while combinations of bactericidal and bacteriostatic drugs are antagonistic when used in combination, responses to many drug combinations are unpredictable. Unless the efficacy of their combined use has been documented, avoid administration of two or more antimicrobial drugs simultaneously. Combinations of trimethoprim with sulfadiazine and amoxicillin with potassium clavulanate represent combinations of drugs that are of established efficacy.

Drug Dosages and Maintenance Schedules for Nonazotemic Patients

Providing safe and effective doses of antibacterial drugs for

TABLE C-4

ANTIMICROBIAL AGENTS THAT MAY REACH THERAPEUTIC CONCENTRATIONS IN PROSTATE OF DOGS WITH CHRONIC BACTERIAL PROSTATITIS

Drug	Lipid Solubility	Chemical Nature	pKa	Plasma Protein Binding (%)	Dose	Route
Carbenicllin indanyl sodium	Yes	?	?	50	15 mg/kg every 8 hours	Intravenous
Chloramphenicol	Yes	NA	NA	53	45–60 mg/kg every 8 hours	Oral, intramuscular, intravenous
Doxycycline	Yes	Ampholyte	3.4, 7.7, 9.7	88	3 mg/kg every 12 hours	Oral
Enrofloxacin	Yes	Ampholyte	6.3, 7.7	15	5.0 mg/kg every 24 hours	Oral, subcutaneous, intramuscular, intravenous
Erythromycin base	Yes	Base	8.8	84	10–15 mg/kg every 8 hours	Oral
Hetacillin potassium	Yes	Base	?	18	10–20 mg/kg every 8 hours	Oral
Minocycline	Yes	Ampholyte	7.8, 9.3	76	3–5 mg/kg every 8 hours	Oral
Tetracycline	Yes	Amphylyte	3.3, 7.7, 9.7	65	25 mg/kg every 12 hours	Oral
Trimethoprim	Yes	Base	7.3	35	3–5 mg/kg every 12 hours	Oral
Trimethoprim-sulfadiazine	Yes	Acid	?	?	15 mg/kg every 12 hours	Oral

NA = not applicable.

TABLE C-5

ANTIMICROBIAL AGENTS THAT MAY NOT REACH THERAPEUTIC CONCENTRATIONS IN PROSTATE OF DOGS WITH CHRONIC BACTERIAL PROSTATITIS

Drug	Lipid Solubility	Chemical Nature	pKa	Plasma Protein Binding (%)	Dose	Route
Ampicillin	No	Acid	2.5	20	20 mg/kg every 6–8 hours	Oral, intravenous, intramuscular
Cefadroxil	No	Acid	?	?	22 mg/kg every 12 hours	Oral
Cephalexin	No	Acid	5.2, 7.3	14	20–30 mg/kg every 8–12 hours	Oral
Cephalothin sodium	No	Acid	2.5	20	35 mg/kg every 8 hours	Intravenous, intramuscular
Cephapirin	No	Ampholyte	2.2	62	20 mg/kg every 6 hours	Intravenous, intramuscular
Sulfadiazine	No	Acid	?	?	100 mg/kg every 12 hours	Oral

TABLE C-6

ANTIMICROBIAL AGENTS COMMONLY USED TO TREAT BACTERIAL URINARY TRACT INFECTIONS IN DOGS AND CATS

Agent	Spectrum of Activity in Urine	Effect	Dose[a] Dog	Dose[a] Cat	Route of Administration
Amoxicillin	Broad	Bactericidal	11 mg/kg every 8 hours	Same	Oral
Amoxicillin trihydrate/clavulanic potassium	Broad	Bactericidal	10–20 mg/kg (combined) every 8 hours	Same	Oral
Ampicillin	Broad	Bactericidal	25 mg/kg every 8 hours	Same	Oral
		Bactericidal	8 mg/kg every 8 hours	Same	Subcutaneous, intramuscular, intravenous
Amikacin	Moderately broad	Bactericidal	10 mg/kg every 12 hours	5–10 mg/kg every 8 hours	Subcutaneous
Cefadroxil	Broad	Bactericidal	10–20 mg/kg every 12 hours	Same	Oral
Cefoxitin[b]	Gram negative	Bactericidal	2.5–5.0 mg/kg every 8 hours	Same	Intramuscular, intravenous
Cephalexin	Broad	Bactericidal	10–30 mg/kg every 8 to 12 hours	Same	Oral
Chloramphenicol	Broad	Bacteriostatic	33 mg/kg every 8 hours	20 mg/kg every 8 hours for 1 week	Oral
Doxycycline	Broad	Bacteriostatic	5–11 mg/kg every 12 hours	Same	Oral
Gentamicin	Broad	Bactericidal	2–3 mg/kg every 8 hours for first day; then ½ mg/kg every 8 hours	Same	Subcutaneous, intramuscular
Enrofloxacin	Broad	Bactericidal	5–10 mg/kg every 24 hours (single or divided dose)	Same	Oral, subcutaneous, intramuscular, intravenous
Hetacillin	Broad	Bactericidal	25 mg/kg every 8 hours	Same	Oral
Kanamycin	Moderately broad	Bactericidal	6 mg/kg every 12 hours	Same	Intramuscular, subcutaneous
Methenamine mandelate; methenamine hippurate	Moderately broad	Bacteriostatic	10 mg/kg every 6–8 hours; urine pH must be below 6	Same?	Oral
Nitrofurantoin	Moderately broad	Bacteriostatic	5 mg/kg every 6–8 hours	Same	Oral
Norfloxacin	Broad	Bactericidal	5–20 mg/kg every 12 hours	Same	Oral
Oxytetracycline	Broad	Bacteriostatic	20 mg/kg every 8 hours	Same	Oral
Penicillin G (Na or K)	Moderately broad	Bactericidal	40,000 units/kg every 8 hours	Same	Oral
Sulfisoxazole	Broad	Bacteriostatic	20–30 mg/kg every 8 hours	Same	Oral
Tetracycline	Broad	Bacteriostatic	20 mg/kg every 8 hours	Same	Oral
Trimethoprim-sulfadiazine	Broad	Bacteriostatic/Bactericidal	15 mg/kg (combined) every 12 hours	Unknown	Oral
Tobramycin	Moderately broad	Bactericidal	1–2 mg/kg every 8 hours	Same	Subcutaneous

[a] Dosage for patients with normal hydration and normal renal function.
[b] Dosage recommended by Dr. David P. Aucoin, Corona, CA.

TABLE C-7
CHECKLIST OF COMPLIANCE PROBLEMS AND SOLUTIONS

Problem	Solution
Forgetfulness	Tailor maintenance intervals to conform with client's life style
Inconvenience of frequent dosing	Use drugs designed for dosing every 12 hours or every 24 hours
Prolonged duration of therapy	Encouragement; regularly scheduled rechecks
Misunderstanding instructions	Simple, clearly written instructions
Drug side effects	Client education; discuss options and alternatives
Premature withdrawal of medication because of apparent cure	Client education; discuss consequences
Apparent nonresponse to therapy	Client education; discuss procedure to follow
Medications too expensive	Provide alternatives if available

TABLE C-8
TOP 10 LIST OF RECOMMENDATIONS TO FOSTER CLIENT COMPLIANCE WITH TREATMENT RECOMMMENDATIONS

DO know the name of the drug(s), and why it is being given.

DO understand when a beneficial response to therapy is expected.

DO be sure you clearly understand all instructions before starting to administer drugs, including exactly how much to give, when to give it, and whether it should be given before, during, or after meals. Also have a clear understanding of how long to give the medication(s) and what to do if problems occur.

DO know what to do if you forget or are unable to give the drug(s) at the prescribed daily intervals.

DO understand important side effects that may be associated with drugs, their likely frequency of occurrence, and what to do if they occur. Before you leave the hospital, obtain a list of side effects that should immediately be reported to the doctor.

DO call your doctor if the symptoms of the disease unexpectedly persist during therapy, especially if they unexpectedly worsen.

DON'T give more or less than the prescribed amount of the drug(s) without first consulting with your doctor.

DON'T suddenly stop giving the drug(s) because the clinical symptoms have disappeared without first checking with your doctor.

DON'T transfer a drug from its original container to another container.

DON'T give the patient old medications without first checking with your doctor; don't give the patient expired medications.

patients with bacterial UTIs depends on several variables. To help eradicate bacterial pathogens from the site(s) of infection, the drug concentration must be maintained at varying concentrations above the MIC for at least a portion of the dosing interval. However, peak drug concentrations and the time drug concentrations remain above the MIC during the dosing interval vary with different antimicrobial agents and different sites of infection. In addition, recall that the MIC varies with different bacterial pathogens, and may vary with different episodes of relapsing infections caused by the same pathogen. Thus the optimum dosage of an antimicrobial drug to treat bacterial UTI varies with the susceptibility of each pathogen, the tissue or organ that it is infecting, and the integrity of host defense and repair mechanisms. These principles justify the value of flexible label dosing of various antimicrobial drugs such as enrofloxacin.

In general, dosage and intervals between maintenance dosages should conform to the recommendations of the manufacturer (Table C-6). Strive to maintain high concentrations of antimicrobial agents in urine to treat lower UTIs and high serum concentrations to treat infections of the renal parenchyma.

Frequency of administration of a drug is based on whether its antimicrobial activity is best correlated with (1) the drug's peak serum concentration (concentration dependent) or (2) the time during the dosing interval that the drug's serum concentration is higher than the MIC (time dependent).[6,7] For example, to maximize the value of drugs whose antimicrobial efficacy is time dependent (such as β-lactams), they should be given more frequently and not just at higher doses. The antimicrobial activity of fluoroquinolones is concentration dependent.

The volume of urine produced by the patient should be considered when selecting doses of antimicrobial drugs. Higher doses are needed to maintain effective urine concentrations of drugs in polyuric patients compared with patients that are producing concentrated urine. Although signs of UTI may subside following administration of suboptimum doses of an antimicrobial agent, bacteriuria may persist.

Because of the short therapeutic half-lives of many antimicrobial drugs used to treat bacterial UTIs and the relatively frequent voiding patterns of most dogs (three to five or more times a day), from a pharmacologic point of view it is ideal to treat lower UTIs by giving most drugs in two to three equal subdoses per day. However, this schedule of administration may be associated with poor owner compliance and thus result in administration of subtherapeutic doses. Therefore the ability of companion animal owners to comply with recommen-

TABLE C-9

CHARACTERISTICS OF FLUOROQUINOLONES THAT ARE DESIRABLE IN PATIENTS WITH COMPLICATED BACTERIAL URINARY TRACT INFECTIONS

- Good tissue penetration into:
  —Kidneys
  —Prostate gland
- High urine concentration
  —Sustained for extended period
  —Urine concentration may exceed MIC in patients with renal failure
- Not nephrotoxic; wide safety margin
- Extended spectrum of activity
- Often effective against resistant bacteria
- Plasmid-mediated resistance extremely uncommon

TABLE C-10

CHECKLIST OF DIAGNOSTIC AND THERAPEUTIC STEPS TO CONSIDER WHEN MANAGING BACTERIAL URINARY TRACT INFECTION IN A PATIENT WITH AZOTEMIC RENAL FAILURE

A. Look for a predisposing cause (Chapter 3, Table 3-9).
B. Select an antimicrobial agent on the basis of bacterial culture and susceptibility tests.
C. For renal infections:
  1. Avoid potentially nephrotoxic drugs.
  2. Select a drug that attains therapeutic concentrations in plasma.
  3. Select a drug with good tissue penetrability (Table C-9).
D. Adjust dose regimen for drugs likely to accumulate as a result of decreased renal clearance.
E. Monitor response to therapy.
  1. Culture urine 3 to 5 days after initiating therapy.
    a. Collect urine by cystocentesis.
    b. Perform urinalysis and quantitative bacterial culture.
      — If urine is sterile, continue treatment for at least 3 weeks.
      — If urine contains any viable bacteria, reevaluate patient to find reasons for treatment failure (Table C-13).
    c. Monitor renal fuction during therapy.
    d. Monitor patient for adverse drug reactions.
  2. Following withdrawal of antimicrobic therapy, perform urinalysis and urine cultures to detect infection recurrence.
    a. If a relapse occurs, continue therapy for a longer period.
    b. If a reinfection occurs, consult Table C-15.

dations must be considered when selecting dose intervals (Tables C-7 and C-8).

To ensure adequate drug concentrations in the urinary tract during treatment intervals, it is recommended that daily doses be administered shortly after micturition, especially just before a period of confinement during which voiding is not permitted (such as overnight).

KEY POINT: Ultimately, practitioners are responsible for balancing the issues of drug safety and efficacy in order to modify the drug dose and maintenance interval according to individual needs.

Modification of Drugs, Dosage, and Maintenance Schedules for Patients With Intrarenal Azotemia

Drugs for treating patients with UTIs and renal failure should be selected only (1) after considering their route(s) of metabolism and elimination and their nephrotoxic potential, (2) on the basis of antimicrobial susceptibility tests, and (3) when there is known potential benefit to be gained from their use. With the advent of fluoroquinolone antimicrobials, the need for nephrotoxic aminoglycosides should be uncommon.

Available evidence suggests that azotemic patients with renal infection should be treated with drugs that obtain a high serum concentration, while patients with lower UTIs should be treated with agents that attain a high concentration in urine (Tables C-3 and C-9).

CAUTION: Special precautions must be taken for patients with azotemic renal failure in order to prevent adverse drug reactions.[8–10] Because the kidneys are the major route of excretion of active and metabolized drugs from the body and because of the inherent nephrotoxicity of some drugs, there is an increase in the frequency and severity of drug intolerance in patients with renal insufficiency.

If renal dysfunction results in retention of urea, creatinine, phosphorus, it is logical to assume that drugs normally eliminated by glomerular filtration will also be retained. Excessive drug concentrations are associated with increased adverse reactions, including nephrotoxicity. Therefore try to avoid drugs that are potentially nephrotoxic or that are dependent on the kidneys for metabolism and/or elimination from the body (Table C-10).

If drugs that are likely to be associated with significant side effects and that are dependent on renal excretion are considered necessary, their dose should be reduced or the maintenance interval between dosages should be increased.[2] The most accurate method of titrating drug dose adjustments in patients with azotemic renal failure is to calculate a dose, administer it, and monitor the resultant peak and trough serum concentrations by direct assay. Adjusted dose calculations are based on measurements of glomerular filtration as determined by creatinine clearance or iohexol clearance. When renal clearance measurements are not available, serum creatinine

TABLE C-11
GUIDELINES FOR DURATION OF TREATMENT WITH ANTIMICROBIC DRUGS

Type	Lower UTI (Days)	Upper UTI (Days)
1. First episode—acute simple UTI	10–14 (female dog; cat)	21+
	21 (intact male dog)	
2. First episode—chronic complicated UTI	14–21	As needed
3. Infrequent reinfection	10–14	21+
4. Relapsing UTI	21+	As needed
5. Persistent UTI	Indefinite	Indefinite
6. Bacterial prostatitis	21+	NA
7. Struvite urolith dissolution	Until dissolution confirmed	
8. Prophylactic	3 to 6 months	As needed

NA = not applicable.

concentration may be considered as an estimate of the magnitude of reduced glomerular filtration rate, as follows:

A. Dose reduction—Constant interval method:

Reduced dose =

$$\text{Normal dose} \times \frac{\text{Normal serum creatinine concentration}}{\text{Patient serum creatinine concentration}}$$

Because the normal serum creatinine concentration is in the numerator, and the elevated patient serum creatinine concentration is in the denominator, the new dose will always be less than the normal dose.

To initiate therapeutic drug concentrations in plasma and tissues, loading is accomplished by giving the usual dose initially, followed by the calculated reduced dose.

The reduced dose – constant maintenance interval of dosage adjustment is associated with lower trough and higher peak concentrations of drug. Periods of subtherapeutic drug concentrations are minimized. Therefore this method is less likely to result in subtherapeutic drug concentrations in the patient. It is a choice to consider when their is a narrow margin between the therapeutic plasma concentration of the drug and the toxic concentration.

B. Constant dose—Interval extension method:

Increased dose interval =

$$\text{Normal interval} \times \frac{\text{Patient serum creatinine concentration}}{\text{Normal serum creatinine concentration}}$$

Because the elevated patient serum creatinine concentration is in the numerator and the normal serum creatinine concentration is in the denominator, the new dose interval will always be greater than the normal dose interval.

The initial two doses should be given according to the usual interval, and subsequent doses given according to the calculated prolonged interval.

The constant dose – increased maintenance interval of dosage adjustment is associated with trough and peak concentrations of drug similar to those seen in healthy patients. However, prolonged periods of potentially subtherapeutic plasma concentrations exist. This method has the advantage of requiring administration of the drug less frequently.

Selection of the method of dosage alteration should be based on whether (1) a drug's antibacterial activity is best correlated with its serum concentration or the time during a dosing interval that serum concentrations are above the MIC of the bacterial pathogen and (2) drug toxicity is correlated to peak, trough, or plasma concentration. The decision should be based on the best balance of efficacy and potential toxicity.

Duration of Antimicrobial Therapy (Table C-11)

Data concerning the minimum and optimum duration of antimicrobial therapy for UTIs are not available. Therefore rigid generalities on the duration of treatment for acute, chronic, and recurrent UTI cannot be stated. Duration of therapy must be individualized on the basis of serial clinical and laboratory findings and therefore depends on patient response to therapy. The goals are to (1) eliminate bacteria from urine and tissue and (2) allow the urinary tract and its defense mechanisms time to recover sufficient function to prevent of UTI recurrence.

Selection of the proper antimicrobial drug, dosage, and frequency of administration usually eradicates bacteriuria within 2 to 5 days. However, if bacteria have gained access to tissue below the urothelium, renal parenchyma, or prostate, a longer course of therapy is usually required to eradicate the infection in these sites.

Remission of clinical signs is not a reliable index of successful eradication of infection nor is reduced white cell, red blood cell, and protein counts detected by urinalysis. Duration of therapy should be based on the persistent elimination of UTI as defined by urine cultures in addition to amelioration of pyuria and clinical signs.

We emphasize that it is not possible to establish rigid gen-

TABLE C-12

EXAMPLES OF PATTERNS OF BACTERIURIA DETECTED BY SEQUENTIAL URINE CULTURES PERFORMED TO MONITOR RESPONSE TO ANTIMICROBIAL PRESCRIPTION

Time and Status of Culture of Urine for Bacteria					
Before Treatment	3 to 5 Days After Initiating Treatment	3 to 5 Days Before Finishing Treatment	7 to 14 Days After Treatment Discontinued	More Than 2 Weeks After Treatment Discontinued	Interpretations
Positive	Positive	Does not apply	Does not apply	Does not apply	Persistent UTI; treatment failure
Positive	Negative	Negative	Positive for same microbe	Does not apply	Relapse (see Table 3-10)
Positive	Negative	Negative	Negative	Negative	Cure
Positive	Negative	Negative	Negative	Positive for different microbe	Reinfection (see Table 3-11)

eralities about the duration of therapy because it depends on patient response. With this perspective, we recommend that the first episode of UTI in females and neutered males be treated for approximately 10 days to 2 weeks, provided bacteria are not isolated from urine during therapy. For intact male dogs at risk for bacterial prostatitis, 3 to 4 weeks of treatment is recommended. If clinical improvement is not noted within 3 to 5 days, the patient should be reevaluated.

For chronic or recurrent UTIs (relapses), treatment should be continued for at least 3 to 6 weeks. The goal is to prevent bacteria from colonizing and reproducing while the damaged site is healing and host defenses regain adequate function to prevent recurrence. Deep-seated or severe infections and infections of the kidney or prostate may require more prolonged therapy (Chapter 3, Table 3-10, and Table C-11).

We recognize that our recommendation regarding duration of therapy may be in excess of that required to eradicate bacterial pathogens in some patients, especially those with uncomplicated lower UTIs. However, until convincing data become available to provide meaningful generalities about duration of therapy, we have chosen to balance our choice in the direction of giving antimicrobial agents for a period that may be too long rather than too short.

Fostering Client Compliance With Treatment Recommendations

In our experience, veterinarians and their staff typically overestimate rates of compliance among their clients and are unable to identify noncompliant individuals. Noncompliance can be expected to be associated with poorer treatment outcomes in patients with chronic or recurrent bacterial UTIs, diabetes mellitus and other endocrinopathies, irreversible heart, renal, and liver failure, and other chronic progressive diseases. Common reasons for noncompliance and suggestions to correct them are

summarized in Tables C-7 and C-8 and in a following section on adverse drug reactions. In most situations, the expectation of full compliance may be unrealistic. In general, less than full compliance is acceptable to us as long as the desired therapeutic benefit can be safely be achieved in an appropriate time.

Most clients understand that bacterial UTIs can often be controlled or eliminated by antimicrobial drugs. However, for treatment to be effective, clients must be able to give (1) the right drugs to, (2) the right patient, (3) at the right times, (4) in the right amounts, (5) in the right dose forms, (6) by the right route of administration, (7) for the right duration of time, (8) with knowledge of the right responses, and (9) knowledge of the right action to take if adverse reactions occur. Where appropriate, clients must also (10) return to the hospital for patient reevaluations on the right date. Providing clients with a list of treatment Dos and Don'ts may help to achieve the right therapeutic outcome (Tables C-7 and C-8).

Monitoring Response to Therapy (Tables C-12 and C-13)

The following recommendations extrapolated from studies in human medicine are based on extensive but uncontrolled clinical observations by veterinary nephrologists and urologists.[11-13] They are guidelines only and should not be interpreted as rigid facts.

1. Select the least expensive, least toxic, and most effective antimicrobial agent and begin therapy.
2. Three to 5 days after initiating therapy, collect a urine sample by cystocentesis and culture it for bacteria. Therapy is considered to be successful only if urine does not contain any pathogenic organisms. Even though there may be viable bacteria in surrounding tissue, the urine should be sterile. Treatment is ineffective and relapse can occur if the bacterial colony count has only been reduced (for example from 10^5 to 10^2). Therefore one cannot rely on examination of urine sed-

TABLE C-13

CHECKLIST OF POTENTIAL CAUSES OF POOR RESPONSE TO ANTIBIOTIC THERAPY

A. Administration of antimicrobial to correct noninfectious disorders causing signs similar to those associated with bacterial UTI.
B. Selection of ineffective drugs and/or ineffective doses.
C. Poor compliance with proper administration of antimicrobial.
   1. Unable or unwilling to adhere to dosing instructions.
   2. Premature withdrawal of drug as clinical signs subside.
   3. Discontinuation of drug due to expense.
   4. Unable to cope with side effects of drug.
D. Impaired action of drug.
   1. Microbes sequestered in inaccessible site.
   2. Host factors that alter concentration of active drug at infection site.
      a. Altered intestinal absorption.
      b. Altered perfusion of infected tissue.
      c. Decreased glomerular filtration reducing urinary excretion.
      d. Diuresis reducing urine concentration of antimicrobial agent.
   3. Other host factors detrimental to drug efficacy.
E. Failure or inability to recognize and eliminate or control a predisposing cause of UTI.
F. Failure to eliminate all microbes in infections caused by more than one pathogen.
G. Iatrogenic reinfection caoused by catheters or surgical techniques.
H. Microbes acquire resistance to antimicrobial agent.

required to detect recurrences at a subclinical stage of development and to determine whether they are due to relapses or reinfections.

Relapses

Relapse of UTI caused by the same pathogenic microbe would be expected to occur shortly after cessation of antimicrobial therapy (Chapter 3, Table 3-10). Relapses are indicative of treatment failure and are of considerable significance in terms of potential morbidity. Therefore urinalysis and culture results should be reevaluated approximately 7 to 10 days after discontinuation of therapy to detect recurrent relapses at a subclinical stage. Recovery of the same organism from urine that was sterile during treatment is presumptive evidence that treatment failed to eradicate the infection and suggests lack of owner compliance with treatment recommendations or deep-seated infection (Chapter 3, Table 3-10).

If diagnostic efforts to find a predisposing cause have not yet been performed, they should be considered as essential at this time. Consult Table 3-10 in Chapter 3 for a checklist of possible events predisposing to relapse infections.

If the relapse occurred after a brief period of therapy, continue treatment for a longer period. If the relapse occurred 10 or more days after therapy, repeat therapy with a different antimicrobial agent selected on the basis of susceptibility tests and continue therapy for a longer period. The procedures to evaluate treatment efficacy described above should be repeated.

Reinfections

Provided the urinary tract has had sufficient time to repair damaged tissues, reinfections caused by different pathogenic microbes would be expected to occur later after discontinuation of treatment as compared to recurrent relapses of infection (Chapter 3, Table 3-11). Therefore urinalysis and culture results should be reevaluated approximately 2 to 3 weeks (and in some instances repeatedly therafter) after cessation of antimicrobial therapy.

Detection of frequent reinfections after antimicrobial therapy is an absolute indication to evaluate the patient for one or more predisposing causes (Chapter 3, Tables 3-6, 3-9, and 3-11). The goal is to correct the predisposing cause. Reinfections should be managed by choosing antimicrobial agents on the basis of antimicrobial susceptibility tests. Each product should be used for a sufficient period (3 to 5 days) to evaluate its effectiveness in sterilizing urine.

> **KEY POINT:** Elimination of bacterial pathogens associated with reinfections may require therapy of shorter duration than recurrences associated with relapses. When recurrences attributable to reinfections occur, the antimicrobial drugs are effectively eradicating bacterial pathogens. The difficulty is associated with impaired host defense mechanisms. Giving therapeutic doses of antibiotics for long periods is usually unwarranted. Infrequent reinfections (two or three times per year) may be treated as single episodes (i.e., short course of a suitable antimicrobial agent). As described in the following sections, frequent reinfections may be managed with prophylactic doses of antimicrobial drugs.

iment to detect elimination of bacteria by therapy because persistence of reduced numbers of bacteria may fall below the limit of detection by light microscopy (see Chapter 11). Although the urine contains no viable microbes, hematuria, pyuria, and proteinuria associated with compensatory inflammation are likely to be detected by urinalysis 3 to 5 days after initiating effective therapy. However, these inflammatory-associated abnormalities may be of lesser magnitude.

3. Consider evaluating culture and urinalysis findings 3 to 5 days (or sooner, if necessary) before therapy is scheduled to be discontinued, especially if prophylactic antibiotics are to be used to prevent frequent reinfection. Therapy may be discontinued if the urine is sterile and the urine sediment normal.

If results indicate persistent infection, reevaluation of therapy is essential. In this situation, initiation of prophylactic low dose antimicrobial therapy is contraindicated.

Management of Recurrent UTIs

If treatment appears to be effective, follow-up evaluation is

TABLE C-14

ANTIMICROBIAL AGENTS WHICH MAY BE EFFECTIVE IN PREVENTING RECURRENT BACTERIAL URINARY TRACT INFECTIONS FOLLOWING ERADICATION OF INFECTION BY CONVENTIONAL ANTIMICROBIAL THERAPY

Agent	Conventional Dose	Prophylactic Dose[a]	Route of Administration
Ampicillin	25 mg/kg every 8 hours	25 mg/kg every 24 hours	Oral
Cephalexin	10 mg/kg every 8 hours	10 mg/kg every 24 hours	Oral
Enrofloxacin	5.0 mg/kg every 24 hours	2.5–3.0 mg/kg every 24 hours	Oral
Nitrofurantoin	4 mg/kg every 8 hours	3–4 mg/kg every 24 hours	Oral
Trimethoprim-sulfadiazine	15 mg/kg (combined) every 12 hours	7–8 mg/kg every 24 hours	Oral

[a]Daily dosage to be administered shortly after micturition and prior to confinement to enhance duration of period during which the antimicrobial agent will be retained in the urinary tract. Patient's urine should be cultured for bacteria at appropriate intervals to be sure that infection has not recurred.

Recurrences Attributable to Bacterial Infections of the Prostate

Chronic infections of the canine prostate gland are a common cause of recurrent UTI. Relapses are apparently related to poor penetration of antimicrobial drugs into prostatic secretions but may also be related to drug resistance (Chapter 3, Table 3-10, and Tables C-4 and C-5). Reinfections may be associated with persistent abnormalities in prostatic defenses against bacterial infections (Chapter 3, Table 3-11).

Prevention of Frequent Reinfections

In some patients with chronic UTI, it may be impossible to identify or correct underlying disorders that permit bacteria to persist in the urinary tract (Chapter 3, Tables 3-8, 3-9, and 3-10). Often the result is frequent reinfections. In such patients, it may be helpful to provide low dose (preventive) antibacterial therapy for an indefinite period (6 months or more) with drugs primarily eliminated in urine (Table C-14). Selection of the drug used for preventive therapy should be based on the results of the most recent antimicrobial susceptibility test. Reduced dosages (about one third to one half of the therapeutic dosage) of drugs excreted in high concentration in urine are acceptable *provided there has been complete eradication of bacterial pathogens by therapeutic doses of appropriate drugs.* Logically, low dose preventive antimicrobial therapy would be inappropriate for managing patients with recurrent bacterial UTIs attributable to relapses.

It is best to give one daily preventive dose of the antibiotic at a time when the drug is likely to be retained in the urinary tract for 6 to 8 hours (e.g., before bedtime). Even though this preventive dosing regimen does not result in MICs throughout the day, low concentrations of some drugs apparently interfere with production of fimbriae by some uropathogens,[14–16] which in turn interferes with the ability of potential pathogens to adhere to and colonize uroepithial cells.

During preventive therapy, urine samples collected by cystocentesis should be recultured at appropriate intervals. Samples should not be collected by catheterization, as catheters may

TABLE C-15

STEPS TO CONSIDER IF A BREAKTHROUGH INFECTION OCCURS DURING PREVENTIVE ANTIMICROBIAL THERAPY

1. Investigate the status of the urinary tract by urinalysis and quantitative bacterial culture.
2. Evaluate owner compliance (Tables C-7 and C-8).
3. Compare bacterial culture results to previous bacterial isolates to determine whether a relapse or reinfection has occurred.
4. Select an appropriate antimicrobial agent on the basis of antimicrobial susceptibility results.
5. Give therapeutic doses of the antimicrobial agent for an appropriate period.
6. When the urine no longer contains evidence of inflammation as detected by urinalysis and is sterile as determined by bacterial culture, resume preventive therapy.

cause iatrogenic infection. Urine samples should not be collected by voiding, as it may be impossible to distinguish bacterial contaminants in voided samples from pathogens.

Surveillence cultures of urine for bacteria should be performed at shorter intervals initially (after the first week of treatment and, if sterile, the fourth week of treatment). If there are no signs of bacteria-induced urinary tract disease and the urine is sterile, surveillance intervals can be extended to every 8 to 12 weeks.

Any time bacteria are identified, a breakthrough infection should be suspected (Table C-15). Recurrences during prophylactic therapy may be associated with poor compliance (Tables C-7 and C-8). The recurrent infection should be treated again with therapeutic doses (so called full dose) of an antimicrobial drug selected on the basis of susceptibility tests. After the infection has been eradicated and the associated inflammatory response subsides, preventive therapy can be resumed.

After 6 to 9 months of consecutive negative urine culture and urinalysis results indicating that the host defenses are functioning adequately, therapy may be discontinued on a trial basis to determine whether reinfection will occur. If abnormalities in host defenses have healed, UTIs may not recur. If a UTI develops within a short period, the procedures outlined above should be repeated

Adverse Drug Reactions

Long-term use of antimicrobial agents is not without risk of adverse effects. For example, sulfadiazine-trimethoprim combinations have been associated with anorexia, lethargy, keratoconjunctivitis sicca, folate deficiency anemia, and immune-complex reactions.[17–20] We have identified sulfadiazine in uroliths.

Practitioners should be familiar with common adverse events associated with antimicrobics to be able to place their significance in perspective with clients. As veterinarians, we have a tendency to overstate the benefits and understate the risks of drugs we prescribe. When unexplained clinical signs occur after treatment was initiated, clients may choose not to comply with further needed treatment if they perceive that these signs are caused by side effects associated with the medication (Tables C-7 and C-8). An effective way to minimize this problem is to list major undesirable side effects known to be commonly associated with the medication(s), the likelihood of their occurrence, and the recommended action to take if they occur.

We have found it beneficial to distinguish between nuisance side effects and those likely to be harmful. We emphasize to clients that not all clinical signs are of equal importance. We have found that it is best to avoid discussion of a laundry list of every potential side effect that might occur because it is possible to unnecessarily heighten anxiety by suggestion. Computer software packages can be used to specify a notation about side effects of drugs to appear on the invoice each time a specific drug is entered. Consult Chapter 4 for further information about the benefits and risks associated with therapy.

> **KEY POINT:** Clients are more likely to be satisfied and compliant if they are educated about what to expect and how to proceed when the unexpected occurs.

STEP-BY-STEP CHECKLISTS OF THERAPEUTIC PROTOCOLS FOR UNCOMPLICATED AND COMPLICATED BACTERIAL UTIs[1,4] (Table C-16 and Figure C-1)

Initial Episode of Untreated Lower UTI

1. Try to determine the nature of uropathogens by examining Gram-stained urine sediment (Chapter 3, Tables 3-12 and 3-18).
2. Select an effective antimicrobial drug (Tables C-2, C-2A, and C-3).
3. Administer the proper dose at the proper maintenance

TABLE C-16

TREATMENT CHECKLIST FOR BACTERIAL UTI

I. **Has bacterial UTI been confirmed?**
    A. Simple or complicated?
    B. First episode or recurrent episode?

II. **Select appropriate drug.**
    A. Antimicrobial susceptibility test?
    B. Upper or lower UTI? Prostatitis?
    C. Status of renal function?

III. **Select appropriate dose and maintenance interval.**
    A. Client compliance?
    B. Status of renal function?

IV. **Select appropriate duration of treatment.**
    A. Upper or lower UTI? Prostatitis?
    B. First episode or recurrent episode?
        1. Relapse?
        2. Reinfection?
    C. Simple or complicated UTI?

V. **Consider need for ancillary treatment.**

VI. **Monitor response.**
    A. Clinical signs.
    B. Urinalysis.
    C. Urine culture.

VII. **Consider prevention.**
    A. Status of host defenses?
    B. Preventive antibiotic treatment (reinfections).
    C. Suppressive antibiotic treatment (persistent infections).

intervals (Table C-6). Ideally, obtain a urine sample for culture 3 to 5 days after initiating therapy. If treatment is to be considered effective, the sample should be sterile.

4. In female dogs and cats, continue treatment for approximately 10 to 14 days (Table C-11). In uncastrated male dogs, continue treatment for 3 to 4 weeks.
5. Discontinue therapy if signs subside, but educate clients about how recurrent UTIs can be recognized.
6. Consider follow-up urinalysis and urine culture 7 to 14 days after completing treatment to verify cure or to detect subclinical recurrent UTI.
7. Consider appropriate diagnostic studies and selection of a different antimicrobial drug on the basis of antimicrobial susceptibility tests if signs of lower UTI persist during therapy.

Infrequent Reinfections (Tables C-12 and C-13)

1. Identify bacterial pathogen(s), preferably by culture (Chapter 3, Tables 3-12, 3-13, and 3-16.)
2. Consider diagnostic procedures to identify the underlying causes of infection (Chapter 3, Tables 3-5 and 3-8).
3. Select an effective antimicrobial drug (Tables C-2, C-2A, and C-3). Pending the availability of bacterial culture and antimicrobic susceptibility results, select antimicrobics to treat patients suspected of having UTI on the basis of Gram

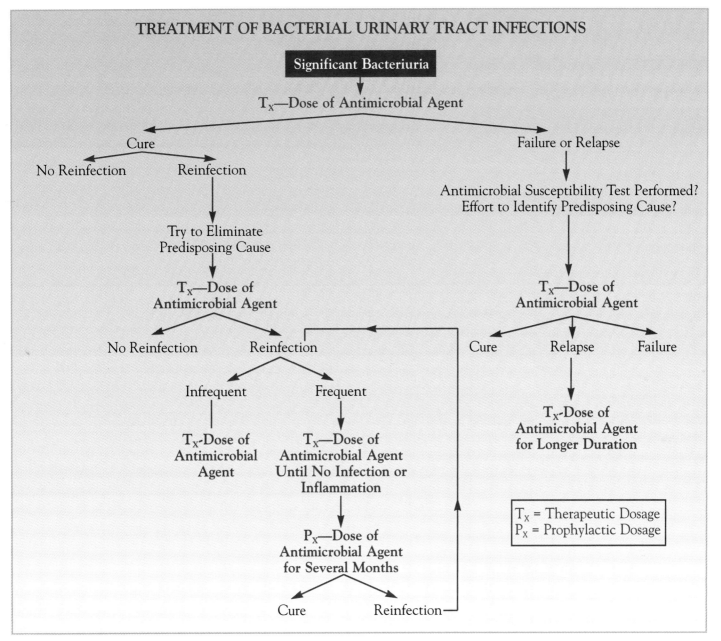

TREATMENT OF BACTERIAL URINARY TRACT INFECTIONS

FIGURE C-1 *Algorithm for treatment of bacterial urinary tract infections. Modified from Osborne CA: Clinical algorithms: Tools that foster quality patient care, in Kirk RW (ed):* Current Veterinary Therapy IX. *Philadelphia, WB Saunders, 1989.*

stain–facilitated identification of bacteria in urine sediment (Tables C-2 and C-2A).

4. If in vitro susceptibility test results indicate bacterial resistance to the antimicrobic initially selected but substantial amelioration of clinical signs have occurred, evaluate a urinalysis to determine the in vivo status of the disease. Decide whether to continue with the initial drug or to select an alternative one on the basis of susceptibility results on relevant available information.

5. Administer the proper dose at the proper maintenance intervals (Table C-6).

6. After 3 to 5 days of antimicrobial therapy, collect a urine sample by cystocentesis for bacterial culture. If the sample is sterile, continue therapy for an additional 7 to 10 days (Table C-12). An inflammatory response may still be detected by urinalysis 3

to 5 days after initiating therapy, even if the sample is bacteriologically sterile. If bacteria are cultured, even in low numbers, therapy should be considered ineffective. If the owner has been compliant in giving therapy, consider appropriate diagnostic studies and select a different antimicrobial drug on the basis of antimicrobial susceptibility tests.

7. Anticipate the probability of recurrence by periodically evaluating urinalysis findings and, when appropriate, urine cultures, after therapy has been discontinued.

Relapses

1. Attempt to identify abnormalities in host defenses by initiating the appropriate diagnostic procedures (Chapter 3, Tables 3-5, 3-9, and 3-10).

2. If possible, control or correct abnormalities predisposing to

TABLE C-17

GUIDELINES TO MINIMIZE RISK OF
CATHETER-INDUCED URINARY TRACT INFECTIONS

1. Avoid unnecessary catheterization, especially in patients with increased risk for bacterial UTI and its sequelae (e.g., patients with diseases of the lower urinary tract, hyperadrenocorticism, diabetes mellitus, and diseases associated with polyuria).
2. Urinary catheterization should only be performed by trained personnel who comprehend associated risks and benefits.
3. Atraumatic intermittent brief catheterization is often preferable to indwelling catheterization.
   a. If single brief catheterization is required for high risk patients, consider prophylactic administration of an antibiotic excreted in high concentration in urine and administer it 8 to 12 hours before and 2 to 3 hours following catheterization. Adequate concentration of the drug should be in the urine prior to catheterization.
   b. Choose antimicrobial agents most likely to be effective against nosocomial pathogens known to be present in the hospital environment.
   c. Collect a urine sample by cystocentesis 2 to 3 days following catheterization to detect nosocomial UTI at a subclinical stage of development.
   d. If UTI is present, select an antimicrobial drug on the basis of susceptibility tests and administer it for an appropriate period.
4. Indwelling transurethral catheters.
   a. Select indwelling urethral catheters constructed of materials least likely to cause irritation and inflammation of the adjacent mucosa.
   b. Thoroughly cleanse the external genitalia, and insert the catheter using aseptic technique.
   c. Avoid overinsertion of catheters to minimize damage to the bladder.
   d. Avoid open catheters; maintain a closed system.
   e. Avoid prolonged use of indwelling catheters.
   f. Prevent retrograde flow of urine from the collection

receptacle by positioning it below the level of the patient.
   g. Try to avoid inducing diuresis during indwelling catheterization, especially if an "open" system is used.
   h. Avoid giving prophylactic antimicrobial drugs in an attempt to prevent UTI unless the duration of catheterization is less than 2 to 3 days. Even when indwelling catheters are used for a short period, waiting until the catheter is removed before instituting antimicrobic therapy is often best.
   i. During longer duration use of indwelling catheters, avoid administration of antibiotics unless evidence of UTI associated with morbidity is detected. Although antibiotics may decrease the frequency and delay the onset of UTI, there is high risk of promoting development of infections by bacteria that are resistant to multiple antimicrobial drugs.
   j. If catheter-induced infection develops and remains asymptomatic, treat the infection following removal of the catheter.
   k. Remove the catheter as soon as possible. At the time of catheter removal, perform a urinalysis, quantitative urine culture, and antimicrobial susceptibility test.
   l. If UTI is confirmed after the catheter is removed, initiate therapy with an appropriate antimicrobial drug and continue giving for at least 10 to 14 days.
   m. If infection with more than one bacterial species occurs and if the pathogens have different susceptibilities to drug, treat the bacteria most likely to be virulent first. Then select the drug most likely to eliminate the remaining pathogens.
   n. Remove and, if appropriate, replace indwelling catheters that are grossly contaminated.
   o. Unless the benefits outweigh the risks, treatment with corticosteroids should not be given to patients with indwelling catheters. In most instances, the risk of UTI outweighs the potential benefit of reducing catheter-induced inflammation with corticosteroids.

UTI recurrences. Pay special attention to client compliance with treatment recommendations.
3. Because by definition, the same type of bacteria is the cause of the relapse, determine its susceptibility to antimicrobial drugs.
4. Select an effective agent, especially one that can attain adequate concentrations in the renal parenchyma, prostate, or tissue surrounding the urinary tract.
5. Administer the proper dose at the proper maintenance intervals (Table C-6).
6. After 3 to 5 days of antimicrobial therapy, collect a urine sample by cystocentesis for bacterial culture. If the sample is sterile, continue therapy for a prolonged interval (6 to 8 weeks or more for renal and prostate infections; Tables C-11 and C-12). If bacteria are cultured, even in low numbers, therapy should be considered to be ineffective. If the owner has been compliant, reevaluate susceptibility of the pathogen by antimicrobial dilution tests to determine the MIC.
7. After therapy has been discontinued, evaluate urinalysis

and urine culture findings at frequent intervals to detect relapses as early as possible.

Frequent Reinfections

1. Attempt to identify abnormalities in host defenses by initiating the appropriate diagnostic procedures (Chapter 3, Tables 3-5, 3-9, and 3-10).
2. If possible, control or correct abnormalities predisposing to UTI recurrences. Pay special attention to client compliance with treatment recommendations.
3. Identify the nature of uropathogens by in vitro culture, and determine their susceptibility to drugs by conducting antimicrobial susceptibility tests (Chapter 3, Table 3-16).
4. Select an effective antimicrobial drug (Tables C-2, C-2A, and C-3).
5. Administer the proper dose at the proper maintenance intervals (Table C-6).
6. After 3 to 5 days of antimicrobial therapy, collect a urine

sample by cystocentesis for bacterial culture. If the sample is sterile, continue therapy for at least an additional 10 to 14 days (Table C-11). An inflammatory response may still be detected by urinalysis 3 to 5 days after initiating therapy, even if the sample is bacteriologically sterile. If bacteria are cultured, even in low numbers, therapy should be considered as ineffective. If the owner has been compliant in providing therapy, consider additional diagnostic studies, reevaluation of antimicrobial susceptibility tests, and alternate forms of therapy to correct predisposing causes.

7. If preventive antimicrobial therapy is to be subsequently used (see below), collect a urine sample by cystocentesis for urinalysis and urine culture before discontinuing therapeutic doses of antimicrobial drugs. The urine should be sterile and have no evidence of inflammation. If infection persists, low dose preventive therapy is inappropriate.

8. If preventive therapy is not to follow withdrawal of antimicrobial drugs, anticipate recurrences by periodically evaluating results of urinalysis and urine culture.

Prevention of Frequent Reinfections

1. Evaluate urinalysis and urine culture results to ensure that bacterial UTI has been eliminated.

2. Select a drug that is excreted in high concentration in urine, and unlikely to cause adverse effects (Tables C-3, C-6, and C-9).

3. Give the drug at approximately one third the normal daily therapeutic dose.

4. Strive to give the drug immediately after the patient has voided and when the drug will be retained in the urinary tract for 6 to 8 hours (before bedtime).

5. Plan to give the drug for 6 to 8 months (Tables C-11 and C-15).

6. Collect urine samples, preferably by cystocentesis (never by catheterization), every 4 to 8 weeks for urinalysis and urine culture. If urine is normal, continue preventive antimicrobial therapy. If bacterial UTI is identified (so-called breakthrough infection), repeat the therapeutic protocol outlined for frequently recurrent UTI (Table C-15). Check owner compliance to determine whether the proper dose is being administered daily (Tables C-7 and C-8).

7. After 6 to 8 months, successful preventive therapy may be discontinued. At this time, the patient's own body may have repaired abnormalities in host defenses. In this situation, anticipate recurrences by periodically evaluating urinalysis and urine culture findings.

Prevention and Treatment of Catheter-Induced UTI
(Table C-17)

KEY POINT: Catheter-induced bacterial UTIs (nosocomial infections) are common and may result in significant morbidity in patients with urinary tract diseases, including pyelonephritis, renal failure, and septicemia. Therefore unnecessary use of urinary catheters should be avoided.

1. Consider administering therapeutic doses of antimicrobial drugs excreted in high concentration in urine, preferably with long elimination half-lives, at an interval of 8 to 12 hours before and 2 to 3 days after single brief catheterization of patients at high risk for UTIs. Choose antimicrobial agents most likely to be effective against nosocomial pathogens. Adequate concentration of the drug should be in the urine prior to catheterization. Collect a urine sample by cystocentesis 2 to 3 days after catheterization to detect iatrogenic UTI at a subclinical stage of development. If UTI is present, select an antimicrobial drug on the basis of susceptibility tests and administer it for an appropriate period.

2. If indwelling urethral catheters must be used, avoid concomitant administration of antimicrobial drugs unless a UTI develops. Although antibiotics may decrease the frequency and delay the onset of UTI, there is high risk of promoting development of infections with one or more bacteria that are resistant to multiple drugs. Use a closed indwelling catheter system. Try to avoid inducing diuresis during indwelling catheterization, especially if an open system is used. Remove the catheter as soon as possible. Obtain a urinalysis, urine culture, and antimicrobial susceptibility test. Initiate therapy with an appropriate drug for 10 to 14 days if UTI is confirmed. If infection with more than one species of bacteria occurs and if the microbes have different susceptibilities to drugs, treat the bacteria likely to be most virulent first, then select the type of drug most likely to eliminate remaining pathogens.

3. Unless there is a very specific indication for administering corticosteroids where the benefits outweigh the risks, they should not be given to patients with indwelling catheters.

REFERENCES

1. Lloyd DH, Lamport AI, Feeney C: Sensitivity to antibiotics amoungst cutaneous and mucosal isolates of canine pathogenic staphylococci in the UK. 1980–1996. *Vet Derm* 7:171–175, 1996.
2. Oluoch AO, Weisiger R, Sirgel AM, et al: Trends of bacterial infections in dogs: Characterization of *Staphylococcus intermedius* isolates (1990–1992). *Canine Pract* 21:12–19, 1996.
3. Ling, GV: Treatment of urinary tract infections with antimicrobial agents, in, Kirk RW (ed): *Current Veterinary Therapy*, vol 8. Philadelphia, WB Saunders, 1983.
4. Ling GV: *Lower Urinary Tract Diseases of Dogs and Cats.* St. Louis, Mosby, 1995.
5. Ling GV, Ruby AL: Cephalexin for oral treatment of canine urinary tract infection caused by *Klebsiella pneumoniae*. *JAVMA* 182:1346–1347, 1983.
6. Aucoin DP: Avoiding antimicrobial failure, in *Selected Scientific Proceeding of the 1998 North American Veterinary Conference*. Orlando, FL, Bayer Corp, 1998, pp 25–27.
7. Papich MG: Optimum strategy for antibacterial therapy, in *Selected Scientific Proceedings of the 1998 North American Veterinary Conference*. Orlando, FL, Bayer, 1998, pp 21–23.
8. Osborne CA, Klausner JS: Adverse drug reactions in the uremic patient, in Kirk RW (ed): *Current Veterinary Therapy*, vol 6. Philadelphia, WB Saunders, 1977.
9. Polzin DJ, Osborne CA, Bartges JW et al: Chronic renal failure, in Ettinger SJ, Feldman EC (eds): *Textbook of Veterinary Internal Medicine*. vol 2, ed 4. Philadelphia, WB Saunders, 1995, pp 1734–1760.
10. Riviere JE: Checklist of hazardous drugs in patients with renal failure, in Kirk RW (ed): *Current Veterinary Therapy*, vol 8. Philadelphia, WB Saunders, 1983.
11. Kunin CM: *Detection, Prevention, and Management of Urinary Tract Infections*, ed 4. Philadelphia, Lea & Febiger, 1987.
12. Smith TW, Roberts JA: Chronic pyelonephritis—Electron microscopic study. II. Persistence of variant bacterial forms. *Invest Urol* 16:154–162, 1978.
13. Stamey TA: *Pathogenesis and Treatment of Urinary Tract Infections*. Baltimore, Williams & Wilkins, 1980.
14. Reid G, Sobel JD: Bacterial adherence in the pathogenesis of urinary

tract infection: A review. *Rev Infect Dis* 9:470–487, 1987.

15. Stengvist K, Sandberg T, Ahlstedt S, et al: Effects of subinhibitory concentrations of antibiotics and antibodies on the adherence of *Escherichia coli* to human uroepithelial cells in vitro. *Scand J Infect Dis* 33(Suppl): 104–107, 1982.

16. Westerlund R et al: Characterization of *Escherichia coli* strains associated with canine urinary tract infections. *Res Vet Sci* 42:404–406, 1987.

17. Collins BK, Moose CP, Hagee JH: Sulfonamide-associated keratoconjunctivitis sicca and corneal ulceration in a dog. *JAVMA* 189:924–926, 1986.

18. Greene CE, Ferguson DC: Antibacterial chemotherapy, in Greene CE (ed): *Infectious Diseases of the Dog and Cat.* Philadelphia, WB Saunders, 1990, pp 461–493.

19. Kunkle GA, Sundlor S, Keisling K: Adverse side effects of oral antibacterial therapy in dogs and cats: An epidemiologic study of pet owner's observations. *JAAHA* 31:46–55, 1995.

20. Wilcke JR: Therapeutic application of sulfadiazine-trimethoprim in dogs and cats. A review. *Compan Anim Pract* 2:3–8, 1988.

BIBLIOGRAPHY

Barsanti JA, Blud J, Edmunds J: Urinary tract infection due to indwelling bladder catheters in dogs and cats. *JAVMA* 187:384–388, 1985.

Barsanti JA, Johnson CA: Genitourinary infections, in Greene CE (ed): *Infectious Diseases of the Dog and Cat*, ed 2. Philadelphia, WB Saunders, 1990, pp 157–183.

Osborne CA, Klausner JS, Hardy RM, Lees GE: Ancillary treatment of urinary tract infections, in Kirk RW (ed): *Current Veterinary Therapy*, vol 7. Philadelphia, WB Saunders, 1980.

Osborne CA, Lees GE: Bacterial infections of the canine and feline urinary tract, in Osborne CA, Finco DR (eds): *Canine and Feline Nephrology and Urology*. Malvern, PA, Williams & Wilkins, 1995, pp 759–797.

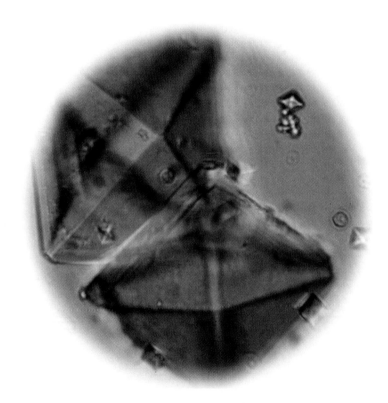

Index

Note: The letter *i* refers to an illustration; *t* refers to a table.

A

Accuracy, diagnostic, in quality assurance, 52–53
  minimizing erroneous test results, 52
Acetaminophen, 110t
Acetazolamide, 92t
Acetest®, 56, 90–91t, 100, 100i
Acetic acid stain, 131t
Acetoacetic acid, *see* Ketones
Acetone, *see* Ketones
Acid urine, urine pH in disorders with excretion of, 92t
Acidification, for urine sample preservation, 60
Acidifiers, urinalysis errors induced by, 62, 92t
Acidosis, respiratory and metabolic, abnormal urine pH in, 92t
  systemic, urinalysis findings in, 42
Acute azotemia, primary, ischemic or nephrotoxic, 66t
Addison's disease, *see* Hypoadrenocorticism
Adrenocorticotropic hormone (ACTH), in diagnosis of polyuria, 67i
Adverse drug reactions, *see* Drug reactions, adverse
Air bubbles, sample contamination with, 149t; Plate 119
Albuminuria, in normal samples, 11t
Albustix®, 90–91t, 113
Alkaline urine, pH in disorders with excretion of, 92t
Alkalinizers, urinalysis errors induced by, 62, 92t
Allopurinol, xanthine crystalluria due to, 144t, 149; Plate 118
Alternaria, contamination with, Plate 123
Amikacin, 193t, 197t
Amino acids, 6
Aminoglycoside antibiotics, 62, 186t
Ammoniacal odor, of urine, 72
Ammonium chloride, 92t, 186t
Amoxicillin, 43t, 197t
Amoxicillin-clavulanate, 193t, 197t
Amphotericin B, 186t
Ampicillin, 193t, 196t, 197t, 203t
Ampicillin crystalluria, 144t, 148
Amyloidosis, glomerular, 127t
Analgesics, 62
Anemia, idiopathic immune-mediated hemolytic, 110t
Anorexia, uremic, factors that may minimize, 187–188t
Antacids, magnesium- and phosphorus-containing, 186t
Antibiotic dilution susceptibility test, 193
Antibiotic treatment, *see also* Antimicrobial therapy
  causes of poor response to, 202t
  prophylactic, 186t
  urinalysis and urine culture results during, 42, 43t
Antidiuresis, 9, 10t
Antidiuretic hormone, effects on clearance, 4
  in urine concentration, 8–9, 10i
  water reabsorption and, 6
Antidiuretic hormone test, in diagnosis of polyuria, 67i
Antimicrobial susceptibility tests, 25, 27t, 191–194
Antimicrobial therapy, for UTI, 191–204
  adverse drug reactions, 203–204
  canine urine concentrations in, 194t
  checklist for azotemic renal failure, 199t
  commonly used agents, 197t
  compliance problems and solutions, 198t
  duration of, 200, 200t
  fluoroquinolones, desirable characteristics of, 199t

for recurrent, 201–203, 203t
in dogs with chronic bacterial prostatitis, 196t
monitoring response to, 201, 201t
poor response to, 202t
step-by-step checklists for, 204–206, 204t, 205i
Anuria, 69
Artifacts, in urine samples, 149t, 150; Plates 119–126
Artifactual turbidity, of urine, 71
Ascorbic acid, effects on urine glucose tests, 97–98
  urinalysis errors induced by, 62, 92t
Asymptomatic bacteriuria, 18
Asymptomatic disease, urinalysis to screen for, 42
Azotemia, causes of, 14t
  classification by causes, 5t
  combinations of prerenal, intrarenal, and postrenal, 84t, 85
  definition of, 13
  diagnostics, 16t
  differentiation between forms of, 74t
  intrarenal, primary, specific gravity value in diagnosis, 84, 84t
  localization of, 5t
    urine specific gravity values and, 82–85
  obstructive postrenal, 66t
  postrenal, urine specific gravity value in diagnosis, 74t, 83–84
  prerenal, urinalysis findings in, 42
    urine volume and specific gravity in, 66t
    urine specific gravity and diagnosis of, 74t, 82–83
  primary acute ischemic or nephrotoxic, 66t
  primary chronic, 66t
  test results in normal samples, 11t
  treatable causes of, in renal failure patients, 186t
  urine volume and specific gravity in types of, 66t
  with glomerulotubular imbalance, 74t, 84–85
Azotemic renal failure, diagnostic and therapeutic checklist, 199t
Azoturia, 110t

B

Babesiosis, 110t
Bacteria, contamination of urine samples with, 57–58
  in urine sediment, 141–143
    appearance, 141; Plates 3, 5, 6, 44–51
    contaminants versus pathogens, 142
    interpretation versus collection method, 141–142
    length of time between collection and examination, 142
    microscopic examination versus bacterial numbers, 142–143
    with sterile culture, 20, 20t, 141t
  normal canine flora, 19t
  prevalence of, in cats with lower urinary tract disease, 26t
    in dogs with UTI, 26t
  urease-producing, urine pH artifacts due to, 92t, 92
  uropathogenic, virulence factors, 22t
Bacterial urinary tract infection (UTI), 17–30
  bacteriuria in, 18
  clinical significance, 17–18
  complicated, 23, 24t
  host defenses against, 23t
  inflammation versus, 20
  prevention of, 190–191
  pyuria in, 18–19
  recurrent, 23–24, 201–202
  recurrent reinfection, 23, 25t, 202

relapsing, 23, 25t, 201–202
superinfections, 24
treatment of (Appendix C), 190–207
  antimicrobial therapy, 191, 192–204
  checklist for, 204–207, 204t, 205i, 206t
  correction of predisposing causes, 191
  objectives for, 192t
  uncomplicated, 21–23
  untreated, sequelae to, 18t
  urinalysis findings in, 41
  urine pH in, 19
  urine specific gravity in, 19
Bactericidal drugs, 195
Bacteriostatic drugs, 195
Bacteriuria, asymptomatic, 18
  covert, 18
  definition of, in UTI, 18
  in diagnostics, 16t
  significant, 19, 27–28
Baruria, *see* Hypersthenuria
Bence Jones protein heat test, 112t, 113
Bence Jones proteinuria, 111, 113
Benzalkonium, 115
Benzocaine, 110t
Benzylpenicillin, 62
Bili-Labstix®, 90–91t, 113
Bilirubin, biochemical analysis, 102–106
Bilirubin casts, 140, 141; Plate 43
Bilirubin crystalluria, 144t, 146; Plates 75, 76
Bilirubinuria, in cats, 105–106
  in dogs, 105
Biliverdin, 104i
Biochemical analysis, of urine, 86–124
  bilirubin, 102–106
  glucose, 92–99
  ketones, 99–102
  leukocytes, 123–124
  nitrituria, 123
  occult blood, hemoglobin, and myoglobin, 106–111
  pH, 88–92
  proteinuria, 111–121
  specific gravity, 124
  urobilinogen, 121–123
Biologic behavior, of disease, urinalysis to monitor, 42
Biopsy, renal, 16t
Bladder, urinary, manual compression of, 47, 47t
Blastomycosis, 143; Plates 59, 60
Blood agar, urine culture results with, 29, 29t
Blood transfusion, incompatible, 110t
Blood urea nitrogen (BUN), 13, 16t
Blood, occult, biochemical analysis, 106–111
  negative chemical test/detection of RBC in sediment, 109
  positive chemical test/lack of RBC in sediment, 109
Bordetella spp., 26t
Boric acid, urine sample preservation with, 60
Bowman's capsule, role in urine formation, 7t
Breakthrough infection, 203, 203t
Broad casts, 140, 141; Plates 23, 37
Burns, severe, 110t
Butyric acid, 102t

C

Cages, metabolism, for urine collection, 2
Calcium carbonate crystalluria, 144t, 146; Plate 77
Calcium oxalate crystalluria, 144t, 146

209